D1488055

From Pink to Green

Critical Issues in Health and Medicine

Edited by Rima D. Apple, University of Wisconsin–Madison, and Janet Golden, Rutgers University, Camden

Growing criticism of the U.S. healthcare system is coming from consumers, politicians, the media, activists, and healthcare professionals. Critical Issues in Health and Medicine is a collection of books that explores these contemporary dilemmas from a variety of perspectives, among them political, legal, historical, sociological, and comparative, and with attention to crucial dimensions such as race, gender, ethnicity, sexuality, and culture.

For a list of titles in the series, see the last page of the book.

From Pink to Green

Disease Prevention and the Environmental Breast Cancer Movement

Barbara L. Ley

Rutgers University Press

New Brunswick, New Jersey, and London

Library of Congress Cataloging-in-Publication Data

Ley, Barbara L., 1972–
    From pink to green : disease prevention and the environmental breast cancer movement /
Barbara L. Ley.
        p.; cm. — (Critical issues in health and medicine)
    Includes bibliographical references and index.
    ISBN 978–0–8135–4530–1 (hardcover : alk. paper)—
    ISBN 978–0–8135–4531–8 (pbk.: alk. paper)
    1. Breast—Cancer—United States—History—20th century.   2. Breast—Cancer—United
States—History—21st century.   3. Breast—Cancer—Environmental aspects.   4. Breast—
Cancer—Prevention.   5. Environmentalism—United States.   I. Title.   II. Series.
    [DNLM: 1. Breast Neoplasms—history—United States.   2. Breast Neoplasms—etiology—
United States.   3. Breast Neoplasms—prevention & control—United States.   4. Consumer
Participation—history—United States.   5. Environmental Exposure—United States.
    6. History, 20th Century—United States.   7. History, 21st Century—United States.
WP 11 AA1 L681f 2009]
RC280.B8L49   2009
362.196'99449—dc22   2008040063

A British Cataloging-in-Publication record for this book is available from the British Library.

Visit our Web site: http://rutgerspress.rutgers.edu

Manufactured in the United States of America

For Paul

Contents

Acknowledgments

I am indebted to the activists and scientists whose efforts first inspired me when I began my research on the environmental breast cancer movement in 1995. I also greatly appreciate the time they took over the years to speak with me about their work. Their devotion and dedication inspires my own work.

Over the years, many individuals have contributed to the development of my book. Scott Gilbert, Steve Piker, and Ken Gergen helped to nurture my budding interest in science studies. Donna Haraway, Nancy Chen, Joan Fujimura, Nancy Stoller, and Barbara Epstein guided my early thinking about the environmental breast cancer movement. I also thank Adele Clarke, Deborah Heath, Rayna Rapp, Karen-Sue Taussig, Susan Bell, Paul Brodwin, Joel Tickner, Devra Davis, Julie Beck, Josie Ramos, Ulrika Dahl, Karen Hoffman, Michael Montoya, Erin Koch, Tim Choy, Mary Gray, Nichole Bennett, Pamela Forman, Susan Halebsky Dimock, and participants at the Science and Democracy Network's 2004 meeting for their feedback, advice, and ideas.

I am grateful to Rutgers University Press for publishing my book and, in particular, to my editor, Doreen Valentine. Her feedback, insights, and guidance were invaluable to my writing process. I also thank Rima Apple, Janet Golden, and the two anonymous reviewers who read the manuscript. Closer to home, Milo Miller, Samuel Hogerton, Bingying Liu, Natalie Jankowski, and Marta Magnuson provided me with excellent research and technical assistance at various stages of my work. I owe particular thanks to Eleanor Anbinder, who facilitated my use of Pat McNabb's artwork for the book cover. Anbinder directs ArtbeCAUSE (http://artbecause.org), a nonprofit foundation that raises funds to advance research on the environmental causes of breast cancer. I initially found McNabb's artwork on the organization's Web site.

The University of Wisconsin–Milwaukee's Center for 21st Century Studies awarded me a faculty research fellowship for the 2006–2007 academic year. This fellowship allowed me to make substantial progress on the book. The Department of Journalism and Mass Communication at UWM also allotted funds to help me prepare the manuscript for publication. Finally, portions of this book were previously published by Routledge as "Disease Categories and Disease Kinships: Classification Practices of the U.S. Environmental Breast Cancer Movement," in *Medical Anthropology: Cross Cultural Studies of Health and Illness* 26, no. 2 (2006): 1–39.

I am especially grateful to my family. Linda Aldrich, Jim and Fran Ley, David Ley and Erica Beck, and Dan and Linda Brewer supported and encouraged me throughout the entire writing process. My golden retriever, Molly, slept by my feet through countless days of writing. Last but not least, I give my biggest thanks to my husband and colleague, Paul Brewer. Paul provided me with much love, patience, feedback, and proofreading through the many stages of my book. My book, as well as my life in general, is better because of him.

From Pink to Green

Chapter 1

A Movement in the Making

While shopping at a San Francisco bookstore in November 2000, I decided to purchase a postcard created by Susan Liroff of Spitfire Graphics, in Oakland, California. On the front of the postcard was a color photo of a topless white woman with short blond hair. A horizontal scar filled the space on her chest where her right breast used to be. With one hand on her hip, she used her other hand to hold a sign that read, "INVISIBILITY EQUALS DEATH." A chronology of the increasing rates of breast cancer incidence filled the space above the woman's head: "1964—1 in 20; 1980—1 in 14; 1994—1 in 8." The text to the left of her sign read, "Since 1971, more than 1 trillion dollars have been spent on cancer research and treatment." The back of the postcard contained the rest of the organization's message: "Breast Cancer is the number one killer of women between the ages of 35 and 50. The cancer industry continues to ignore the link between epidemic cancer rates and the contamination of air, food and water. We demand that our lives be valued over financial profit and that adequate health care be available to all!"[1]

When I took the postcard to the counter, the cashier—a white man in his late twenties—picked it up and paused, looking at both sides. Then he placed it on the counter and said, "I can't charge you for this. This is for breast cancer. There shouldn't be a charge for this." Receiving the postcard for free left me feeling pleasantly surprised, yet it also spoke to the powerful resonance of breast cancer and the political culture surrounding it in contemporary American life. Liroff's postcard focuses on a small but increasingly influential facet of this political culture: the environmental breast cancer movement.

1

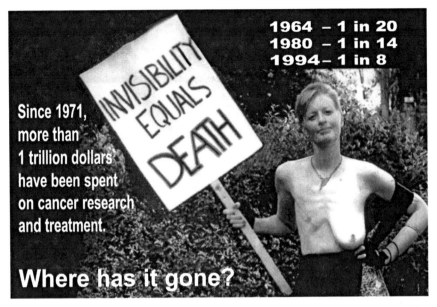

Figure 1.1 A postcard of activist and breast cancer survivor Raven Light created by Susan Liroff in 1994. Courtesy of Susan Liroff (Spitfire Graphics) and Raven Light.

In one sense, the postcard reflects social and political themes that are as central to the U.S. environmental breast cancer movement today as they were in 1994 when Raven Light, the postcard's model, boldly showed her mastectomized body. The postcard highlights activists' concerns about the overall increase in breast cancer incidence rates over the past thirty (now forty) years and the failure of the nation's "War on Cancer" to halt this growing problem through predominantly biomedical research and interventions. It also condemns the cancer industry for deflecting attention away from what activists view as the solution to the breast cancer problem—disease prevention, especially the reduction of everyday toxic exposures. Additionally, the postcard embodies the feminist and lesbian activist roots of environmental breast cancer activism by demanding that more attention be paid to a disease that primarily affects women, as well as by depicting a woman defying cultural standards of femininity with her short hair, cosmetic-free face, and publicly displayed mastectomy. The fact that a queer bookstore sold the postcard further highlights these sociopolitical roots. Finally, the postcard reflects—perhaps unintentionally—how the environmental breast cancer movement is structured in many ways by the social, political, and public health concerns of white women.

Yet much has changed since 1994. A growing number of not only breast cancer organizations but also women's health, environmental justice, environmental health, and public health groups advocate for increased attention to suspected environmental causes of breast cancer. Activists extend their political and economic critiques of the cancer industry to other forms of corporate power and cultural practices that deflect attention from such causes and from breast cancer prevention more generally. They regularly push for scientific research and policy reform as part of their prevention efforts. They also embrace a particular theory of disease causation—endocrine disrupter theory—that shapes the movement's social, cultural, political, and scientific landscape in compelling ways.

With its focus on toxic exposures, the environmental breast cancer movement seeks to transform the dominant paradigm for addressing the breast cancer problem. The "future imaginaries" that guide these efforts, however, not only provide a new vision for public health, biomedicine, science, and environmental policy.[2] They also require a new vision for social, cultural, political, and everyday life. Just as important, the movement's efforts highlight the ways in which the breast cancer problem is inextricably entwined with other health problems facing human and nonhuman populations alike. In many respects, preventing breast cancer goes hand in hand with improving the environmental health of all beings.

Understanding the Breast Cancer Problem

Breast cancer is one of the most—if not the most—feared diseases among women in the United States.[3] Given that many women have a personal history with it, know someone with it, or both, this fear is not surprising. Yet social and cultural factors contribute to this fear, as well. Breasts function as cultural symbols of female sexuality and motherhood; thus, the disease can complicate women's sense of identity and self-worth. Breast cancer is also one of the most prominent diseases in contemporary society. Indeed, it is difficult to go for even a few days without coming across a magazine article about the disease; a news story about it; a brochure for a breast cancer walk or running event; a pink ribbon attached to someone's backpack or jacket; or an announcement of a company's pledge to donate a percentage of its sales of its food products, cars, appliances, cosmetics, clothes, or other consumer goods to a breast cancer organization.

Although often referred to as a single disease, breast cancer actually comprises a series of related diseases. In situ carcinomas are cancers confined to either the ducts (ductal carcinoma in situ) or the lobules (lobular carcinoma in situ) of the breast. In contrast, invasive breast cancers are those that have spread into surrounding breast tissue. When confined to this tissue, the cancer is considered local. When it has spread beyond the breast to nearby tissue or lymph nodes, the tumor is considered regional stage. Cancer that has metastasized to distant organs is considered distance stage.[4] Another form of the disease is inflammatory breast cancer, which accounts for 1 to 6 percent of new breast cancer cases. This rare but highly aggressive form of the disease is characterized not by distinct tumors but by sheets of cancer cells that are not easily detected by mammogram or ultrasound.[5]

Breast cancer is an old affliction, with reports of its existence going back thousands of years to places such as early Egypt, the Byzantine Empire, and ancient Greece.[6] In many respects, however, it is a disease of the contemporary industrialized world. Currently, one in seven U.S. women will develop invasive breast cancer at some point in her lifetime—a rate that is almost three times as high as it was in 1964.[7] As of January 2004, 2.4 million women living in the United States had breast cancer or prior histories of the disease. More women are diagnosed with breast cancer than with any other cancer except skin cancer. In 2007, an estimated 178,480 women were newly diagnosed with invasive breast cancer, and 62,030 women were newly diagnosed with in situ breast cancer. Behind lung cancer, breast cancer is the second leading cause of cancer deaths for all U.S. women, with an estimated 40,460 women expected to die from it in 2007.[8] White women suffer the highest overall incidence rates, followed by African Americans, Asian Americans/Pacific Islanders, Hispanics/ Latinas, and American Indians/Alaska Natives. Age further complicates the pattern: white women over the age of forty face higher incidence rates than those of their African American counterparts, but African American women under the age of forty face higher incidence rates than those of white women from the same age group.[9] African American women suffer the highest overall mortality rates, followed by white women, Hispanic women, Native Americans, and Asian Americans.[10]

Across the country and around the world, biomedical and research centers, government agencies, health organizations, pharmaceutical companies, and other entities devote significant resources to end what many view as a breast cancer epidemic. The dominant paradigm that guides most of their efforts emphasizes a biomedical approach by addressing the disease after it initially develops. This approach includes screening and detection measures in the form of clinical breast exams, self–breast exams, mammography, ultrasound, and magnetic resonance imaging (MRI). It includes diagnostic techniques such as surgical and needle biopsies. It also consists of treatment modalities such as mastectomies, lumpectomies, radiation, chemotherapy, and other therapies to remove the cancer from the body, halt its growth, prevent it from metastasizing to other organs, decrease its chances of reoccurrence, and ultimately cure it. In recent years, this focus on treatment has expanded somewhat to include complementary approaches such as psychosocial support, acupuncture, and relaxation practices.

The dominant paradigm also extends to factors that heighten a woman's risk of developing breast cancer and strategies for reducing these risks. Identifying such factors can be a long and complicated process. Breast cancer, like many other cancers and chronic diseases, is caused by a complex interplay of factors at work over the course of a woman's life. Being a woman and getting older are two of the most significant established risk factors. Another set of important factors relate to a woman's reproductive history. The earliest suspicion of reproductive factors occurred in 1713 when Italian research Bernardo Ramazzini observed that nuns had higher rates of breast cancer than those of married women. Ramazzini's hypothesis that nuns' celibacy caused their higher rates was not too far from the truth. Many years later, researchers determined that never giving birth increased the risk of developing the disease. Other reproductive factors identified over the years include starting one's period before the age of twelve, beginning menopause after the age of fifty-five, giving birth to one's first child after the age of thirty, and never breastfeeding.[11]

The 1980s ushered in an increased focus on behavioral factors (sometimes called lifestyle factors) that heighten breast cancer risk, including moderate to heavy alcohol consumption, diet, overweight and obesity, and the use of certain synthetic hormone drugs. This increased focus came on the heels of two articles written by prominent cancer researchers advocating for an increased focus on "avoidable" causes of cancer.[12] This decade also brought advancement in the genetics of cancer, especially with regard to "oncogenes," that is, "disfigured genes that may underlie the gene abnormalities of cancer." Proto oncogenes stimulate the growth of cancer cells, whereas recessive oncogenes suppress the development of tumors. Damage sustained by tumor suppressor genes over the course of one's lifecycle, however, can lessen their protective qualities.[13] In the following decade, scientists built on this body of research by locating and identifying BRCA1 and BRCA2, called the "breast cancer genes." It is estimated that 65 percent of women with BRCA1 and 45 percent with BRCA2 will develop breast cancer by the age of seventy. Together, these inherited genes are responsible for 5 to 10 percent of all breast cancer cases. Scientists are currently studying other types of "low risk variations" in genetic susceptibility to breast cancer, as well as gene-environment interactions.[14] Furthermore, a number of clinical factors—such as having high breast tissue density and a personal history of assorted benign breast conditions—increase the risk of breast cancer.[15]

Despite its growing emphasis on risk factors and risk reduction, the dominant paradigm's approach to these features is still limited. Overall, research to address them receives less public and private funding and fewer resources than what is given to basic research and biomedical approaches to the disease. In addition, the dominant paradigm emphasizes reproductive, behavioral, clinical, and genetic factors over environmental factors.[16] Consider, for example, ionizing radiation, the only established environmental cause of breast cancer. Researchers first discovered its link to the disease after the 1945 bombing of Hiroshima and Nagasaki. In the years following this catastrophe, studies found increased breast cancer incidence among women who had been exposed to the radioactive fallout, especially those exposed before the age of twenty. Since then, exposure to ionizing radiation from assorted medical procedures, among them excessive chest X-rays and certain radiation treatments; nuclear research and production facilities; military weapons testing; and other occupational conditions have also been shown to cause breast cancer.[17] Still, ionizing radiation does not garner the degree of attention paid to those other factors noted above. Further, the dominant paradigm tends to minimize a growing body of research linking breast cancer to other types of environmental exposure, such as to electromagnetic fields (nonionizing radiation) and to toxic compounds found in common chemicals, household products, synthetic materials, and industrial pollution.

The inattention to environmental factors linked to breast cancer has not gone unnoticed. A growing number of health professionals, scientists, policymakers, activists, and citizens now demand that public, private, and nonprofit sectors devote more resources to these areas. Perhaps more than any other individual or group, the environmental breast cancer movement leads many of these efforts.

Transforming the Dominant Paradigm

The environmental breast cancer movement is one of many "health social movements" that have formed in recent decades to address the social, political, biomedical, emotional, and economic needs of particular disease constituencies. Such movements have developed in response to the increased scientization of regulation and policy; the rise of medical authority; and the cultural transformation of citizens, particularly patients, from recipients of expert knowledge to critics of such knowledge.[18] More specifically, environmental breast cancer activism is what sociologist Phil Brown and his colleagues call an "embodied health movement," a type of health social movement that addresses "disease, disability, or illness experience by challenging science on etiology, diagnosis, treatment, and prevention of disease." Embodied health movements ground their analyses in the lived experience of afflicted persons and emphasize collaboration between activists, on the one hand, and health professionals and researchers, on the other.[19]

Environmental breast cancer activism functions as a "culture of action," as the sociologist Maren Klawiter calls it, within the broader breast cancer movement.[20] For the past three decades, the broader breast cancer movement has worked to raise awareness about the disease; increase the financial resources devoted to it; provide more services and support for women struggling with it; demand a voice in biomedical, research, and policy decisions; and ultimately eradicate the breast cancer problem. In turn, the movement has gained momentum, strength, and legitimacy from the growing political and public focus on the disease. Not all organizations that work on breast cancer issues, however, approach the disease in the same way. The majority—including some of the largest and most prominent in the country—tend to espouse the dominant paradigm. Indeed, this paradigm is central to many of the breast cancer "awareness" efforts that have become so prevalent and popular in contemporary society since the mid-1990s, in the form of runs, television specials, pink ribbon merchandise, and corporate advocacy. In contrast, a smaller—albeit increasing—number of groups seek to transform the dominant paradigm, as well as the broader cultural milieu that sustains it. The environmental breast cancer movement, with its focus on environmental factors and disease prevention, exemplifies this latter perspective. It is perhaps the most active and outspoken critic of the dominant breast cancer paradigm and the broader disease culture surrounding it.

Certainly, environmental breast cancer activists acknowledge the importance of working toward better treatments and more effective detection measures. Many even devote efforts to advancing them. They do not believe, however, that a biomedical approach should guide breast cancer science, policy, and care. This perspective reflects a basic principle of public health: that it is better to prevent the disease from occurring than to confront it after it has already developed. It also reflects troubling facts. Despite recent drops in overall breast cancer incidence and mortality, rates for both are still high. Given that the ample resources devoted to biomedical strategies have yielded limited progress toward eradicating the breast cancer problem, an increased focus on prevention is the next logical step. At the same time, the dominant paradigm's focus on reproductive, behavioral, clinical, and genetic risk factors is not enough. Up to 50 percent of all breast cancer cases cannot be attributed to established factors, including the types mentioned above.[21] The question of what accounts for the remaining cases serves as an incentive for considering the possible role of toxic exposures, especially from chemicals, in the development of the disease. Such exposures take place in utero, as well as in homes, outdoor spaces, workplaces, schools, health care settings, and other "geographies of exposure."[22] Indeed, many activists argue that environmental factors lie at the heart of true breast cancer prevention.

In a broader sense, attention to environmental factors challenges the dominant construction of breast cancer as an individual problem that requires individualistic solutions. This construction is evident in the biomedical emphasis on the detection and treatment of the disease in individual women, as well as in the focus on risk factors that link the disease to a woman's biological and genetic makeup, reproductive history, and behavioral choices. The construction of risk reduction strategies—such as increased exercise, chemoprevention drugs, and even prophylactic mastectomies in women with the breast cancer gene—as choices that women can make to protect their health further exemplifies this tendency. When it comes to addressing toxic exposures, however, the approach is limited at best. Such exposures are often faced not only by individual women but also by larger communities and populations. The dominant approach also obscures the ways in which environmental exposures can influence individual risk factors. For example, recent research indicates that exposure to certain chemicals may influence the age at which a girl begins to menstruate. Finally, the focus on individuals places the responsibility for dealing with the breast cancer problem on women themselves rather than on the institutions responsible for exposing them to harmful substances in the first place.

In constructing environmental links to breast cancer as a societal problem, activists do not completely reject the importance of individual efforts. After all, they encourage women to take action in their own lives through strategies such as eating organic food and using nontoxic personal care products. They do believe, however, that working toward prevention requires structural changes on the part of policymakers, industries, and other societal institutions to reduce the risks faced by women in general. Such measures include banning the manufacture and use of harmful chemicals; developing safer products; and passing legislation to protect the health of workers, neighborhoods, and consumers. To promote these prevention efforts, activists work to transform not only social and cultural norms regarding sustainability, environmental stewardship, health advocacy, corporate responsibility, consumerism, and gender politics but also conceptions of what constitutes the environment, an environmental health risk, and disease prevention. From this perspective, healthy bodies go hand in hand with healthy communities, and eradicating environmental links to breast cancer necessitates the revamping of the social, cultural, political, and economic foundations of society itself.

Strategic Science

The environmental breast cancer movement expresses concern about an array of toxic substances found in the air we breathe; the water we drink; the food we eat; the products we use; and the indoor and outdoor spaces in which we live, work, and play. Of course, concerns about environmental risks are not new. Throughout the past century, scientists, citizens, activists, public health professionals, and policymakers have worked to reduce health risks associated with contaminated drinking water, industrial pollution, occupational exposures, poor sanitation, and agricultural practices. Yet concerns about toxic exposures have grown especially strong in recent decades, partly as a response to the growing body of evidence linking increasing rates of numerous diseases and disorders to the chemical revolution that took place after Word War II. In the name of social progress and modernization (as captured by DuPont's slogan "Better Things for Better Living . . . through Chemistry"), this revolution led to the massive production of tens of thousands of new chemicals and other synthetic materials that were widely—and often indiscriminately—used for assorted agricultural, technological, health care, industrial, and other everyday purposes. Thus, the linking of breast cancer to toxic exposures is one aspect of a bourgeoning trend that cuts across many public health arenas, including environmental justice, environmental health, and children's health.

As part of their efforts, environmental breast cancer activists work to raise public awareness about harmful exposures, pass more stringent environmental regulations, improve scientific understandings of environmental causes of breast cancer, and promote prevention of the disease more generally. From the start, they paid attention to an array of suspected environmental causes of the disease. In the mid-1990s, however, they became increasingly concerned with a particular group of chemicals known as xenoestrogens. Named from the Greek root, *xeno*—meaning "foreign, alien, or strange"—these substances share chemical properties with the hormone estrogen and can act on the body's cells and tissues as false estrogen molecules, disrupting the ability of natural estrogen to function normally. Xenoestrogens, which include well-known chemicals such as DDT, dioxin, and PCBs, as well as the more recently publicized phthalates and bisphenol A, are found in plastics, cosmetics, pesticides, car exhaust, growth hormones, and industrial pollution, among other sources. Today, they rank among the movement's top environmental health concerns.

Despite activists' calls for action, the body of evidence linking breast cancer to most environmental factors is uncertain and subject to scientific and public debate. Although a growing body of research demonstrates a connection between such factors and the disease, many studies show no link. Moreover, the evidence linking particular environmental factors to breast cancer generally does not meet the high standard of proof needed to take regulatory action in the United States. Thus, a significant part of activists' efforts revolve around making the case for why concern about environmental exposures is warranted given that uncertainty is present. To bolster their argument, activists highlight epidemiological, experimental, and ecological research showing an association between toxic substances and breast cancer. Likewise, they note how the majority of breast cancer clusters across the nation are located in heavily industrialized and often polluted areas. They also situate the evidence connecting chemicals to breast cancer in broader patterns of evidence linking the same types of chemicals to assorted health problems afflicting humans and wildlife. Furthermore, activists work to make sense of—and explain—the uncertainty that surrounds environmental exposures. To this end, they point to the political and economic factors that lead industries, biomedical institutions, research institutions, government agencies, and health organizations to downplay suspected environmental causes. They describe the scientific and technical limitations of existing research, and they challenge the very idea that proof of harm should be the basis for prevention-based policies.

For these reasons, environmental breast cancer is as much a scientific problem as it is a social, cultural, and political one. Activists critique the authority of science and biomedicine while simultaneously drawing on these fields to legitimate their claims and efforts. In doing so, they challenge—and help to transform—the social, cultural, and political institutions that support and are shaped by the domains of science and biomedicine. I use the term *strategic science* to describe the ways in which activists engage science as part of their efforts to bolster their argument that toxic exposures cause breast cancer and to promote disease prevention more generally. More broadly, the term refers to the array of scientific discourses, values, and practices embraced by social movements to further their political agendas regarding public health, the environment, technological development, and other issues for which scientific knowledge and expertise matter.

In one sense, the concept of strategic science highlights the ways in which the production of knowledge about environmental causes of breast cancer—and arguably the production of scientific knowledge in general—is what the sociologist Steven Epstein describes as "impure," that is, shaped by social and political factors as much as scientific ones.[23] By taking on the role of lay experts, environmental breast cancer activists promote local, state, and federal research on possible environmental causes of breast cancer. They participate in scientific agenda setting, study design, data interpretation, and the public dissemination of scientific knowledge. Activists make the case for why they should play an active role in scientific and policy decision making, positioning themselves as key actors in the "credibility struggles" that both shape and reflect the debates surrounding suspected environmental causes of breast cancer.[24]

Just as important, the concept of strategic science emphasizes the influence of science on the environmental breast cancer movement itself. To begin with, activists integrate science into their prevention efforts. Such practices include decisions by activists to embrace particular theories of disease causation over others, as well as the ways in which activists incorporate scientific theories, data, and discourses into their health education materials, awareness campaigns, policy initiatives, speeches and conversations, meetings with elected officials, membership drives, grant applications, and other work. These practices also refer to the impact of particular bodies of scientific knowledge on activists' political values, movement culture, and coalition-building efforts. Additionally, the concept of strategic science foregrounds the central role that scientists play in the environmental breast cancer movement. A growing number of scientists support activists' political efforts and the latter's desire to participate in the research process. Some even position themselves as allied scientists who actively situate their work within the broader political and public health terrain of the movement.

Ultimately, the concept of strategic science emphasizes how environmental breast cancer activism and environmental health science "mutually construct" one another.[25] By *mutual construction*, I mean the ways in which the two fields shape and evolve together over time. In the case of environmental breast cancer, activists and scientists influence one another's beliefs, values, epistemologies, practices, workplace cultures, social networks, professional identities, and institutional boundaries. Moreover, many "citizen-science alliances" take place in hybrid spaces such as not-for-profit environmental health research centers, environmental policy think tanks, and advisory committees.[26]

Disease Categories and Disease Kinships

Environmental breast cancer activism may constitute one culture of action within the broader breast cancer movement, but it is also true that the movement is multifaceted and diverse in its own right. The organizations and political networks that constitute the movement exist in numerous regions across the country. Activist groups often approach the environmental breast cancer problem in different ways and, consequently, rely on different social, cultural, and political strategies for addressing it. Moreover, environmental breast cancer activism, like other embodied health movements, is a "boundary movement," its boundaries overlapping other professional and political arenas. In this regard, environmental breast cancer activism's "movement field" consists not only of its own activists but also of those working in the similarly porous fields of environmental health, women's health, environmental justice, wildlife health, and children's health.[27] The same movement field also includes an array of scientists, health professionals, policymakers, funders, journalists, business leaders, and concerned citizens who align themselves and their work with its values and objectives.

The concept of disease classification provides a useful framework for thinking about the heterogeneity of environmental breast cancer activism's movement field and its public health efforts. Classification is a practice that takes place in all facets of daily, professional, and institutional life. Indeed, sociologists Susan Leigh Star and Geoffrey Bowker argue that "to classify is human."[28] In particular, classification plays a central role in the life sciences, biomedicine, and other health-related fields, where diseases, illnesses, and disorders are classified into one or more broad disease categories. Such categories are based on common characteristics such as affected population (for example, children's health or women's health), seat of illness (heart conditions or eye conditions), type of illness (cancer or dwarfism), and cause of illness (inherited genes).[29] Like others diseases, illnesses, and disorders, breast cancer is often, if not always, classified in multiple ways by activists, scientists, health professionals, mass media, policymakers, and industries. From this perspective, the environmental breast cancer problem is never just about breast cancer.

Classification, however, is not simply a taxonomical practice. It is also a meaning-making practice that carries social, discursive, and material implications for the classified diseases, disorders, or illnesses at hand. In other words, the decisions to classify breast cancer in relation to various categories structure how activists define and navigate the social, cultural, political, organizational, and epistemological terrain of the disease. Such practices shape the ways in which they conceptualize and work to address the scientific uncertainty surrounding environmental causes of breast cancer, as well as the form and content of their organizational objectives, political analyses, educational campaigns, research agendas, and policy initiatives. Furthermore, activists' classification practices helped to catalyze their initial interest in environmental causes of breast cancer.

Just as important, disease categories link the diseases, disorders, and illness that are classified within them. Such linkages, which I call *disease kinships*, produce what science studies scholar Donna Haraway describes as "the material and semiotic effect of natural relationship, of shared kind"—an effect, in turn, that helps to "refigure provocatively the border relations among specific humans, other organisms, and machines."[30] In some respects, a disease kinship shares characteristics with anthropologist Paul Rabinow's notion of a "biosociality," which refers to the cultures, communities, and collective identities that form in relation to particular diseases or perceived sets of biological similarities.[31] It also resonates with what Maren Klawiter calls a "disease regime," namely, the "institutionalized practices, authoritative discourses, social relations, collective identities, emotional vocabularies, visual images, public policies and regulatory actions through which diseases are socially constituted and experienced."[32]

Yet a disease kinship differs from these concepts in that it emphasizes the ways in which broader classification practices shape the construction, experience, and enactment of particular diseases, as well as the social, discursive, material, and institutional terrain surrounding them. Specifically, disease kinships shape the cultures, communities, and identities that form among affected persons and their loved ones; the political alliances that work across diseases, affected populations, and professional disciplines; and the social, discursive, and institutional spaces in which these assorted personal, political, and professional arenas intersect. As a result of such kinships, activists make important allies, with whom they develop joint political agendas and collaborative campaigns. Such campaigns, in turn, foster "synergistic reactions," enabling breast cancer activists and their allies to accomplish more together than they would have been able to on their own.[33] Furthermore, disease kinships play a key role in the production of political, scientific, and embodied knowledge about environmental causes of breast cancer, with particular kinships going hand in hand with linkages between cell cultures, epidemiological data, animal studies, blood samples, and other bodies of evidence.[34]

Activists situate breast cancer in numerous disease categories, including cancer, women's health, children's health, and environmental health. Each of these categories emerged as a salient classification at a particular moment in the movement's development. Newer categories, however, were not replacements for earlier ones. Rather, activists added these later constructs to their growing classification repertoire, with each category providing a specific yet flexible framework through which to assemble and reassemble the past, present, and future terrain of environmental breast cancer science, politics, and activism.[35]

A particularly salient disease category is based on endocrine disrupter theory. This groundbreaking theory links hormone-disrupting chemicals, including xenoestrogens, to an array of cancerous and noncancerous disorders affecting humans and wildlife. In many respects, activists' growing focus on science over the years has developed in tandem with their increased concern about endocrine disrupters. With its linkages between cancerous and noncancerous disorders afflicting women, men, children, and wildlife, endocrine disrupter theory also complements and in some cases complicates the biopolitical landscape of a social movement largely rooted in a feminist and women-centered approach to cancer activism, education, and care. Additionally, the focus on endocrine disrupters carries complex implications for the movement's racial and class politics—which have in many ways been based on the values, vantage points, and experiences of white and economically advantaged women. Furthermore, endocrine disrupter theory serves as a central trajectory along which the environmental breast cancer and environmental health movements co-evolve.

A Movement in the Making

This book, based on research I conducted between 1995 and 2008, presents a cultural history of the U.S. environmental breast cancer movement and its efforts to promote disease prevention. The environmental breast cancer movement provides a compelling case for examining the significance of health science movements in general and embodied health movements in particular. This case highlights the complex set of negotiations and contestations that take place for an array of intersecting social, cultural, political, and scientific domains related to a disease that affects a vast number of women and holds a prominent place in the public imagination. Additionally, the case of environmental breast cancer activism illuminates the negotiations and contestations within the broader breast cancer movement in regard to the different cultures of action that help to define what constitutes the breast cancer problem and how best to address it.

In conducting my analysis, I approach this body of activism as a movement in the making. Given that I began my research during the movement's early years and continued it for more than a decade, I had the opportunity to track this body of activism—and to some extent participate in it—as it developed over time. Specifically, I followed the evolution of its political objectives, campaigns, and action strategies. I traced its ever changing social relationships with other movement fields, professional communities, political bodies, and the public at large. I assessed the multifaceted—and sometimes contradictory—set of cultural politics that guided activists' everyday efforts, professional relationships, and long-term goals. I examined the organizational development of particular groups that emerged and dissolved at different points in time. Finally, I observed the movement's developing relationship to science in terms of the specific theories of disease causation that activists embraced, as well as the ways in which activists positioned themselves in relationship to science, policy, and other movement fields, especially those focusing on environmental health.

To these ends, I conducted semistructured interviews with almost fifty activists, scientists, and policymakers. I collected and analyzed activist texts such as films, newsletters, action alerts, fact sheets, reports, pamphlets, resource guides, campaign materials, transcripts from press conferences, postcards, posters, buttons, and Web sites run by activist organizations. I read popular and scholarly accounts of environmental breast cancer politics, the breast cancer movement, the scientific and social dimensions of endocrine disrupters, and other relevant environmental health issues. At the same time, I kept abreast of the scientific literature on environmental causes of breast cancer in general and on endocrine disruption as it related to both breast cancer and other disorders afflicting humans and wildlife.

A significant portion of my research consisted of participant observation ethnography in various organizational settings. As part of this "multi-sited" fieldwork, I volunteered twice a week for a year at two cancer organizations in Santa Cruz, California.[36] I worked part time as a research associate for eighteen months in the Environment and Health program at World Resources Institutes (WRI), a nonpartisan environmental policy think tank in Washington, D.C. I attended activist conferences, meetings, press conferences, and public fundraising events across the country. In addition, I worked for nine months as the coordinator of the Safe Drinking Water program at a public health advocacy organization in Washington, D.C. Although this job did not focus on environmental breast cancer per se, it provided me with a deeper understanding of environmental health politics, activism, and policymaking at the federal level.

These experiences shaped my understanding of the bourgeoning environmental breast cancer movement and its efforts to transform the dominant breast cancer paradigm. In particular, I came to understand that transforming the dominant paradigm from a biomedical focus to a preventative one is more than a conceptual enterprise. New paradigms come into being through continual enactment and reenactment in social, discursive, material, and institutional contexts. During my fieldwork, I learned about the ways in which activists help to facilitate these processes through their daily work. Such efforts include developing newsletters and other education materials for the public about ways to reduce one's risk; participating in planning sessions with activists, scientists, and health professionals to establish policy campaigns, research projects, and other initiatives; holding public events to gain media coverage of their work; cultivating relationships via e-mail, phone calls, and face-to-face meetings with representatives from grant foundations to garner funds for their activities; and meeting with elected officials to encourage them to author and support bills that promote breast cancer prevention.

My eighteen months at WRI exerted a particularly strong influence on my thinking. While with the organization, I worked for Devra Lee Davis, an environmental health scientist who specializes in endocrine disrupters and breast cancer. Davis self-identified as a scientist, yet she positioned herself and her work at the crossroads where science, activism, and environmental health policy meet. Indeed, she spent much of her time working with activist organizations across the country on environmental breast cancer–related projects. As a result, my study of Davis's scientific work dovetailed with my study of the activist groups. I learned a great deal about not only individual breast cancer organizations but also the relationships between activists, scientists, and policymakers that partially constitute the broader terrain of environmental breast cancer activism. Of course, had I spent those eighteen months at another organization, I would have viewed the movement and its engagements from a different perspective. Thus, my account presents only a facet of the multidimensional and evolving fields of environmental breast cancer science, politics, and activism.

My focus on environmental breast cancer activism—prompting my decision to spend time at the organizations noted above—resulted from both my scholarly interests and my long-standing personal and political commitment to improving the state of women's health. Consequently, my decision to conduct fieldwork on the U.S. environmental breast cancer movement reflected my desire not only to develop a better intellectual understanding of the topic at hand but also to do activist work. As much as I wanted to describe and theorize about the movement and its engagements with environmental health science and policy, I also wanted to do my part to further them. Accordingly, I came to see my research and writing as what the anthropologists Akhil Gupta and James Ferguson call "location work"—that is, work casting the political task of anthropology not as " 'sharing' knowledge with those who lack it but as forging links between different knowledges that are possible from different locations and tracing lines of possible alliance and common purpose between them."

In this sense, my research area was not only a " 'field' for the collection of data" but also "a site for strategic intervention."[37]

At times, however, I found the practice of merging my activism and scholarly research troublesome. For example, the new director of a cancer organization at which I volunteered asked me to describe my research to her. In doing so, I related some of the criticisms made by activists about her organization's long-standing inattention to environmental causes of cancer. She was somewhat surprised by this revelation because she had assumed that her organization worked to minimize environmental risks. For the next thirty minutes, I showed her the organization's literature (which she had not yet read) that dismissed or remained silent on environmental links to cancer. This new knowledge shaped some of her subsequent thoughts and actions—which, in turn, shaped my analysis of the organization and her role within it. Although such "modest interventions" fulfilled my political desires, they also made me uneasy, as if I had rigged my data.[38] To compensate, I made countless attempts over the course of my fieldwork to protect the so-called purity of my data by not intervening, even when I found it difficult to remain silent. Yet these decisions also made me uncomfortable because I felt that I had missed opportunities to make a difference.

Such experiences recall the anthropologist Rayna Rapp's own mixed feelings about helping the women whom she studies. "While I painfully learned when to hold myself back and when to intervene to give information or suggest how a woman might gain access to needed resources," she writes, "I also came to accept the inevitable contamination of data that serious interactive feedback entails. The issue was not simply 'establishing rapport' with informants. The issue was how I might contribute. . .to their empowerment in a world where scientific and medical services are inequitably distributed."[39] My own experiences and Rapp's account led me to realize that influencing those whom I study is to some degree inevitable, whether or not that influence is deliberate. When I have intervened, I have done my best to remain accountable to my informants. Likewise, I work to remain accountable to my readers by making such interventions "visible" and discussing the impact that they had on my analysis and, perhaps, on myself.[40]

The environmental breast cancer movement has come a long way from its early days as a handful of locally based groups seeking to raise awareness about the cancer industry in their communities. Over the past twenty years, the movement has evolved into a national entity that has shaped the cultural, political, and public health landscape for breast cancer, environmental health, and disease prevention in significant ways. Moreover, it has provided women,

men, and even children with a new framework for protecting themselves, their family members, and their communities from breast cancer; for supporting the breast cancer cause; and for improving the environmental health of all living beings in the process. Even so, the environmental breast cancer movement continues to develop, both on its own and in tandem with other scientific, activist, policy, and cultural domains. Thus, my analysis of the movement's first two decades sets the stage for reflecting on the directions that the movement may take—and perhaps should take—in the years to come.

Chapter 2

"End the Silence"

Uncertainty Work and the Politics of the Cancer Industry

On a Monday morning in October 1995, I walked the mile and a half from my apartment to WomenCARE to begin my twice-a-week volunteer work. WomenCARE—short for Women's Cancer Advocacy, Resources, and Education—was located in a small duplex on Soquel Avenue in Santa Cruz, California, about a half mile from the downtown Pacific Garden Mall. Its office consisted of one room, a closet, and a tiny bathroom. With its couch, several coffee tables covered by assorted cancer literature, shelves of books, and a teapot, the front part of the room functioned as a meeting space for support groups, a library, and a place for women to relax and talk. The back part of the room, which contained two desks, a computer, and two metal filing cabinets, served as WomenCARE's administrative space.

At the time, the organization's paid staff consisted of two part-time co-directors. Amber Coverdale Sumrall, a tongue cancer survivor, was in her early fifties and a well-known local author and writing instructor. She lived with her partner in Santa Cruz. Lynn Boulé was in her late thirties and a mother of two young children. She resided on the west side of town. Several years before moving to the area, Boulé was diagnosed with lymphoma, and soon after, the doctors told her that she would die within the year. When I met Boulé, she drove a large green SUV to work. "A relic of the cancer," she told me one day while giving me a ride home from my volunteer shift. "After my doctor told me the cancer was terminal, my husband and I decided to go wild and buy an SUV for the hell of it. Why not? I was supposed to die. But then I didn't die, and now we're stuck with this huge, gas-guzzling thing."

My volunteer work at WomenCARE marked the beginning of my foray into the culture and politics of the U.S. environmental breast cancer movement. At the time, WomenCARE brought attention to breast cancer's environmental links by addressing the social, political, and economic forces that marginalized these links. Indeed, such critiques lay at the heart of the broader environmental breast cancer movement; they exemplify the primary strategy that activists took in the movement's early days not only to bring attention to suspected environmental causes but also to bolster their position for why, despite the uncertainty surrounding them, public concern is warranted. Ultimately, the movement relied on—and continues to rely on—these critiques as the foundation for its efforts to transform the dominant breast cancer paradigm.

An Emerging Social Movement

On my first day at WomenCARE, Boulé and Sumrall gave me a crash course on the organization's history and mission. Michelle Hobbs, Wendy Traber, and Deborah Abbott founded the organization in 1992, with Abbott serving as its first executive director. Hobbs and Traber were recovering from cancer—Hobbs had Hodgkin's disease and Traber had Hodgkin's disease and breast cancer— and felt that they knew few other women with whom to talk about their experiences living with the disease. Abbott, a therapist with a background in women's health activism, got involved after realizing that Santa Cruz had few resources to help one of her young friends with cancer.[1] When I met Boulé and Sumrall in 1995, WomenCARE was operating on a small budget consisting primarily of private donations from individuals and local businesses, as well as proceeds from community fund-raisers. Although the resultant budgetary constraints meant that Boulé and Sumrall could afford to staff the office only from 9:00 A.M. to 12:00 P.M. on Mondays, Wednesdays, and Fridays, they still managed to accomplish a good deal. To women with cancer, the center offered free holistic health services, including massage, tai-chi in the park, and yoga. It published a quarterly newsletter about cancer issues, newly published books, and upcoming events. It held drop-in support groups open to all women with cancer, as well as more structured groups that served specific populations— lesbians with cancer, Spanish-speaking women with cancer, and terminally ill women. Sumrall and Boulé also recently had started to develop a bilingual outreach program in nearby Watsonville for the town's Latina residents, many of whom did not speak English and did not have access to cancer education, support, or services.

WomenCARE did not have the resources to make environmental issues one of their top priorities. However, the organization managed to address these issues in various ways. Boulé, Sumrall, and clients who visited the office often talked about their suspicions that exposure to toxic substances in food, water, the air, and household cleaning products caused breast and other cancers. WomenCARE also discussed environmental issues in some of its public events and publications. For instance, the winter 1994 issue of the organization's newsletter included Wendy Traber's article "My Body, the Planet," which Traber had originally presented as a talk at a fund-raising event. Traber writes, "People have often asked me (and many more wondered out of earshot) why do you think you got cancer? Women in my support groups ask themselves, what did I do to get cancer? Did I eat the wrong things? Did I think the wrong thoughts? Did I have a bad or incorrect attitude? Did I live the wrong life? If I die, is it because I didn't 'do cancer' right? As if the diagnosis and disease, the treatments and losses aren't enough, women are ashamed. We are blaming ourselves. We blame our mothers for inheriting their cancers. We are blamed and judged by others for having cancer. The victims are being blamed, *not* the carcinogens and the producers of carcinogens."[2]

The feminism that motivated Traber and Hobbs to establish WomenCARE situated the organization within a long history of women's health activism, which, evolving out of the broader feminist movement of the 1970s, seeks to eradicate the social, cultural, political, and economic barriers that hinder women's abilities to achieve well-being. Further, women's health activists position themselves as health experts in their own right. By drawing on their individual and collective experiences as women, feminists, and marginalized citizens, these activists have developed alternative forms of medical treatment, care, research, and knowledge that they believe help to heal and empower women in ways that established biomedicine and social institutions, as well as the dominant culture, do not.[3]

The early women's health movement worked on a range of issues, from improving access to birth control and legal abortion, to empowering women to become informed patients, to encouraging them to attend medical school. The movement also provided the social, cultural, and political sparks for the development of breast cancer activism, which emerged after First Lady Betty Ford announced her diagnosis in 1974. Until then, breast cancer had been a taboo subject, viewed as a private matter not appropriate for public discussion. Fortunately, Ford's declaration challenged this social stigma and inspired other women to do the same. In 1975, Rose Kushner, diagnosed in the previous year, founded the first breast cancer organization, the Breast Cancer Advisory Council, which offered a hotline and mail service that provided newly diagnosed women with information about what to do next. That same year, she wrote *Breast Cancer: A Personal History and Investigative Report*, the first book that divulged a personal account of breast cancer and discussed the political dimensions of the disease. Over the following few years, other breast cancer organizations, along with the first wave of breast cancer support groups, continued the efforts to encourage women with the disease to discuss their experiences and bring the topic of breast cancer into public discourse.[4]

In the late 1970s and early 1980s, activists turned their attention to treatment. Initially, they focused on "overturning the orthodoxy" of radical mastectomy. Developed by William Halstead in the 1880s, this procedure remained the breast cancer surgery of choice well into the mid-1970s. Criticized for its disregard of women's bodies and needs, the surgery involved removing the entire breast, as well as the chest wall muscles, the fat under the skin, and lymph glands. The procedure left many women physically and emotionally debilitated, and it was shown to be unnecessary: research conducted in the early 1970s demonstrated that less invasive procedures, such as a simple mastectomy or a lumpectomy with follow-up radiation, was just as effective at halting the cancer. Historically, surgeons had performed the Halstead procedure in part because they viewed breast cancer as a localized disease; if they could remove the cancerous tissue and lymph nodes from a woman's body, she would be cancer free. By contrast, in the 1970s, oncologists began to view breast cancer as a systemic disease that could be spread through circulatory systems. The growing advocacy for less invasive surgeries recognized that for many women, removing their tumors was only one step toward eradicating their cancer.[5]

In addition to promoting less invasive procedures, activists helped to pass legislation requiring doctors to obtain informed consent from their patients before conducting breast cancer surgery. Previously, many women who went in for a surgical biopsy awoke with a mastectomy—the surgeons had assumed complete authority for what to do next when they found cancerous tissue. Activists challenged this, arguing that women had the right to make their own treatment decisions.[6] Since then, "treatment activism" has shifted to breast cancer drugs, with activists intervening in the development of such drugs, the clinical trials used to study their efficacy, and the policies and procedures designed to increase their accessibility.[7]

Early detection, particularly through mammography, became another important issue in the 1980s. Developed in 1913 by radiologist Robert Egan, mammography has become a primary—and perhaps the most important—method of early detection promoted by the health care profession. Even so, there is controversy over its use. Some activists have criticized the wide promotion of mammography by the National Cancer Institute and other cancer organizations because women diagnosed with the disease were not given ample follow-up treatment and care. In the early 1990s, activists began to question the popular assumption—perpetuated by the media, cancer organizations, and the mammography industry—that regular mammograms would prevent not only death, but also the disease itself, as evidenced by the slogan "Early detection is the best prevention." Another point of contention was the age at which women should get their baseline mammogram. Although a number of health organizations recommended that women should get a baseline mammogram at the age of forty, some breast cancer activists cited studies demonstrating that mammography does not prevent extra deaths in women under the age of fifty. They further challenged the use of mammography among younger women, stressing that too many mammograms may hurt such women more than help them, as the ionizing radiation that mammography machines emit is an established cause of breast cancer.[8]

The 1980s and early 1990s brought increased attention to access to care. Activists worked to break down social, cultural, political, and economic barriers to support services, educational resources, treatment, and early detection that were faced by all women but especially by marginalized and disadvantaged groups such as lesbians, poor women, and women of color. Some organizations, such as WomenCARE, serve a broad array of women. Others are directed toward a specific population. For example, Susan Hester founded the Mautner Foundation in 1990, a year after her partner, Mary-Helen Mautner, died of breast cancer. The only national lesbian health organization in the country, the foundation provides support services for local women, trains health care professionals in the health needs of lesbian women, and helps lesbians with breast cancer navigate obstacles to health care with which they may have to contend upon being newly diagnosed.[9] The sexism that has historically shaped the scientific, clinical, and advocacy domains related to breast cancer and women's health more generally has also perpetuated homophobia and subsequent discrimination against lesbians.[10] Compared with heterosexual women, lesbians face greater financial and sociocultural barriers to obtaining adequate health care, including breast cancer early detection and treatment. Moreover, lesbians may suffer from higher rates of breast cancer than those of heterosexual women.[11] In many ways, then, the struggle to eradicate breast cancer goes hand in hand with the battle to end homophobia and heterosexism.

In the early 1990s, activists became increasingly concerned about what they saw as a breast cancer "epidemic," alarmed by the incidence of the disease and mortality rates. At the beginning of the decade, the chance that a woman would develop breast cancer in her lifetime was one in nine, with rates having risen 1 percent each year since 1975. Mortality rates had decreased only marginally from the early 1970s. Two political factors intensified activists' concern. First, women's health needs did not receive as much federal funding as men's, especially in biomedical research.[12] In the summer of 1990, the Congressional Caucus for Women's Issues organized hearings on the federal government's inadequate attention to women's health, including to breast cancer. Second, the growth of HIV/AIDS activism prompted a dramatic increase in HIV/AIDS research during the early 1990s and sparked a move to increase funding for breast cancer research. Both established and newly formed breast cancer groups began to argue that the federal government, state governments, and biomedical institutions should devote more resources to the breast cancer problem.[13] Such groups demanded increased federal and state funding for basic breast cancer research and research to find a cure, better treatments and early detection methods, and greater access to breast cancer care. Some also began to push for breast cancer prevention, especially pertaining to possible environmental causes.

The environmental breast cancer movement that has evolved over the past two decades is not so much a clearly defined set of organizations as it is a diverse collection of knowledge, beliefs, values, ideologies, discourses, practices, artifacts, individuals, and relationships that crosscut a number of groups to varying degrees and in different ways. At one end of the spectrum are organizations that address environmental breast cancer as one issue among their broader women's cancer, environmental health, environmental justice, women's health, and public health agendas. Indeed, women's cancer activists were among the first to identify and discuss the environmental breast cancer problem. In the middle of the spectrum are breast cancer groups that address environmental issues along with their other health care and support efforts. At the other end are organizations that focus primarily on environmental breast cancer and disease prevention. The political strategies that groups take to address environmental breast cancer vary, as well. Across the broader movement, activists promote environmental health policy reform, push for increased scientific research, educate the public about suspected environmental causes, and mobilize public support for the cause. These activities, in turn, take place at the local, state, national, and even international levels. The majority of groups work across most, if not all, of these political and geographical domains, but some organizations emphasize specific domains over others.

The organizations that make up the environmental breast cancer movement are scattered across the nation in cities and towns such as Minneapolis; Washington, D.C.; and San Diego. The most prominent, oldest, and largest networks of environmental breast cancer activism are located in the San Francisco Bay Area, Greater Boston, and Long Island. Indeed, the groups within these regions are among the most active and influential in the country. To be sure, it is important not to reduce the broader environmental breast cancer movement to the work that takes place in these areas. After all, groups from other locations have contributed to the movement in important ways. Yet one cannot understand the movement's development and ongoing efforts without also examining the social, cultural, political, and public health contexts in which these three networks of activism developed and continue to flourish. Understanding the movement's emergence also requires attention to the various movement fields that shaped activists' early focus on the political and economical dimensions of environmental breast cancer issues.

Political and Economic Critiques

Wendy Traber's view that "the victims are being blamed [for their cancers], *not* the carcinogens and the producers of carcinogens," reflects one of earliest approaches—if not the first approach—that activists used to challenge the dominant breast cancer paradigm. Specifically, they argued that this paradigm's disregard for breast cancer prevention, especially relating to environmental factors, results from political and corporate malfeasance. One of the first women to articulate this position publicly was poet and activist Audre Lorde, author of the 1980 *The Cancer Journals.* From her perspective as a self-identified black lesbian feminist, Lorde gave voice to the physical, emotional, and political dimensions of living with breast cancer; the loss of a breast; and her decision to live as a "one-breasted woman." She asserted that social pressures faced by postmastectomy women to reconstruct their breasts make the existence of breast cancer invisible to society at large. By creating a cultural silence around the disease, especially among affected women, these social pressures also lead to political inaction around the disease, particularly regarding suspected environmental causes. Lorde wrote, "When other one-breasted women hide behind the mask of prosthesis or the dangerous fantasy of reconstruction, I find little support in the broader female environment for my rejection of what feels like a cosmetic sham. But I believe that socially sanctioned prosthesis is merely another way of keeping women with breast cancer silent and separate from one another. What would happen if an army of one-breasted women descended upon Congress and demanded that the use of carcinogenic, fat-stored hormones in beef-feed be outlawed?"[14]

Lorde was not the only woman with breast cancer in the 1980s to speak publicly about its possible environmental causes. Judy Brady, a San Francisco

Bay Area cancer activist, was diagnosed with breast cancer in 1980 at the age of forty-three. From the start, she believed that environmental pollution played a role in her cancer, as well as in most cancers. "I had read Rachel Carson many years ago," Brady explained, "and it just seemed liked common sense to me."[15] Several years after her diagnosis, Brady and other members of her women's cancer support group, including Jackie Winnow, participated in a nuclear disarmament march in San Francisco to bring attention to the link between ionizing radiation and breast cancer. They carried a banner that read, "People against Cancer," receiving many confused stares from the crowd.[16] In 1986, Winnow, a lesbian diagnosed with breast cancer who also participated in the early HIV/AIDS movement, co-founded the Women's Cancer Resource Center (WCRC) in Berkeley (now in Oakland) because no local services were directed at the needs of women with cancer, especially low-income women, lesbians, and women of color. What began as an answering machine in someone's living room grew into an organization offering information, support, financial help, and other outreach services to women with cancer and their families. Winnow's bourgeoning awareness about environmental politics shaped WCRC's objective of "working for a life-affirming, cancer-free society."[17]

Similar efforts took place on the East Coast. In September 1989, the feminist newsletter *Sojourner: The Women's Forum* published Susan Shapiro's essay "Cancer as a Feminist Issue." Shapiro, a freelance writer with breast cancer from Lexington, Massachusetts, expanded on many of the topics—especially the environmental politics of breast cancer—that Lorde discussed in *The Cancer Journals*. At the end of her article, Shapiro invited the public to attend a meeting at the Cambridge YWCA later that month to discuss the formation of the Women's Community Cancer Project. Around two dozen women showed up, among them Rita Arditti, a researcher in microbial genetics who was diagnosed with breast cancer in 1974 at age thirty-nine. From the time of her diagnosis, Arditti had sought to determine what had caused her cancer. She also wondered why she did not know more women with the disease. Although Shapiro died two months later, the group continued to meet, with Arditti taking a prominent role. From the start, the community-based and volunteer-only organization emphasized direct support, political action, and education, with cancer prevention and a cancer cure as its two primary objectives. Several years later, the group narrowed its focus to prevention.[18]

Despite these early efforts, most activists did not begin to write about and advocate on behalf of environmental issues substantively until the 1990s. Not surprisingly, activists drew from earlier feminist critiques of societal norms, biomedical practices, barriers to care, and federal research policy to highlight the ways in which sexism—and racism, homophobia, and classism—helped to perpetuate the disregard for breast cancer prevention and environmental causes of the disease in health care, research, advocacy, policy, industry, and public discourse. These feminist values also empowered breast cancer activists to mobilize around environmental issues in the first place. Indeed, feminism and environmentalism have complemented one another within a number of social and cultural arenas: ecofeminist movements that hold masculinist ideologies and institutions responsible for environmental destruction; environmental justice movements that highlight the disproportionate toxic burden faced by low-income women and women of color; antitoxics movements spearheaded by women; professional women's health and environmental organizations that work to reform local, national and international environmental policy; and women's movements in developing countries that resist the negative impacts of globalization on their local cultures, social relations, economies, human health, and natural and built environments.[19]

The feminist movement is not alone in shaping the emergence of these political and economic critiques or the formation of environmental breast cancer activism more generally. The politics of cancer have also been instrumental. Cancer is often constructed as a specific disease, but it is actually a disease category that links an array of disorders that, notwithstanding variations in their causes and sites of manifestations, share a set of characteristics related to the uncontrolled growth of abnormal cells.[20] This complex disease category came to dominate the focus of biomedical research, clinical practice, environmental health science, and environmental health policy in the twentieth century. In 1937, Congress established the National Cancer Institute (NCI), which since 1977 has been the largest and most heavily funded institute within the National Institutes of Health (NIH).[21] Since President Richard M. Nixon's signing of the National Cancer Act of 1971, authorizing $625 million for the nation's first "War on Cancer," the U.S. government has allocated more than $75 billion to the NCI for its cancer research and programs.[22]

Many nongovernmental organizations, pharmaceutical companies, and private institutions have directed their own financial resources toward the problem of cancer. Starting with the founding in 1913 of the American Society for Cancer Control—which several years later became the American Cancer Society—hundreds of local, regional, and national advocacy and support groups formed across the country to address the social, cultural, political, medical, psychological, and scientific dimensions of specific cancers (National Breast Cancer Coalition, National Prostate Cancer Coalition), cancer in general (American Cancer Society, National Coalition for Cancer Survivorship), and even specific populations affected by cancer (Women's Cancer Resource Center, National Childhood Cancer Foundation). Thousands of books, articles, television shows, and Internet sites have documented the many dimensions of cancer. Given that one in two men and one in three women in the United States will develop cancer at some point in his or her lifetime, it is little wonder that Americans consider cancer the "dread disease."[23]

Despite public consensus on the need to alleviate human suffering from cancer, individuals and institutions have not always agreed on how best to understand and approach the disease. During the past twenty-five years, these disagreements have revolved around issues such as the efficacy of conventional versus alternative cancer treatments, the health benefits of chemotherapy, and the relationship between diet and cancer.[24] To some extent, uncertain and contradictory bodies of scientific evidence have sparked these debates. Yet the positions that individuals and institutions take in relation to such debates, including the contrasting ways in which they make sense of the bodies of scientific evidence at hand, also reflect differences in their social, political, economic, organizational, and epistemological vantage points.

Debates also surround the topic of environmental causes of cancer. Samuel Epstein's *The Politics of Cancer* (1979) and Ralph Moss's *The Cancer Syndrome* (1980) were among the first books to address these debates.[25] Both had a strong influence on the feminist cancer activism that emerged during the 1980s. In *The Cancer Journals*, Lorde draws on Epstein, an academic researcher in the field of environmental and occupation medicine, to develop her critique of the medical establishment's inattention to environmental causes of the disease and prevention more generally. Epstein's book also resonated with Judy Brady. Following her breast cancer surgery in 1980, she found it at Modern Times, a political bookstore in San Francisco. Though she had already come to the conclusion on her own that toxic exposures caused cancer, Epstein's book validated her belief as well as her desire to take political action. Brady states, "Sam's book gave me the vehicle that I needed to really begin pushing it because now it wasn't just the ravings of an old leftist; now I had an 'expert' giving testimony to what was actually happening to us."[26] Similarly, members of the Women's Community Cancer Project read *The Cancer Industry* (the updated version of *The Cancer Syndrome*) to better understand the political and economic dimensions of cancer medicine, research, and policy.[27]

Taken together, Epstein's and Moss's books highlighted how, at the time, incidence rates for most cancers continued to increase, and overall cancer mortality rates had not declined—despite the array of scientific, biomedical, and advocacy efforts to eradicate the disease in the wake of Nixon's War on

Cancer.[28] Failure to reduce these rates resulted from the biomedical approach that guided the funding priorities and professional agendas of mainstream governmental, health, advocacy, and research institutions. Epstein and Moss argued that these institutions should devote more money and other resources to cancer prevention, especially regarding possible environmental causes, rather than find ways to deal with the disease after it developed.

In a broad sense, the dominant cancer paradigm reflects the ideology of individualism that structures biomedicine and disease prevention policy in the United States. This individualism is largely rooted in the classic liberalism and laissez-faire philosophy that have historically structured the country's social, cultural, political, and economic fabric.[29] Yet Moss and Epstein also claimed that the dominant paradigm's entrenchment grew from the political and economic interests of the "cancer industry." Coming together on boards, committees, and panels, the group of loosely connected government agencies (including the National Cancer Institute and the Food and Drug Administration), cancer advocacy organizations (including the American Cancer Society), industry entities, and pharmaceutical companies hold financial stakes in promoting a biomedical approach over disease prevention and environmental exposures in particular. After all, drug therapies, surgical interventions, and technologies that treat and detect cancer make money; preventing cancer, especially by restricting the production, marketing, and use of harmful—yet often profitable—synthetic products, does not.[30]

Along with the women's health movement and political analyses of cancer, a third set of movement fields that provided an early foundation for environmental breast cancer activism and its critiques of the cancer industry were the antitoxics and environmental justice movements. These diverse movements and their practices draw attention to the environmental exploitation of local communities, especially those that are home to socially, politically, and economically marginalized populations such as people of color and low-income workers. In this regard, they highlight the ways in which environmental problems brought on by industrial practices, corporate malfeasance, inadequate regulations, and lack of governmental oversight disproportionately affect marginalized communities in the form of excess pollution, toxic contamination, and human health problems. Further, they promote "ecological democracy."[31] Among other things, this set of principles argues that all people, including marginalized groups, have the right to healthy workplaces and living spaces. It also demands that such groups play an active role in determining the environmental fate of their communities by participating in industrial, governmental, and environmental policy decision-making processes, especially at the local level.

The antitoxics and environmental justice movements signify the coming together of the environment, civil rights, and other social justice movements that bourgeoned in the 1960s and 1970s. One of the earliest—and perhaps best-known—cases of the antitoxics movement arose in 1978, when chemicals from a toxic waste dump leaked into the Love Canal neighborhood of Niagara Falls, New York. In the aftermath of this event, resident Lois Gibbs—now the director of the Citizen's Clearing House for Environmental Health in Falls Church, Virginia—became concerned about the incident, its possible health effects, and the seeming inaction of local officials to address it. She took action by documenting the scope of the problem and its impact on community members, forming the Love Canal Homeowners Association, drawing public attention to the problem, and demanding that officials rectify the problem. Not only did the state buy out the homes closest to the leakage site; the federal government also passed the Comprehensive Environmental Response, Compensation, and Liability Act of 1980 (generally known as Superfund).[32]

Environmental justice activism truly came into its own in the 1980s as an increasing number of low-income communities, indigenous communities, and other communities of color across the country confronted health risks in their neighborhoods and workplaces. A particularly significant moment in the movement's development was the 1987 publication of *Toxic Wastes and Race in the United States* by the United Church of Christ. This report documented environmental racism by showing the disproportionate presence of toxic waste dumps in communities of color, particularly low-income areas.[33] Another milestone was the First National People of Color Environmental Leadership Summit, held in Washington, D.C., in October 1991. This three-day event, which brought together more than seven hundred activists, academics, and others from across the country, helped to solidify and legitimate environmental justice as a bona fide social movement.[34]

By the mid-1990s, environmental justice concerns had garnered notable public recognition. Journalists and social critics increasingly wrote about environmental racism and the social movements that sought to eradicate it. As a response to environmental justice critiques of traditional conservation and environmental groups for the latter's limited conceptions of nature and inattention to the needs of marginalized populations, established organizations such as the Sierra Club expanded their historical focus on the protection of wilderness, land, and waterways to include the protection of urban and other human-inhabited communities. Even the federal government became involved. In 1990, the Congressional Black Caucus charged the U.S. Environmental Protection Agency (EPA) with failing to address the heightened environmental risks of minority and low-income communities. To address these concerns, the EPA convened the Environmental Equity Workgroup to examine whether—and, if so, to what extent—such communities faced higher environmental burdens. The group determined that such burdens existed. In 1992, the EPA established the Office of Environmental Equity (later renamed the Office of Environmental Justice) to incorporate environmental justice concerns and perspectives into the agency's policies and programs.[35] The following year, the agency created the National Environmental Justice Advisory Committee, representing environmental groups, academia, industry, and tribal nations, to help set the EPA's environmental justice agenda.[36] In February 1994, President Bill Clinton signed Executive Order 12898, which established the Interagency Working Group on Environmental Justice, bringing together representatives from eleven federal agencies and several White House offices with the goal of incorporating environmental justice initiatives across the federal government.[37]

Cancer activism and the antitoxics and environmental justice movements influenced the environmental breast cancer movement's development in important ways. Cancer activism provided a broader disease context in which to situate critiques of the dominant breast cancer paradigm. Activists melded their feminist and economic perspectives to argue that the cancer industry's disregard of environmental factors resulted from the industry's desire to put profit over women's health. With their concern for the exploitation of marginalized groups, the antitoxics and environmental justice movements complemented environmental breast cancer activism's feminist critiques of the ways in which sexism pervaded breast cancer research, care, advocacy, and policy. They also pushed activists to pay closer attention to the intersection of race and class with gender in the context of environmental breast cancer politics. The movements further provided environmental breast cancer activists with a local perspective in regard to so-called breast cancer clusters, as well as reinforced the feminist and consumer health roots of breast cancer activism by encouraging women to participate in environmental decision making. Finally, the antitoxics and environmental justice movements' focus on corporate and governmental malfeasance complemented breast cancer activism's growing concerns with the cancer industry and its willingness to downplay environmental factors to bolster its profits. Although breast cancer activists targeted an array of institutions for malfeasance, they singled out the American Cancer Society for particular scrutiny.

Critiques of the Cancer Industry

In April 1996, six months after I started my work at WomenCARE, I began to volunteer at the Santa Cruz chapter of the American Cancer Society (ACS).

Although the two cancer organizations were located less than a mile apart, their financial and material statuses were quite different. Located in a wealthy, tree-lined historical district downtown, the Santa Cruz ACS was housed in a five-room late nineteenth-century Victorian registered with the Santa Cruz County Historical Society—a far cry from WomenCARE's one-room office in a stucco duplex at the back of a large parking lot on the outskirts of downtown. Inside, the two offices, meeting room, and front desk area contained many cabinets, tables, and bookshelves piled high with cancer materials. It also had a sizable kitchen. The chapter, which held regular business hours, had an ample staff, including a full-time office assistant, headed by a full-time executive director.

The ACS, which has become the largest nonprofit cancer organization in the country, bills itself as the oldest "nationwide community-based voluntary health organization dedicated to eliminating cancer as a major health problem by preventing cancer, saving lives, and diminishing suffering from cancer, through research, education, advocacy, and service."[38] Headquartered in Atlanta, Georgia, it has thirteen state-level offices, more than thirty-four hundred local chapters, and more than 2 million volunteers across the country. The organization runs an office in Washington, D.C., that deals with cancer policy. With an annual budget of more than $600 million, the ACS devotes significant resources to four program areas: research, prevention, patient support, and detection/treatment.[39] Although most of its work takes place in the United States, the organization increasingly reaches out internationally by collaborating with overseas cancer organizations that share its mission and by establishing new groups in other countries.[40]

Historically, the ACS has devoted significant resources to breast cancer. The organization earmarks more money to research on tumors of the breast than to studies of any other solid tumors. Since 1972, it has spent about $323 million on breast cancer research grants, the largest amount given by any nonprofit health organization. As of July 1, 2007, the ACS was funding 197 extramural research grants, totaling $106 million.[41] In 1977, the ACS, in collaboration with the National Cancer Institute, established the Breast Cancer Detection Demonstration Project, a nationwide program to promote the use of mammography among physicians and women.[42] In addition, the ACS provides outreach and support for women with the disease. In the mid-1950s, breast cancer survivor Therese Lasser started the Reach to Recovery Program, which continues to be the largest and most popular ACS program. This program "matches newly diagnosed breast cancer patients with trained volunteers who have survived breast cancer to help them cope with their disease by providing emotional support and information." In the mid-1980s, the Look Good ... Feel Better program was established to "teach [women] beauty techniques to help restore their appearance and self-image during chemotherapy and radiation treatments."[43] The noncompetitive five-kilometer Making Strides Against Breast Cancer fund-raiser walk, begun in 1993, is held annually in thirty-eight states and has drawn 4 million walkers and raised $280 million for the ACS's early detection and prevention programs.[44] Indeed, the majority of current volunteer programs at the organization are targeted at women with cancer, especially breast cancer.

Despite the ACS's breast cancer efforts, many feminist breast cancer activists view the organization's approaches to the disease as problematic. They critique the Reach to Recovery and Look Good . . . Feel Better programs for their tendency to reduce breast cancer to a cosmetic problem; to stigmatize women who choose not to wear prosthetic breasts or get reconstructive surgery after their mastectomy; and to gloss over the anger, sorrow, and the pain, both physical and emotional, that women with the disease often feel. Moreover, the fact that these programs focus on cosmetic makeovers, the restoration of women's bust lines, and the diminishment of women's negative feelings about the disease perpetuates the traditional—and sexist—notions of womanhood that feminist activists challenge.[45] Such critiques extend to particular ACS chapters. In fact, Michelle Hobbs and Wendy Traber established WomenCARE partly because the Santa Cruz branch of the ACS did not meet their needs. Whereas the Santa Cruz chapter tended to attract older and more conservative women invested in traditional forms of medical care, WomenCARE sought to reach out to younger and more progressive women who wanted a less conventional, and perhaps more feminist, healing experience. Further, WomenCARE offered a wider range of support groups for women with cancer and their families than its ACS counterpart.[46]

Breast cancer activists condemn the ACS for its stance on environmental links to the disease. Although the bulk of its breast cancer efforts go toward diagnosing and addressing the disease after it has already developed, the ACS devotes some resources to prevention. For the most part, however, its preventative approach is geared toward biogenetic and behavioral factors while downplaying environmental factors such as toxic chemicals. Much of the research that it does conduct on environmental factors are on a woman's genetic susceptibility to their effects, rather than the potential harm that they pose in and of themselves. In 2007, the organization listed the following breast cancer risk factors on its Web site: gender, race, age, family history of breast cancer, personal history of breast cancer and abnormal breast biopsies, genetic inheritance, reproductive history, alcohol consumption, obesity, exercise habits, and the usage of three synthetic drugs (diethylstilbestrol [DES], birth control pills, and postmenopausal hormone replacement therapy). The organization does not dismiss environmental factors outright, but neither does it take them seriously. The ACS clumps them together as "uncertain risk factors," along with "smoking, antiperspirants, underwire bras, abortion history, miscarriage history, silicon breast implants, [and] working night shifts." The ACS also states, "At this time, research does not show a clear link between breast cancer risk and environmental pollutants such as pesticides and PCBs."[47] The organization's *Breast Cancer Facts and Figures, 2007–2008* report takes a similar position by emphasizing the lack of evidence linking "environmental pollutants, such as organochlorine pesticides" to the disease rather than evidence that does show a link. The report mentions "high-dose radiation to the chest" as a risk factor, yet it provides no explanation of what this risk factor specifically entails. Nor does it mention other possible sources of medical, occupational, or industrial exposure to ionizing radiation that may increase the risk of breast cancer.[48]

The ACS devalues environmental causes of cancer in more general terms, as well. Although the organization's Web site provides a lengthy discussion about what constitutes a carcinogen, the methods used to determine whether a substance is a carcinogen, and information on chemicals that the International Agency for Research on Cancer and the National Toxicology Program list as known or probable carcinogens, it does not advocate reducing the public's exposure to these chemicals. Instead, the organization states, "Carcinogens do not cause cancer in every case, all the time. Substances classified as carcinogens may have different levels of cancer-causing potential. Some may cause cancer only after prolonged, high levels of exposure. And for any particular person, the risk of developing cancer depends on many factors, including the length and intensity of exposure to the carcinogen and the person's genetic makeup."[49] Given this ambivalence, it is not surprising that the organization only discusses about a dozen known or possible environmental causes of human cancer, including ionizing radiation, benzene, diesel, tetrachlorethylene (PERC), secondhand smoke, hormone replacement therapy, and diethylstilbestrol (DES).[50] The organization refused to support environmental measures such as the 1978 and 1983 Clean Air acts; occupational safety standards; proposed regulations in 1977 and 1978 on hair coloring products linked to breast cancer; and the 1958 Delaney Clause, an amendment that banned the deliberate use of any substance in food that has been shown to cause cancer in human and animals. In 1992, the ACS teamed up with the Chlorine Institute to issue a statement supporting the "global use of organochlorine pesticides" and dismissing the evidence linking these pesticides to breast cancer.[51]

During my time there, the Santa Cruz chapter of the ACS tended to replicate the national organization's stance on environmental causes of breast cancer. The chapter's approach to this issue was especially evident in the array of fact sheets, pamphlets, and booklets that it provided community members about the disease. Few of these materials—produced, for the most part, by the ACS's national organization—discussed environmental breast cancer issues, focusing instead on topic such as treatment, early detection, and the organization's support programs. The materials that mentioned environmental factors downplayed—and in some cases explicitly dismissed—the role of these contaminants in breast cancer development. Consider the Special Touch program, which the organization's California Division established in the mid-1990s. The goal of this program is to teach women about the importance of breast cancer early detection and proper techniques for conducting monthly self-breast exams. Consequently, the program devotes only five minutes of its forty-five-minute to two-hour presentations (the length depending on the needs of the program facilitator and participants) to risk reduction and prevention. In that five minutes, women are taught that "breast cancer has no one single cause, and is probably caused by a number of factors. ... Breast cancer does not seem to be associated with hormone use, and it is not caused by trauma, fondling, and chemical pollution in the environment. ... Until the causes of the disease are known and it can be prevented, the best way it can successfully be treated is through early detection when the cancer is small and has not spread."[52]

Activists argue that the position of the ACS that environmental chemicals pose little or no threat to human health has less to do with a lack of scientific evidence and more to do with its own political and economic interests: previous ACS board members have included a president of the American branch of Hoffman–La Roche, an ex-president of the Warner-Lambert pharmaceutical company, a former official of the Johns-Mansville company, and a Sun Oil executive.[53] In 1992, the organization established the American Cancer Society Foundation to bring in donations of one hundred thousand dollars or more. Its board of trustees has included corporate executives from the chemical, pharmaceutical, biotech, and financial industries.[54] The ACS also receives corporate funding for its specific programs and events; the Special Touch program, for example, is funded by DuPont—a corporation that produces not only mammography film but also synthetic materials and chemical byproducts, such as 1,3-butadiene, that are linked to breast cancer.[55] The fact that DuPont produces mammography film is particularly revealing, given that the Special Touch program's discussion on risk factors does not mention ionizing radiation, the one known environmental cause of breast cancer. Such radiation is emitted from such sources as X-ray and mammography machines. In a related fact, along with General Electric, DuPont tops the EPA's list of corporations responsible for causing the highest number of Superfund waste sites across the country.[56]

Uncertainty Work

Critiques of the cancer industry play an important role in the "uncertainty work" that environmental breast cancer activists conduct. Such work consists of the social, discursive, and material strategies deployed to make the case for why public concern is warranted about possible environmental causes of breast cancer despite the controversies and debates surrounding them. Indeed, uncertainty work constitutes one of the most significant set of practices that the movement undertakes.

To understand the significance of this uncertainty work, it is important to recognize that uncertainty not only causes scientific debate but also functions as a tactical element within it. Instead of detracting from the credibility of those who acknowledge it, uncertainty sometimes legitimates it.[57] For example, individuals and institutions associated with the cancer industry often label particular bodies of evidence linking toxic substances to breast cancer as uncertain as a way to cast doubt on their validity. Environmental breast cancer activists also construct uncertainty in ways that legitimate their own claims. Although they recognize that the evidence does not prove that toxic substances cause breast cancer, their acknowledgment of uncertainty allows them to argue that the evidence does not disprove this premise, either. Moreover, they argue that the cancer industry produces uncertainty for its own political and economic gain. Its strategies for doing so include dismissing, downplaying, and even stifling studies that find links between chemicals and cancer; pointing to inconclusive and negative studies as proof that environmental toxins do not cause cancer; holding back adequate funds for research on environmental causes of cancer; designing studies that will find inconclusive or negative evidence of causation; dismissing evidence from animal studies; not accounting for the additive or synergistic health effects from multiple chemical exposures when designing studies and risk assessment models; and basing regulatory action on standards of proof of human causation that are virtually unobtainable.[58]

Just as uncertainty functions as a strategic element within a debate, the particular meanings given to uncertainty have consequences for social action. For example, scientists, policymakers, and other actors invoke uncertainty to bolster their credibility in expert disputes, manage professional relationships, and negotiate disciplinary boundaries.[59] Similarly, activists' constructions of uncertainty shape their understanding of the environmental breast cancer problem and their efforts to resolve it. Uncertainty has made it difficult, if not impossible, to justify more stringent environmental policies within a regulatory system that demands proof of harm before taking action. By highlighting the political and economic stakes that certain corporations, government agencies, and health organizations have in creating uncertainty, activists can call for accountability and cooperation from these institutions as necessary steps in making environmental causes of breast cancer and disease prevention a federal priority.

One of the earliest strategies that activists took to achieve corporate and political accountability was to expose publicly the cancer industry's stakes in downplaying breast cancer prevention and environmental risks in particular. This strategy is evident in activists' texts from the 1980s and 1990s. Early on, various collections of personal essays functioned as forums for activists and women with cancer to discuss the ways in which sexism, racism, classism, corporate greed, and government malfeasance contributed not only to women's exposures to cancer-causing chemicals but also to the social, political, and scientific disregard for environmental causes of women's cancers.[60] In the wake of these personal narratives about women's cancers, a number of volumes from the mid-1990s focused exclusively on breast cancer, covered the debates surrounding environmental breast cancer and analyzed the controversies over treatment options, early detection, and research, among other breast cancer issues.[61] The second half of the decade saw the publication of books that honed in on environmental links to breast cancer, with in-depth coverage of the toxic substances suspected of causing the disease and the reasons why they received little attention from most biomedical, research, governmental, and advocacy institutions.[62] Activist organizations made these books available to their constituents. WomenCARE, for example, ran a small but frequently used small library out of its one-room office, where its entire collection, containing many of the books referred to above, fit onto four shelves.

Besides disseminating advocacy information through books, organizations raised awareness about the cancer industry through their newsletters. One of the first groups to do so was Breast Cancer Action. BCA was founded in 1990 by Elenore Pred and Linda Reyes, two San Francisco women with histories of breast cancer who decided to bring breast cancer survivors and their supporters together to challenge the government's inattention to the growing breast cancer epidemic. Despite Pred's death from the disease in late 1991, the organization continued to grow and flourish, working on issues related to treatment, access to care, alternative medicine, prevention, and the environment.[63] In its October 1990 newsletter, its second issue, BCA included a short exposé documenting controversies surrounding the ACS's limited approach to the disease. Among other things, the report discussed the organization's "stand against environmental carcinogens." Also in this issue, in the Books to Read section, was a review of Ralph Moss's *The Cancer Industry*, as well as a brief summary of the "possible causes of breast cancer under investigation," including electromagnetic fields, oral contraceptives, and artificial light.[64] In the following years, BCA's newsletter continued to highlight environmental issues.

Another strategy was to demand that the cancer industry take responsibility for its decision to put profit over women's health. Cambridge's Women's Community Cancer Project (WCCP), for example, protested the National Breast Cancer Conference that the ACS held near Boston in August 1993. About forty people participated in the protest, including members of WCCP, Greenpeace/Boston, and Women's Action. Protestors carried signs reading, "End the Silence" and "Hey ACS! Confront Those Polluters," and "Target the Real Causes of Cancer," and "No More Business as Usual, Fighting to Save Women's Lives." "The ACS claims to be 'leading the fight against cancer,'" WCCP wrote in a recap of the event, "yet have consistently remained silent on possible environmental links to breast cancer such as DDT and other pesticides, PCBs, low-level radiation exposure, and electro-magnetic fields." Earlier that year, WCCP and Greenpeace held a similar protest outside ACS's Massachusetts headquarters.[65]

The Massachusetts Breast Cancer Coalition (MBCC) chose another strategy for holding the cancer industry accountable. The MBCC was founded in 1991 by several women who had attended some of the early WCCP meetings. Although they supported the community-based work of WCCP, they wanted to focus on policy issues at the state and national level. In fact, MBCC's early efforts led Massachusetts to become the first state to describe breast cancer as an epidemic.[66] In line with its mission, in October 1993, MBCC organized a two-day conference, "Breast Cancer and the Environment: Your Health at Risk," one the group's first events devoted to environmental causes of breast cancer. MBCC invited representatives from the Food and Drug Administration (FDA), EPA, and the state government to participate in a panel discussion on the first day. The representatives sat at the front of the room and faced the audience, which consisted of scientists, activists, and others affected by the disease. Rather than answering questions posed by these audience members, the representatives listened to their personal and professional testimony about environmental links to breast cancer.[67]

As exemplified by this conference, many groups challenged the cancer industry during National Breast Cancer Awareness Month (NBCAM), an annual monthlong event held each October since 1985.[68] NBCAM's founder, Imperial Chemical Industries (ICI), aimed to spread the message that "early detection is your best protection" and to encourage women to "get a mammogram now," through public service announcements, pamphlets, and public events. AstraZeneca Pharmaceuticals, a subsidiary of ICI, took over the event in 1993.[69]

Other key sponsors have included the ACS, the National Cancer Institute, Cancer Care, and the American College of Radiology.[70] Since its inception as a monthlong awareness event, NBCAM has spawned its own organization that works throughout the year to promote the use of screening services.[71]

Although its sponsors asserted that NBCAM worked to improve women's health and prevent breast cancer deaths, activists felt that the campaign's emphasis on early detection and mammography deliberately deflected public attention from preventative efforts, particularly relating to environmental causes of cancer. For example, ICI produced acetochlor, a carcinogenic herbicide implicated in breast cancer that brought in $300 million a year during the early 1990s. The company was named in a 1990 federal lawsuit for dumping several other chemicals linked to breast cancer into Southern California harbors. Meanwhile, AstraZeneca was producing tamoxifen and marketing this controversial synthetic hormone as a treatment to prevent the recurrence of breast cancer, generating $470 million a year by 1994.[72]Likewise, other corporations, as well as cancer organizations and agencies, that supported NBCAM downplayed environmental causes of breast cancer and prevention in their daily work. Reflecting on this, Jeanne Marshall of WCCP, before her death of spinal cord cancer in April 1995, suggested a new name for NBCAM: National Cancer Industry Awareness Month, highlighting what she and other activists viewed as "the true motive behind National Breast Cancer Awareness Month: corporate greed."[73]

A particularly compelling series of NBCAM protests took place in 1995. On Friday, October 27, activists across the country celebrated National Cancer Industry Awareness Day by holding candlelight vigils outside their local ACS chapters. They protested the institution's contribution to the cancer epidemic through its denial of cancer's environmental links and of the importance of disease prevention more generally. San Francisco's Breast Cancer Action, WCCP, Massachusetts Breast Cancer Coalition, Greenpeace, and the National Coalition for Health and Environmental Justice were among the groups that helped to organize these protests. This last group organized a two-day conference, "Make the Link: Health and Environmental Justice," on October 27 and 28 in Atlanta, the home of the ACS's national headquarters.[74]As a follow-up to these efforts, WCCP co-sponsored the International Conference on Breast Cancer and the Environment in Ontario in early November. This two-day event, organized by the Canadian Breast Cancer Research and Education Fund, presented environmental breast cancer researchers Devra Lee Davis and Harlee Straus and other speakers and featured a panel discussion of activists, including WCCP's Arditti and Lise Beane.[75]

The general public was encouraged to participate in these 1995 events. A one-page flier with the headline "October: National Cancer Industry Awareness Month," written by Greenpeace, Breast Cancer Action, and National Coalition for Health and Environmental Justice, announced the failure of the nation's War on Cancer, the problems with NBCAM, and the economic stakes held by AstraZeneca, the ACS, and other NBCAM sponsors in promoting early detection over breast cancer prevention. In addition to encouraging people to participate in these local ACS protests and the Atlanta conference, the flier listed a number of other strategies that citizens could take, including "hold[ing] an education workshop to discuss the links between polluting corporations, the environment and cancer . . . writ[ing] an op ed piece for your local newspaper explaining the conflicts of interest between corporate polluters and Breast Cancer Awareness Month . . . organiz[ing] a National Cancer Industry Awareness Day at the local shopping mall to distribute literature." The flyer further encouraged citizens to call their local ACS chapters to insist that they "relinquish their role as a 'silent accomplice' and publicly take a stance on cancer's environmental links."[76] The ACS took these actions seriously, sending a memo to its local chapters on the subject. Wary of further protests, ACS headquarters listed responses that its local chapters should give individuals who asked questions about the organization's suspected corporate ties and its policies regarding environmental causes of breast cancer.

Other events organized to critique NBCAM revolved around educating residents about the presence of polluters in their communities and beyond. The Toxic Links Coalition in Oakland, California, was established in 1994 by local community organizations, women's health organizations, and environmental justice groups. This coalition worked to educate the community about the links between environmental contamination in the San Francisco Bay Area and public health problems—particularly cancer—facing the region's inhabitants. The goal was to alleviate the social, political, and economic conditions that gave rise to environmental racism, especially the disproportionate burden of environmental risk that "people of color, immigrants, and workers bear." By the time the coalition became inactive in 2004, it consisted of three dozen environmental, consumer, and public health organizations, among them Marin Breast Cancer Watch (now Zero Breast Cancer), Breast Cancer Action, and the Women's Cancer Resource Center; these last two were among its founding members.[77]

The Toxic Links Coalition used various strategies to educate the public about the cancer industry. Its Web site—which is still running—provides an overview of the federal government's failed War on Cancer, a description of the cancer industry, and facts on the economic stakes that this entity holds in downplaying environmental causes of the disease and cancer prevention. Most compelling was the annual Cancer Industry Awareness Tour of San Francisco that the coalition organized every October between 1995 and 2002. The tours walked participants through the city's financial district to point out companies that contributed significantly to local, national, and global pollution levels. During the tour there were protests against these companies in the city's downtown district.[78] Throughout the year, groups affiliated with the coalition sponsor tours of local communities facing environmental justice problems. These events allow residents and other concerned citizens to learn firsthand about environmentally hazardous sites and their locations, neighborhoods with unusually high rates of cancer or other suspected environmental health problems, and local companies that activists believe contribute to these community environmental health problems. For example, Green Action for Health and Environmental Justice, the group that oversaw the Toxic Links Coalition and continues to manages its Web site, conducts tours of toxic sites (among other environmental justice work) in Bayview Hunters Point, the most polluted area of San Francisco. Some research suggests that this low-income—and primarily African American—neighborhood has the highest breast cancer incidence rate in the city. Many activists and community leaders link this to the area's various sources of indoor and outdoor contamination.[79]

The Late 1990s and Beyond

Early efforts to hold the cancer industry accountable for its silence on environmental factors produced some results. The public became more aware about the cancer industry and the environmental links to breast cancer, and a growing number of health-related organizations began to address the issues. Additionally, some policymakers, health care professionals, and individuals affiliated with mainstream cancer organizations began to acknowledge that environmental factors may cause the disease. Nevertheless, the dominant paradigm remained entrenched a decade after activists began their campaign to challenge the cancer industry.

In September 1998, I attended a two-day event called the March, in Washington, D.C. A coalition of national and local cancer groups, including the ACS, the National Coalition for Cancer Survivorship, and the Intercultural Cancer Council, organized the event to protest the lack of progress in lowering overall cancer incidence and mortality in the United States. In "coming together to conquer cancer," the coalition's members called not only for improved treatment and early detection in general but also for better access to adequate health care for individuals from ethnic minority, low-income, and other disadvantaged backgrounds. The main event began early Saturday morning with a march around the district, followed by a rally on the Mall featuring Hilary Clinton, Al and Tipper Gore, Jessie Jackson, and other speakers. Even with such a diverse coalition of participating cancer organizations, no speaker, rally cry, or sign mentioned anything about environmental risks, much less cancer prevention. Instead, the speeches and signs and slogans were about fighting cancer, beating it and curing it—goals that, although important and necessary components of a cancer program, did nothing to prevent cancer from occurring in the first place. Not surprisingly, the pharmaceutical companies Bristol-Myers Squibb, Glaxo-Welcome, and Pharmacia and Upjohn were the presenting underwriters of the March.

Most of the booths offering cancer information to the public embodied this dominant cancer paradigm. Some booths were set up by pharmaceutical companies: representatives from AstraZeneca Pharmaceuticals handed out pink cloth ribbons attached to business cards reminding people of the upcoming National Breast Cancer Awareness Month, while Novartis Pharmaceuticals passed out literature on its chemotherapy and immunotherapy treatments. For their part, many cancer organizations, among them the Melanoma Research Foundation, National Kidney Cancer Association, National Prostate Cancer Coalition, and Ovarian Cancer Research Fund had on offer written materials that touted the importance of early detection. The breast cancer organizations that participated in the event—particularly Susan G. Komen for the Cure and the National Breast Cancer Coalition—espoused these conventional approaches as well. Several groups even promoted products that environmental breast cancer activists have criticized for having suspected links to the disease. The National Beef Association, for instance, had a tent—at least three times as big as most of the booths—in which representatives passed out fact sheets lauding the health benefits of red meat.

Environmental discussions were not completely absent from the event, however; bits and pieces took place in the rally's social and spatial margins. Consider the ten-foot-high cardboard writing walls that organizers set up for event attendees to express their thoughts about cancer. Hundreds of notes written in different-colored pens covered their surfaces. For the most part, the notes described their authors' personal ordeals with cancer, their family members' experiences with the disease, and the need for more research. Several writers, however, stressed the importance of examining possible environmental causes. Environmental discussions also occurred in two booths on the far edges of the rally's boundaries, quite a distance from the main stages where public figures such as Cindy Crawford (who lost her younger brother to leukemia when she was ten) emceed events. The National Coalition against the Misuse of Pesticides organized one of these booths. The young woman running it observed that most of the event's attendees did not know about her booth because of its location. Thirty minutes later, I visited the table run by a children's environmental health organization. As I collected the group's literature, Nancy Evans, a San Francisco breast cancer survivor and activist, stopped by to say hello to the woman who ran the booth.

Evans was, and still is, one of the best-known environmental breast cancer activists in the country. After her breast cancer diagnosis in 1991, she left her position as a science writer and the following year joined the fledgling group Breast Cancer Action, in San Francisco. She was elected president of the organization two years later.[80] In 1997, she left Breast Cancer Action to become health science consultant at the Breast Cancer Fund, also located in San Francisco (she remained a member of Breast Cancer Action's board). Ex-lawyer and restaurant owner Andrea Martin founded the Breast Cancer Fund in 1992 after receiving two breast cancer diagnoses between January 1989 and May 1990. Under Martin's directorship, the organization sought to "transform breast cancer into a public health priority" in the areas of early detection, treatment, access to care, and prevention, especially pertaining to environmental issues. After receiving, in 2001, a diagnosis of brain cancer (from which she died in 2003), Martin stepped down as executive director of the organization. Jeanne Rizzo, a longtime consultant and advisor to the Breast Cancer Fund, took over the position. During its leadership transition, the organization revamped its mission statement, becoming the only national breast cancer organization solely focused on breast cancer prevention and environmental health issues.[81]

Both Evans and the children's environmental health representative noted the lack of environmental presence at the rally and particularly the relegation of environmental groups to the outskirts of the Mall. Although they did not think that there had been a deliberate effort by the March's organizers to silence environmental health advocates, they did believe that the organizers, with their focus on different issues, most likely did not know what to do with the environmental groups that wanted to participate in the event. Consequently, these groups wound up in the event's margins by default. To counter the disregard of environmental issues, Evans organized, separate from the March, a public showing of the documentary *Rachel's Daughters: Searching for the Causes of Breast Cancer* two days later at the National Museum for Women in the Arts in downtown D.C. On September 11, 1997, the film premiered at the Castro Theatre in San Francisco, and on October 1, it premiered on HBO. It documents several San Francisco Bay Area breast cancer survivors, including Evans, who acted as "detectives," investigating why so many younger women were developing breast cancer. As part of their investigation, the detectives met with twenty-one scientists across the country whose research focused on breast cancer, particularly the disease's environmental connections. They also met with a number of women living with breast cancer who thought that environmental factors played a role in the development of their disease. Filmmakers Allie Light and Irving Saraf directed and edited the documentary as a response to their thirty-nine-year-old daughter's diagnosis of breast cancer, with Evans serving as the film's co-producer. After chatting with the children's health representative for a few more minutes, Evans left to meet up with a friend.

Because of the dominant paradigm's continued entrenchment, criticism of and challenges to the cancer industry guided much of breast cancer activism throughout the late 1990s and into the early 2000s. In particular, they continued to shape how activists conceptualized the economic dimensions of breast cancer politics, the debates surrounding environmental causes, and strategies for promoting disease prevention. Such understandings of and approaches to the cancer industry have broadened over time, most notably in response to the environmental breast cancer movement's evolving social, political, and scientific terrain. Activists now expose the political and economic interests of environmental health research institutions that do not focus primarily on cancer. In some cases, they go beyond the cancer industry to focus on the "pharma-chem" industry, especially in relation to the growing biomedical trend toward chemo-prevention drugs. They also target an array of corporations and social organizations outside the cancer industry that perpetuate the dominant paradigm through their charitable giving, funding-raising efforts, and sponsorship of breast cancer–related events.

Challenging the cancer industry and other forms of corporate power is not the only strategy that activists take to rethink the dominant breast cancer paradigm and push for prevention. By the mid-1990s, they had begun to intervene in the scientific-research process by influencing the production, interpretation, and dissemination of research examining environmental causes of breast cancer. Although activists' scientific efforts did not replace their political and economic critiques, they provided them with another framework for conceptualizing the politics of environmental causes of breast cancer, the uncertainty surrounding these causes, and strategies for implementing disease prevention. Such scientific interventions now rank among the movement's best-known and most innovative set of practices.

Chapter 3

From Touring the Streets to Taking On Science

In February 1999, I began my job as a research associate for Devra Lee Davis, an environmental health scientist who had spent the past fifteen years researching and writing about environmental causes of breast cancer. At the time, Davis was a senior scientist and the director of the Health, Environment, and Development Program at the World Resources Institute (WRI), a nonpartisan environmental policy think tank located at Seventeenth and G Streets Northwest, a few blocks from the White House. In contrast to WomenCARE's small stucco duplex and the American Cancer Society Santa Cruz chapter's five-room Victorian house, WRI's setting for its offices was two floors of a ten-story office building that spanned almost half a city block. On my first day, I checked in at the front desk. Several minutes later, Davis came out to meet me, wearing a blue dress, stockings, and heels. If clothing styles help to delineate cultures of action within the broader breast cancer movement, as sociologist Maren Klawiter claims, it is also the case that they help to delineate different cultures of action within the terrain of environmental breast cancer activism. Rather than the casual outfits worn by Lynn Boulé and Amber Sumrall at WomenCARE, dresses and suits turned out to be Davis's standard garb.[1]

Davis's scientific work at WRI was part of a developing culture of action within the environmental breast cancer movement. Although the movement's earlier efforts to challenge the cancer industry's stance on environmental links to breast cancer included critiques of the uncertainty surrounding these causes, this set of political strategies did not necessarily emphasize direct participation in the scientific process itself. In fact, some activists who embraced this approach discouraged the promotion of further research, as they viewed it as a regulatory stall tactic within a system that demanded levels of proof that were difficult, if not impossible, to achieve.[2] By the mid-1990s, however, a growing number of activists began to call for more research on environmental causes of breast cancer as a way not only to better understand the disease but also to further their prevention agenda.

A Growing Focus on Xenoestrogens

My arrival at WRI coincided with its move to another office building across town, next to Union Station and several blocks from Capitol Hill. As Davis led me through the halls toward her office, people were filling Dumpsters with unwanted books, journals, and papers and packing their office supplies into moving boxes. Davis should have already started to do so as well, but because of her perpetual business trips and meetings, she had barely begun. As we sat in her office, attempting to talk in the midst of incoming phone calls and visits by WRI staff who were hoping to catch her before she left for another appointment, Davis told me that one of my first jobs would be to help pack up her files, books, and other office things.

Davis's interdisciplinary background gave her with ample experience in science, politics, and policy. In 1972, Davis received her PhD in sociology of science from the University of Chicago. She then completed a postdoctorate in epidemiology at the National Cancer Institute, receiving a Master's of Public Health from the Johns Hopkins University in the process. From 1983 to 1993, she worked at the National Academy of Sciences—first as the director of the National Research Council's Board on Environmental Studies and Toxicology and several years later as its scholar in residence. In 1994, President Bill Clinton appointed her to the newly established National Chemical Safety and Hazard Investigation Board. She also held affiliated faculty positions at Mount Sinai Medical Center, George Washington University, and Strang Cornell Cancer Prevention Center of Rockefeller University. In her position at WRI, which she took up in 1995, Davis continued her work on breast cancer; she also took on new projects relating to children's environmental health, reproductive health, air pollution, and climate change.

In her breast cancer work, Davis is perhaps best known for her research on xenoestrogens. In contrast to the more widely studied carcinogens (such as ionizing radiation) that cause normal cells to become breast cancer cells by directly mutating their DNA, xenoestrogens are believed to increase breast cancer risk by mimicking natural estrogen function. Among the xenoestrogens that are of particular relevance to breast cancer are the organochlorine pesticide

Table 3.1 Xenoestrogens in Common Indoor and Outdoor Environments

Chemical Name and Function	Source/Site of Contamination	Also a Known Breast Cancer Carcinogen?
Atrazine (pesticide)	Water, radishes, carrots	Yes
Bisphenol A (packaging material)	Plastic food packaging, lining of food cans	No
Chlordane (pesticide)	Beef, lamb, chicken, freshwater and saltwater fish	Yes
Cyanzine (pesticide)	Water	Yes
DDT (pesticide)	Beef, lamb, chicken, freshwater and saltwater fish	No
Dieldrin (pesticide)	Beef, lamb, chicken, freshwater and saltwater fish	Yes
Diethylstilbestrol (DES) (animal and human medicine)	Beef and poultry	Yes
Dioxin (chemical byproduct)	Pesticides and industrial pollution in air, food, water, earth	No
Endosulfan (pesticide)	Fruits, vegetables	No
Growth hormones (animal drugs)	Beef, lamb	Yes
Heptachlor (pesticide)	Beef, lamb, chicken, freshwater and saltwater fish	Yes
Lindane (pesticide)	Beef, pork, lamb, chicken, freshwater and saltwater fish	No
Phthalates (plasticizer; cosmetic dye)	Hair dyes, cosmetics, aluminum foil, printing inks, plastics	Yes
Polycyclic aromatic hydrocarbons (PAHs) (industrial pollutants)	Seafood, meats and seafood heavily grilled on charcoal, cigarettes, products of fuel combustion	Yes
Polychlorinated biphenyls (PCBs) (industrial pollutants)	Freshwater and saltwater fish, European meat	No
Polystyrene (packaging material)	Plastic food packaging, lining of food cans, plastic tubing	No
Polyvinyl chloride (PVC) (plastic)	Plastic tubing, clothing material	No
Red dye no. 3 (food coloring)	Processed foods	Uncertain
Simazine (pesticide)	Water	Yes

Sources: Devra Davis, *When Smoke Ran Like Water: Tales of Environmental Deception and the Battle against Pollution* (New York: Basic Books, 2002); Deborah Cadbury, *The Estrogen Effect: How Chemical Pollution Is Threatening Our Survival* (New York: St. Martin's Press, 1997); Samuel S. Epstein, David Steinman, and Suzanne LeVert, *The Breast Cancer Prevention Program* (New York: Macmillan, 1997); Theo Colborn, Dianne Dumanoski, and John Peterson Myers, *Our Stolen Future: Are We Threatening Our Fertility, Intelligence, and Survival? A Scientific Detective Story* (New York: Plume Books, 1997); Ted Schettler, Gina Solomon, Maria Valenti, and Annette Huddle, *Generations at Risk: Reproductive Health and the Environment* (Cambridge, Mass.: MIT Press, 1999).

DDT; industrial pollutants known as polychlorinated biphenyls (PCBs); bisphenol A, a found in plastic goods and packaging materials; and dioxin, a chemical byproduct present in certain pesticides and industrial pollution. Some toxic chemicals are both xenoestrogenic and carcinogenic; among them are the pesticide dieldrin; phthalates, found in plastics and personal care products; and polycyclic aromatic hydrocarbons (PAHs), pollutants in cigarette smoke and in the byproducts of fuel combustion. (See table 3.1.)

Xenoestrogens play a significant role in the environmental breast cancer movement. In the movement's early days, activists frequently talked about bona fide carcinogens, including ionizing radiation and benz(a)pyrene. Some even applied the term *carcinogen* to hormone-mimicking chemicals. Their use of the term in this way may have partly resulted from the fact that knowledge about hormone disruption was still emerging, yet it also related to the tendency to situate environmental breast cancer within the broader framework of cancer politics. Thus, the term *carcinogen* not only referred to actual carcinogenic chemicals but also symbolized the movement's challenges to the cancer industry's disregard for environmental causes and disease prevention. By the mid-1990s, however, activists paid more attention to xenoestrogens and the scientific theory of how they work. As activist and breast cancer survivor Sharon Batt wrote in *Patient No More: The Politics of Breast Cancer*, "Suddenly, it's not wildly speculative to discuss breast cancer and environmental contaminants—and to talk about actually trying to prevent breast cancer through changes to the way we live. The theory that fat-soluble synthetic chemicals mimic or amplify the effects of estrogen is so frequently discussed it now has a name—the xenoestrogen hypothesis."[3]

This increased awareness of and concern about xenoestrogens came on the heels of a growing number of studies that shed light on the impact of the chemicals on breast cancer development. The impetus for some of the earliest studies was a case of serendipity. In the late 1980s, Tufts University biologists Ana Soto and Carlos Sonnenschein noticed breast cancer cells that inexplicably started to divide and multiply in their plastic tube. The scientists soon realized that a chemical from the plastic had leached into the cells. They found that this chemical, *p*-nonylphenol, mimicked estrogen and, in doing so, caused the cells to grow. In subsequent experiments, Soto and Sonnenschein exposed breast cancer cells to a number of other hormonally active compounds, both separately and in combination with one another, to determine whether they, too, would cause these cells to divide and multiply. They found not only that the compounds led to increased breast cancer cell growth but also that the potency of individual chemicals was much stronger after the scientists combined them.[4]

In the early 1990s, researchers at Cornell University's Strang Cancer Prevention Center studied how different kinds of natural estrogen affect breast cancer cell growth. They found that "good" estrogens, called 2-hydroxyestrones, promote healthy cell development and can help to fix damaged cells. "Bad" estrogens, by contrast, promote breast cancer cell development, in two ways: the 16-a-hydroxyestrones can increase the division and multiplication of breast cancer cells that already exist, as well as hinder the capacity of these cells to be repaired, and the 4-hydroxyestrones are carcinogenic, meaning that they may have the capacity to damage the DNA of healthy cells directly and turn them into cancer cells.[5]

In 1992, Davis teamed with H. Leon Bradlow, a biochemist then at Rockefeller University who was researching the differences between good and bad estrogens, to test the impact of hormone-mimicking chemicals such as DDT and atrazine on the production of these natural estrogens. Upon their finding that these chemicals caused increased bad estrogen, Davis and Bradlow developed xenoestrogen theory, which hypothesizes that xenoestrogenic chemicals increase the risk of breast cancer.[6] As other scientists subsequently observed, hormone-mimicking compounds are more dangerous than endogenous ones because they tend to be more potent than their natural counterparts. To make matters worse, the amount of xenoestrogens found in the body, primarily in breast fat, is often higher than that of natural estrogens. Once in the body, hormone mimickers do not leave it as quickly as do endogenous estrogens, often remaining and accumulating in fat cells for many years.[7] In later articles, Davis further developed xenoestrogen theory, claiming that "good" xenoestrogens, which include "phytoestrogens" such as those in broccoli and soy, may decrease the risk of breast cancer. Indeed, Davis and other scientists hypothesize that the consumption of a high-soy diet contributes to low rates of breast cancer among Asian women.[8]

Although Soto, Sonnenschein, Davis, and Bradlow demonstrated that xenoestrogens increase the production of breast cancer cells in the laboratory, their research did not offer evidence of increasing breast cancer risk in humans. In 1993, Mary Wolff and her colleagues offered the first epidemiological evidence when they compared levels of PCBs in the blood serum of women with and without breast cancer. By demonstrating that PCB levels were higher in women with breast cancer, the study corroborated Davis and Bradlow's theory.[9] Then, in 1994, Nancy Krieger, Wolff, and several other researchers found no statistically significant difference between the levels of DDE and PCBs in the blood of women with breast cancer and the levels of these toxins in women without the disease. When analyzing the results by race, however, the findings looked different. Although Asian women with and without breast cancer showed no significance difference in their blood levels of both toxins, African American women and white women with breast cancer had higher blood levels of DDE than those of African American and white women without the disease.[10]

Concerns about xenoestrogens were based partly on the fact that many—if not most—of the established risk factors for breast cancer relate to high levels of exposure to natural estrogens. These factors include early onset of menstruation, delayed menopause, giving birth to one's first child after the age of thirty or not giving birth at all, never breastfeeding, obesity, and moderate to heavy alcohol consumption. Among other possible risk factors connected to high estrogen levels are high bone density; excess weight that is carried in the abdomen; high insulin levels; and a diet high in fat, meats, and simple carbohydrates. (Studies on these dietary factors, however, are still in their early stages, and results are tentative.) Many factors known to reduce women's risk of the disease, in turn, decrease a woman's estrogen levels; such factors include breastfeeding for a year and a half or longer, giving birth to one's first child before the age of nineteen, and regular exercise.[11] Some research also indicates that a low-fat diet and the consumption of soy and broccoli and other foods containing "good" estrogens (phytoestrogens), as well as fruits and vegetables more generally, may decrease breast cancer risk by lowering estrogen levels.[12]

Xenoestrogen theory was further strengthened by the identification of drugs delivering synthetic hormones—including birth control pills—as possible breast cancer risk factors. Although the overall body of research on the relationship between birth control pills and breast cancer has produced mixed results, many researchers and health organizations take the position that current or recent use of birth control pills slightly increases a woman's chance of developing the disease.[13] Another synthetic hormone drug is diethylstilbestrol (DES), an estrogen prescribed to pregnant women from 1938 to 1971 to prevent miscarriages. The Food and Drug Administration banned the use of DES in response to findings that it caused a range of health problems, especially for the daughters (and to a lesser extent, the sons) of women who took the drug during their pregnancies. More recently, researchers have found that DES increased the risk of developing breast cancer not only in women who took it during their pregnancies but also in women who had been exposed to it in utero.[14]

The most compelling evidence regarding synthetic drugs surrounds the use of hormone replacement therapy. In July 2002, investigators for the Women's Health Initiative, a ten-year Harvard University study examining the health effects from hormone replacement theory among 16,608 postmenopausal women aged fifty to seventy-nine, halted the project early because they found that the drug, which contained a combination of estrogen and progestin, increased the incidence of invasive breast cancer among their study population by 26 percent.[15] Four years later, another study found that overall incidence rates for invasive breast cancer dropped by 7 percent in 2003, marking the first age-adjusted decline in such rates since the 1970s. Of particular note was the decline in estrogen-receptor-positive breast cancers, which are fueled by exposure to estrogen. Whereas the number of estrogen-receptor-positive tumors declined by 8 percent, estrogen-negative tumors decreased by 4 percent. Among women between the ages of fifty and sixty-nine, the rates of estrogen-receptor-positive breast cancer tumors declined by 12 percent. Many researchers attribute this sharp decline in overall invasive breast cancer rates and estrogen-positive tumors in particular (especially in older women) to the decreased use of hormone replacement therapy (HRT) after the Women's Health Initiative released its results. In the decade before the study came out, 30 percent of postmenopausal women took HRT. By late 2002, half of these women had stopped the regimen.[16]

The emergence of endocrine disrupter theory provided yet another scientific context for understanding the links between xenoestrogens and breast cancer. The most advanced explanation of endocrine disruption theory is in *Our Stolen Future: Are We Threatening Our Fertility, Intelligence, and Survival?—a Scientific Detective Story* (1996) by Theo Colborn, Dianne Dumanoski, and John Peterson Myers. In this account, the release of hormone-disrupting chemicals—most of which were developed after World War II—into the environment have contributed to recent increases in reproductive, developmental, neurological, immunological, thyroid, and cancerous conditions found in wildlife and humans. Many of the most intensively studied chemicals disrupt estrogen production; other compounds, however, are believed to alter the production of androgen, progesterone, and thyroid hormones, among other hormones. Chemicals can disrupt the endocrine system in four ways. First, they can mimic or block naturally occurring hormones. Second, they can alter the levels of the carrier proteins that transport naturally occurring hormones through the bloodstream or interfere with the hormone's attachment to the receptor. Third, they can interfere with natural hormone production and, in some cases, can permanently alter baseline levels of hormones. Finally, they can affect the number of hormone receptors to which natural hormones bind.[17] Although evidence of harm to health is more conclusive for wildlife than for humans, Colborn and her co-authors assert that enough data exist on the latter to warrant serious public concern.

On its release, *Our Stolen Future* was heralded as the sequel to Rachel Carson's 1962 classic, *Silent Spring*, the first book to take a scientific and ethical stand against the widespread and indiscriminate use of DDT and other pesticides, insecticides, and herbicides on crops and in neighborhoods. Carson argued that these compounds killed not only unwanted weeds and insects but also birds and fish. She raised concern about possible effects on humans, especially children, and noted some of the chemicals' potential estrogenic effects. Picking up where *Silent Spring* left off, *Our Stolen Future* grouped Carson's targeted compounds, among others, into a new class of chemicals, provided a theory of disease causation that explained how these chemicals worked, and expanded on Carson's list of health disorders linked to them. In doing so, the book highlighted how pervasive these chemicals are in the environment, our bodies, and the synthetic materials used in daily life. In addition to affirming Carson's call for increased public health protection from such chemicals, Colborn and her co-authors explicated some of the industrial, agricultural, technological, institutional, and consumer changes that this protection would require.

Endocrine disrupter theory emerged as a "scientific hypothesis" of concern to the scientific community in the early 1990s. After the 1996 release of *Our Stolen Future*, the theory also emerged as a "public hypothesis" of concern not only to the media but also to advocacy groups, policymakers, health professionals, and the public at large.[18] Environmental breast cancer activists were among those who embraced this theory. To be sure, some of them had begun talking about it prior to the book's release. In the months and years following the book's scientific and public hype, however, many more activists joined and helped to perpetuate the endocrine disrupter theory "bandwagon."[19] Most notably, they helped to legitimate the theory through increased participation in scientific research and analysis.

The Blurring of Science and Activism

Although Devra Lee Davis conducted environmental health research during my tenure at the World Resources Institute, she spent increasing amounts of time working with breast cancer, environmental health, and women's organizations to bring attention to environmental causes of breast cancer. As part of these efforts, she sat of the boards of various groups, advised them on their publications, spoke at their conferences and events, and helped to plan their health campaigns and agendas. In addition, Davis collaborated with such groups on her own public health projects. Hadassah, a Jewish women's organization in New York City, was among these groups. "Jewish women of Ashkenazi descent have a higher risk of breast cancer than other women do because the BRCA1 gene is more frequent in this population," Davis explained when I once asked her why she did so much breast cancer work with the organization. "Having the gene does not automatically lead to breast cancer. Instead, the gene predisposes women to getting the disease. Therefore, it is important to educate those with the gene or who are suspected of having the gene about dietary and environmental risk factors that can trigger breast cancer to develop. You can't control your genes, but you can control many dietary and environmental risk factors."

The work that Davis did in conjunction with health organizations and other groups exemplifies a broader trend within the environmental breast cancer movement: namely, the social, material, and conceptual "blurring" of science and activism.[20] Along with Davis, a growing number of other breast cancer scientists have become involved in the movement. Such scientists draw on their knowledge, skills, and expertise to develop a better understanding of environmental links to the disease and raise awareness about such links. Some even sit on the advisory boards of activist groups, help to develop educational materials for the groups; speak at their conferences; appear in their films; and collaborate with them on policy, research, and public health initiatives. On the flip side, activists have increasingly become involved in matters of science. Not only do they continue to critique the lack of scientific attention to environmental causes of breast cancer and the political and economic factors that have perpetuated this inattention; they also demand an active role in decisions about research funding, the health issues that scientists examine, the design of research studies, and the interpretation and dissemination of scientific results. Ultimately, activists realize that to bolster public concern about environmental causes of breast cancer, they cannot simply argue that the cancer industry has stakes in downplaying such causes and demand that it "end its silence." Rather, they must also "work from the inside out," as anthropologist Mary Anglin puts it, and participate in the research and policy process. In doing so, activists immerse themselves in the culture, discourses, everyday practices, and technical knowledge that are integral facets of these specialized fields.[21]

Environmental breast cancer activism's growing focus on science was part of a scientific turn taken by the broader breast cancer movement—a turn that was directly influenced by the research efforts of AIDS activists in the late 1980s and early 1990s. Indeed, AIDS activism was arguably the first and one of the most influential embodied health movements to engage science in a significant way. Influenced by the feminist health movement's efforts to eradicate the sexism embedded in biomedicine, AIDS activists challenged the homophobia and other social prejudices that led the federal government, research institutions, and pharmaceutical companies to ignore this growing public health problem. In addition to demanding more research funding for the disease, they focused on getting "drugs into bodies." Specifically, AIDS activists helped to determine which drugs researchers study, design clinical research trials, assess the safety and efficacy of particular therapies, and influence the regulatory process so that patients had quicker access to new—and in some cases controversial—drugs.[22]

The 1991 founding of the Washington, D.C.–based National Breast Cancer Coalition (NBCC) by Philadelphia lawyer and breast cancer survivor Fran Visco marked one of the earliest examples of the breast cancer movement's foray into science. The organization launched its first campaign, Do the Write Thing, in October that year during National Breast Cancer Awareness Month. Many environmental breast cancer activists and organizations—such as Breast Cancer Action, Massachusetts Breast Cancer Coalition, 1 in 9: The Long Island Breast Cancer Action Network, and Women's Community Cancer Project—participated in this research campaign. Its goal was to deliver 175,000 letters (a figure representing the number of women who die from the disease each year) to Congress and the president demanding more federal breast cancer research funding. With the help of citizens and breast cancer activists across the country, NBCC collected more than six hundred thousand letters. These efforts led to a $132 million (almost 50 percent) increase in the National Cancer Institute's budget for breast cancer research. The same year, the NBCC helped to establish a breast cancer research program within the Department of Defense that would fund external projects. Since its inception in 1992, the program has received more than 26,500 proposals and spent $1.9 billion on its research projects. As part of the department's program, NBCC oversees the participation of consumer advocates in the proposal review process.[23]

Another body of "citizen science" shaping the scientific direction of environmental breast cancer activism was the bourgeoning environmental health movement.[24] The advent of the environmental movement in the 1970s gave rise to different types of political action. Whereas some environmental groups worked at the local level, others sought to implement more stringent state and federal policies for issues such as safe drinking water, clean waterways, clean air, and the cleanup of hazardous waste. As part of these regulatory efforts, the Natural Resource Defense Council, Environmental Defense, the Sierra Club, and other national organizations hired lawyers, policy analysts, and scientists who could go head to head with officials from the EPA, other federal agencies, state agencies, Congress, and industry. In the late 1980s and 1990s, however, the boundaries between this "traditional environmentalism" and public health began to blur, as many environmental groups intensified their examination of the relationship between pollution and other toxic substances, on the one hand, and human diseases and disorders, on the other.[25] From the other direction, many professional public health and consumer health organizations, especially those at the state and federal levels, increasingly began to address the environmental dimensions of human health. In addition, an array of new organizations focusing solely on environmental health issues formed. Notably, the environmental health movement helped to stir public and scientific concern about endocrine disrupter theory—a theory of disease causation that, in and of itself, played an important role in environmental breast cancer activists' increasing participation in science.

The theories laid out in *Our Stolen Future* received much public and scientific support, yet they also drew ample criticism, especially from representatives of industry. Skepticism arose from the theory's general inability to draw a definitive link from hormonally active agents to any one disorder, including breast cancer. Critics argued that *Our Stolen Future* drew too heavily on questionable evidence, ignored studies that disproved its claims, and relied on faulty understandings of toxicological processes.[26] To counter these critiques, proponents of endocrine disrupter theory constructed the uncertainty surrounding it in political and economic terms. That is, they argued that many debunkers had economic incentives in downplaying the potential harm from endocrine-disrupting chemicals. Yet proponents also legitimated the theory by constructing its uncertainty as a problem arising from inadequate and misapplied scientific methods.[27]

Throughout the twentieth century, cancer has been more than an organizing principle for the fields of biomedical research, clinical practice, and health advocacy. It has also been the organizing principle for the fields of environmental health science and policy. In addition to serving as the primary disease of concern to researchers who study the impact of chemicals and other toxic substances on human health, the development of cancer has been the primary biological measure that toxicologists have used to determine whether specific chemicals pose a threat to human health. Moreover, cancer has been the primary endpoint for the risk assessment models for environmental regulations, meaning that decisions to regulate specific chemicals have been based primarily on the number of cancer deaths predicted to result from specific levels of toxic exposure.[28]

When endocrine disrupter theory emerged in the early to mid-1990s, it posed a challenge to cancer's status as an organizing principle. The new theory broadened the scope of environmental epidemiology, toxicology, and risk assessment to consider noncancerous health risks posed by endocrine-disrupting chemicals (and other types of chemicals, for that matter). It also broadened the scope of environmental cancer research itself. Before the emergence of endocrine disrupter theory, most researchers assumed that cancer-causing chemicals were carcinogenic, meaning that they caused the disease by directly mutating DNA. In the wake of the new theory, however, researchers started to realize that some cancers—especially breast cancer and others for which established risk factors already included exposure to increased levels of natural hormones—may also be caused by chemicals that disrupted hormone production. Consequently, this emerging theory provided new research questions for scientists to answer, new issue areas for environmental health, public health, and consumer activists to politicize, new scientific and health topics for the media to cover, and new health concerns for the public to consider.[29]

As researchers continued to piece together the theory of endocrine disruption, they began to realize that the widely established methods and scientific paradigms used within the fields of environmental health research to study the health effects from carcinogens might not accurately assess the health effects from their hormone-disrupting counterparts. This is because the toxicological principles of endocrine disrupters differed from those of carcinogenic compounds.[30] The environmental health sciences have long grappled with methodological limitations when it comes to understanding the impact of toxic exposures on human health, but the emergence of endocrine disrupter theory added a new dimension to an existing set of problems. Moreover, the recognition that established research methods might be inappropriate for the study of endocrine disrupters provided the theory's proponents with a new strategy for justifying its scientific merits to skeptics.

Given the growing importance of endocrine disrupter theory to breast cancer activists, it is not surprising that they started to construct the uncertainty associated with past research on environmental causes of breast cancer as a result of scientific limitations. It is also not surprising that their increased focus on endocrine disrupters went hand in hand with their bourgeoning interest in science. Just as holding the cancer industry responsible for uncertainty led activists to demand that it "end its silence" and start doing its part to reduce public exposure to toxic substances, holding misapplied methods and other scientific inadequacies responsible for this uncertainty encouraged activists to address the problem through further research. Of particular note are activists' efforts to establish community-based studies on Long Island; in Greater Boston; and in Marin County, California. These studies investigated—and in some cases, continue to investigate—the possible role that environmental exposures, especially to xenoestrogens, play in the regions' high rates of breast cancer incidence. All the projects rank among activists' earliest, most innovative, and most influential scientific work.

The Establishment of Community-Based Research

When it comes to activists' scientific efforts, many of them focus on toxic exposures in local communities. In a general sense, this research consists of what sociologist Sabrina McCormick and her colleagues call "popular epidemiology"—that is, "the interaction between a lay population and medical/pubic health professionals that has a consequent effect on research and policy."[31] Yet the specific research practices that constitute popular epidemiology are diverse. Some of them consist of environmental health studies initiated, designed, and carried out primarily by lay citizens, who turn to scientists when they need particular forms of expertise. For the most part, however, community-based research efforts occur within the context of professional science, whereby activists and scientists work together to ensure that opportunities for community participation are built into the social, material, and institutional structure of the actual projects. At one end of the spectrum, activists participate—often in small but significant ways—in studies already designed and approved by research officials. At the other end, activists are involved in "community-based participatory research," an innovative approach that emphasizes "active and equal" collaboration between lay citizens and scientific investigators from the very beginning of a study's design to the dissemination of its results and the development of interventions.[32] As illustrated by the studies carried out on Long Island and in Greater Boston and Marin County, environmental breast cancer activists participate in different ways and to varying degrees in the community-based research process.

Long Island

The earliest community-based research took place on Long Island. A report released in the mid-1980s by the New York State Department of Health found that Long Island had the highest breast cancer incidence rates in the state. In Nassau County, 112.6 women per 100,000 women developed breast cancer every year, a rate that was 18.9 percent higher than the state average and 30 percent higher than the national average. Suffolk County followed at 103.6 cases per 100,000 women and 9.4 percent above the state average. In the initial aftermath of the report, concerned citizens pressured local political officials to fund research to assess the causes of these high rates, particularly possible environmental factors. Such concerns stemmed from several other sets of local issues—namely, the extensive use of pesticides on Long Island's farmlands and golf courses, various cases of contaminated drinking water in the region, and prior suspicions about the health effects from local landfills and other toxic dumpsites. Over the following few years, the New York State Department of Health looked into possible environmental factors. By 1990, the agency determined that these factors did not contribute to the breast cancer problem in Nassau and Suffolk counties. Rather, it argued that traditional risk factors were the cause of the area's high incidence rates. The agency stated that no further studies on the topic were warranted.[33] Concerned residents were unhappy with the agency's position because the study only examined the 25 percent of afflicted women who fell into the high-risk category and did not consider the factors involved in the other 75 percent of women who developed the disease. They decided to take matters into their own hands.[34]

The first of the region's breast cancer groups, called 1 in 9: The Long Island Breast Cancer Action Coalition, was established in November 1990 by Fran Kritchek and Marie Quinn, two teachers with breast cancer. Fifty-eight women showed up to the first meeting. Kritchek and Quinn served as co-presidents for the first year. After Quinn died, Geri Barish, who had attended the first meeting, was elected co-president, in 1992. Barish joined 1 in 9 because she felt that she "had to do something" about the disease. Her mother was diagnosed with breast cancer in 1974 around the same time that her son was diagnosed with Hodgkin's disease. Twelve years later, Barish developed breast cancer herself, motivating her to act on the promise she had made to her son before he died to find the cause of his cancer (and other cancers, especially breast cancer). She always felt that the environment was a factor; in particular, she remembers how kids in her neighborhood used to run after the "fog man" when he sprayed the area with DDT. When Kritchek retired from her leadership position in 1997, Barish became sole president, a position she still holds.[35]

In the years that followed, an array of other breast cancer organizations formed in the region. They promoted the importance of early detection, provided support services for women with the disease, and raised community awareness about breast cancer issues. A number worked to identify and eliminate the possible causes, especially environmental, of Long Island's high breast cancer rates. In addition to 1 in 9, these organizations included the West Islip Breast Cancer Coalition, Babylon Breast Cancer Coalition, Huntington Breast Cancer Action Coalition, Great Neck Breast Cancer Coalition, and Long Beach Breast Cancer Coalition. In many ways, their early efforts resonated with those of the other environmental breast cancer groups formed during this time in other parts of the country, particularly the San Francisco Bay Area and Greater

Boston. Like these groups, the Long Island organizations wrote about environmental issues in their newsletters, organized rallies and conferences, and garnered attention from the media. However, Long Island's activists were arguably the first to embrace community research as a political strategy. Consider the original goals of 1 in 9: "To raise the consciousness level and to increase public awareness of the epidemic of breast cancer by keeping the disease at the forefront; to obtain more funding for research; to investigate the role of pesticides, since Long Island was, and continues to be, a farming area; to increase early detection of breast cancer; to find the causes, prevention, and cure for breast cancer."[36]

The first scientific effort established and carried by Long Island activists was a community mapping project. In early 1992, Lorraine Pace, a breast cancer survivor from West Islip, Suffolk County, who wanted understand why so many women in her ZIP code had the disease, initiated the project. Pace, along with family members, town residents, local health officials, and nearby researchers, developed and carried out a survey to determine the geographic patterns of breast cancer incidence in West Islip. Beginning in August 1992, they disseminated the survey by publishing it in the regional paper, *Suffolk Life*, mailing it to residents' homes, going door to door, asking church leaders to include copies of it in their weekly bulletins, and even getting a dry cleaning store to enclose it with the garments that customers picked up. The activists also designed a ten-foot-wide street map and with a felt-tip marker denoted houses with cases of breast cancer. That same year, Pace helped to found the West Islip Breast Cancer Coalition. In addition to participating in the mapping project, the group addressed the environmental breast cancer problem through education and community outreach, legislation, corporate reform, and research.[37]

In December 1993, the West Islip mapping project completed its data collection, with more than 62 percent of the town's 8,750 homes participating in the study. Among other things, the study found that breast cancer incidence rates were higher on streets with cul-de-sacs. Although the cause of this incidence pattern was never officially determined, the activists speculated that drinking water contaminated by industrial dumping and pesticides—which was more prevalent on cul-de-sacs with dead-end water mains—might be to blame.[38] Inspired by the West Islip mapping project, other Long Island groups established similar studies in their own towns. The Suffolk County groups that conducted these projects included the Brentwood/Bayshore Breast Cancer Coalition, South Fork Breast Cancer Coalition, North Fork Breast Cancer Coalition, Babylon Breast Cancer Coalition, and Huntington Breast Cancer Action Coalition. In Nassau County, the groups included Great Neck Breast Cancer Coalition and

Manhasset Breast Cancer Coalition.[39] Although Pace left the West Islip Breast Cancer Coalition in 1994 to help found Breast Cancer Help, Incorporated, she continued with her mapping efforts, both on Long Island and beyond. Indeed, Breast Cancer Help has worked with breast cancer groups in the region, across the nation, and even around the world in developing mapping projects in their communities.[40]

During this time, Long Island activists pushed for federal research to examine possible environmental causes of breast cancer in their communities. In conjunction with many of the breast cancer organizations noted above, 1 in 9 used a several strategies to achieve this goal. In October 1991, members held a rally and press conference on the steps of the Nassau County courthouse, calling on the public to recognize that the epidemic proportion of breast cancer on Long Island was unacceptable. Three hundred and fifty people showed up; numbered among them was every state politician.[41] The event made the cover of *Newsday*. Activists also organized several conferences, in 1993 convening a symposium titled "Breast Cancer and the Environment." This event brought together twenty-three scientists and a host of concerned citizens from across the country to discuss the research linking breast cancer to environmental factors, as well as the steps that activists and scientists needed to take to pursue the matter further.[42]

Just as important, activists engaged federal officials. Soon after the symposium, Kritchek and Barish met with David Broder, then director of the National Cancer Institute (NCI), to discuss the prospect of an NCI-funded study on environmental causes of breast cancer on Long Island. Devra Davis, who participated in the symposium and encouraged the activists to push for a federal study, also attended the meeting. Broder said that the NCI would need $5 million to conduct such a study but did not know from where the money would come. When Kritchek and Barish suggested that Congress allocate the funds, Broder told them, according to Barish, "not to mix politics with test tubes." Unfazed by his reaction, they decided to contact their congressional representatives.[43] Over the following few months, activists from the region met with U.S. legislators, particularly Representative Gary Ackerman and Senator Alphonse D'Amato, both of New York, in an effort to procure federal funds for an environmental breast cancer study. Sympathetic to their cause, Ackerman and D'Amato convened a public hearing at Huntington Town Hall, in Ackerman's congressional district. Activists, families, public officials, and the media, as well as representatives from the NCI, the National Institute of Environmental Health Sciences, and other federal agencies, participated. Ultimately, the hearing led to the Long Island Breast Cancer Study Project

(LIBCSP), under Public Law 103–43, in 1993. The bill allocated more than $30 million from the NCI and the National Institute of Environmental Health Sciences for extramural and intramural studies between 1993 and 2004.[44]

Broadly speaking, the LIBCSP consisted of epidemiological studies, laboratory research on the mechanisms of breast cancer causation, the establishment of a family breast and ovarian cancer registry, a plan to reduce barriers to breast cancer screening, and research on methodological issues. The project also funded the development of a geographic information system to monitor past and present environmental exposures on Long Island. Marilie Gammon, originally from Columbia University's School of Public Health and later based at the School of Public Health at the University of North Carolina–Chapel Hill, conducted the LIBCSP's centerpiece study, Breast Cancer and the Environment on Long Island. This population-based, case control study examined the relationship between breast cancer incidence and exposure to organochlorine compounds such as DDT/DDE, PCBs, dieldrin, and chlordane, as well as polycyclic aromatic hydrocarbons (PAHs). To carry out the study, Gammon recruited 1,508 women from Nassau and Suffolk counties who were newly diagnosed with in situ or invasive breast cancer between August 1996 and August 1997 and a similar number of women from those counties who did not have the disease. In 2001, she received funding from the NCI to conduct a four-year follow-up study examining whether exposure to PAHs and organochlorine compounds, as well as various lifestyle factors, affected survival rates of Long Island women with breast cancer. The LIBCSP's other environmental studies examined possible associations between the disease's incidence and women's residential proximity to past and present farmland, hazardous waste sites, and toxic release inventory sites, as well as exposures to organochlorine compounds, especially DDT/DDE and PCBs; electromagnetic fields; and drinking water contaminants such as pesticides, solvents, volatile organic compounds, nitrates, and metals.[45]

Long Island activists participated at various stages of the LIBCSP's research process. Early on, they helped to decide which epidemiological studies the NCI should fund. When it came time for the NCI to decide which of the more than one hundred extramural research proposals it should fund, it asked Karen Joy Miller to participate on the peer review committee. In 1987, Miller, an interior designer, mother of three, and avid runner, was diagnosed with invasive breast cancer at age forty-one. Given that the disease had not spread to her lymph nodes, she elected to have a mastectomy instead of a lumpectomy with adjuvant therapy, as she did not want to expose her body to radiation. Soon after her diagnosis, she started to meet regularly with other women with the disease whom she met at the hospital. Calling themselves the "Tit for Tatters," they not only provided one another with support but also discussed the need to take public action to address Long Island's breast cancer problem. Miller's foray into breast cancer activism led her to help establish 1 in 9 and, several years later, the Huntington Breast Cancer Action Coalition. She also played a key role in the rally and press conference held at the Nassau County courthouse, the 1993 breast cancer and environment symposium, the meeting with Representative Ackerman, and the subsequent hearing that he and Senator D'Amato organized. Once Miller agreed to sit on the peer review committee, she received scientific proposals to review, a month before the committee was convened for a meeting in Manhattan.[46]

Miller's presence on the committee marked an early instance of the NCI's allowing a lay citizen to participate in the peer review process. When she walked into the meeting room, she said, "you could have heard a pin drop." Nonetheless, both Miller and the researchers were fully prepared to work together. Although they knew that she did not have the expertise to assess the scientific merits and technical details of the proposed projects, they asked her to identify which proposal best met the needs of her fellow Long Island activists and members of the community. She chose Marilie Gammon's proposal, as it outlined an examination of many of the chemicals about which residents had the most concern. Gammon's project ended up winning the contract for the LIBCSP's centerpiece study.[47]

The LIBCSP also developed ways to involve community members in the studies themselves by having them sit on the project's various advisory boards. Kritchek and Miller, among others, sat on the LIBCSP's ad hoc advisory board. Board meetings took place in 1995, 1996, and 1997 with around one hundred citizens and scientists attending each. The two case control studies— Gammon's centerpiece study and M. Christina Leske's project on breast cancer and electromagnetic fields—had their own external advisory committees. The scientists affiliated with both studies met regularly with their community partners to discuss the research process. The geographic information system project included five community members on its oversight committee, which met four times a year, either physically or through conference calls.[48]

As members of the advisory boards, activists participated in the studies in various ways. They provided input into cancer epidemiologist Ruth Allen's Integrated Chemical List, a compilation of one hundred suspected xenoestrogens on which the EPA had conducted toxicological studies. This list was based on Ana Soto's earlier group of one hundred chemicals, known and suspected xenoestrogens, that Soto believed warranted further research. It also served as the basis for many of the LIBCSP's studies.[49] Activists on the advisory board for Gammon's study helped to design the questionnaire that assessed the study participants' past and present exposures. For inclusion in the package that went to homes to solicit volunteers for Gammon's study, the Long Island Breast Cancer Network—a coalition of all Long Island breast cancer groups—wrote a letter encouraging women to participate. Furthermore, the advisory board members for Gammon and Leske's studies helped to procure funds to pay for added research costs.[50]

The LIBCSP encouraged community involvement through other public meetings. In 1995, the project sponsored a town hall meeting to kick off its launch. Throughout the project's duration, the NCI and the National Institute of Environmental Health Sciences met with Long Island groups to discuss the status of the overall project. NCI staff and scientists met with residents every other month to discuss the status of particular studies and listen to the community's thoughts and concerns about the research. In 1996, NCI staff held three workshops to garner community members' reactions to the NCI's request for proposals for the geographic information system project. In a 1999 follow-up, the researchers who received the contract for the system ran seven meetings to solicit from residents information about local pollution sources not listed in existing databases.[51] The information provided by community members allowed researchers to develop a better understanding and analysis of the region's past and present environmental exposures.[52]

Greater Boston

In 1994, activists from the Massachusetts Breast Cancer Coalition (MBCC) began their own community-based research efforts after the Massachusetts Department of Health reported that Cape Cod had unusually high breast cancer incidence rates. Between 1982 and 1994, incidence rates in this region were 20 percent higher than elsewhere in the state. Indeed, Cape Cod was home to seven of the state's ten towns with the highest incidence rates and had rates above the national average.[53] Soon after the release of the 1993 report, MBCC decided to push the state legislature to allocate funds for research into possible environmental causes of the disease on Cape Cod. Activists' suspicion about environmental factors was based on prior concerns about the environmental health impacts from the local Otis air force base and the pesticides used on the cranberry bogs that covered parts of the cape. MBCC had already begun to address environmental breast cancer issues by the time it decided to push for state research funds. Although later research demonstrated that the base and bogs were not necessarily the causes of Cape Cod's high breast cancer rates, MBCC helped to spark initial concern about environmental factors and led to the investigation of other potential factors.[54]

MBCC worked with several state officials, among them state representative John Klimm of Cape Cod, who introduced and helped to pass legislation dedicating state funds to an examination of environmental causes of the disease in the region. As a result of these efforts, the Massachusetts legislature inserted into the state budget an annual allocation of $1 million for such research, stipulating that research institutions had to apply and compete for the funds. At the same time that it worked to develop this legislation, however, MBCC realized that simply asking state officials to provide this money was not enough. The activist group also wanted to influence the types of research that this money would go toward. To this end, they spearheaded the Silent Spring Institute, a nonprofit research organization that examines environmental links to women's health disorders, especially breast cancer, in Massachusetts, and hired the scientists who would direct and staff it. Given that activists created the institute with the call for research proposals in mind, they knew that the institute had a good chance of receiving the money. They were right. The institute won the grant it sought, and soon after, it began a three-year process to define the scope of its research and plan the specific studies.[55]

Although the Long Island Breast Cancer Project inspired MBCC activists to establish the Silent Spring Institute, the two community efforts differed in structure. The LIBCSP, which was funded and overseen by the NCI and NIEHS, consisted of a series of studies conducted by investigators at various institutions for a specific duration of time. In contrast, Silent Spring functions as "a lab of our own," from the perspective of the scientists and activists affiliated with it.[56] In July 2008, the nonprofit consisted of one office, an executive director, three staff scientists, two postdoctoral researchers, two research assistants, an information specialist, several other administrative and project coordinators, and an advisory board.[57] Although it faces certain funding constraints, the institute, as much as possible, makes its own decisions on the lines of research to pursue and the methodologies for pursuing them. Furthermore, the institute will remain open indefinitely, as long as it continues to receive the necessary funds.[58] Currently, it functions on a $2 million annual budget from grants and awards it receives from federal agencies, state agencies, private foundations, corporations, universities, breast cancer organizations, other nonprofits, and individuals.[59]

Harlee Strauss, a molecular biologist, served as the institute's first director until 1995. Julia Brody, who holds a PhD from the University of Texas at Austin, took over as executive director in 1996. When Silent Spring offered Brody the position, she asked the mothers on her street whether she should take it, as she felt a bit daunted by the prospect of the job. They said yes, and so did she.

Prior to her work at Silent Spring, Brody did environmental policy and consulting work for the Massachusetts Department of Environmental Management and the Texas Department of Agriculture. Her interest in environmental health began much earlier, however: her father died of cancer in his forties, and she attended high school in Richmond, Washington, next to the Hanford nuclear production facility.[60] The facility opened in 1943 as part of the Manhattan Project, and most of its reactors were shut down in the 1960s and early 1970s. The final reactor was shut down in 1987. The most contaminated nuclear site in the country, Hanford has been linked for decades to many health problems, including cancer, facing local residents, site workers, and farm animals.[61]

In 1994, Silent Spring began its first phase of the Cape Cod Breast Cancer and Environment Study, a phase entailing environmental data collection; the review of plausible hypotheses for the region's high breast cancer rates; the mapping of such rates; meetings with community members; and the development of exposure assessment methods, including a geographic information system to integrate information about environmental exposures on the cape and health problems afflicting residents.[62] Several years later, the institute began the second, two-part phase of the study. For the first part, a case control study was enacted of 2,171 women, 1,165 of whom had personal histories of breast cancer. Investigators conducted fifty-minute telephone interviews with these women to learn about their established and suspected breast cancer risk factors. They were especially interested in exposures to toxic chemicals, particularly endocrine disrupters found in products in the home.[63] The second part of the phase was the Household Exposure Study. This honed in on 120 homes from the Breast Cancer and Environment Study that were deemed to have particular environmental risks. Specifically, researchers looked for the presence of eighty-nine endocrine disrupters and mammary carcinogens found in common household products such as pesticides, cleaning substances, plastics, and health care items.[64] As part of its broader body of research, Silent Spring assessed the presence of endocrine disrupters and other contaminants in local groundwater and drinking water supplies.[65]

Silent Spring also conducted two studies of communities other than Cape Cod. A report released by the Massachusetts Department of Health noted that the Boston suburb of Newton had unusually disparate breast cancer rates. Whereas the town's neighborhoods with the lowest incidence rates were 20 percent below the state average, neighborhoods with the highest rates of breast cancer were 55 percent above the state average. In 1999, researchers conducted the Newton Breast Cancer Study to examine whether reproductive, lifestyle, familial history, and environmental factors contributed to the disparate breast cancer rates in the different parts of the town.[66] More recently, the institute has embarked on the Breast Cancer and Environmental Justice project in collaboration with Brown University and Communities for a Better Environment. Designed as an extension of the Household Exposure Study, the project examines toxic exposures, particularly from endocrine disrupters, in and around homes located in the California towns of Richmond and Bolinas.[67]

The founders of Silent Spring envisioned the institute as a collaborative venture by activists and scientists. In addition to establishing the institute and procuring state funds for its research activities, activists play other roles in its scientific work, along with the lay public. They sit on the institute's board of directors along with scientists, lawyers, and health professionals. Currently, four of the Silent Spring board's eight members—Ellen Parker, Bev Baccelli, Amy Present, and Cathie Ragovin—have ties to MBCC. The board meets several times a year and has the authority to hire and fire the lead investigator of the Cape Cod Breast Cancer and Environment Study.[68] The institute also formed a science advisory committee and a public advisory committee to help oversee the Cape Cod Breast Cancer and Environment Study. Members from both groups helped to determine the study's research priorities, and the study's investigators sought input from both groups, as well as from community members, women with breast cancer, and health professionals to determine the questions that would guide their research project. Although the Public Advisory Committee no longer meets, the Scientific Advisory Committee, as well as the institute's National Advisory Committee, does.[69] Moreover, the institute sponsors community events such as film showings, lectures, town hall meetings, and poster sessions as a way not only to update residents on the latest scientific developments but also to gather public feedback on the institute's research activities. Along this line, in 2004 the institute surveyed leaders from fifty-six breast cancer organizations across the country and Canada to ascertain their interest in environmental breast cancer issues and their specific priorities when addressing such issues. The institute will use the information it gained in developing its future research and public education agendas.[70]

Lay citizens have not only influenced what research scientists have conducted; they also have helped to shape how scientists have conducted it. On the basis of feedback that the institute received from the advisory boards and the community at large, the investigators for the Cape Cod study decided to examine the levels of endocrine-disrupting chemicals found in homes. Few methods existed for studying these types of exposures. The idea that many conventional methods for studying environmental exposures and health impacts may not work in the case of endocrine disrupters, along with the dearth of methods for assessing exposures to and health risks from endocrine disrupters and other chemicals found at home, has led these scientists to develop more effective testing strategies. For example, the Silent Spring researchers have studied environmental exposures at home by using vacuum cleaners to collect dust and other potentially contaminated materials found in carpets, in furniture, and on household surfaces.[71] Indeed, developing new exposure assessment methods has become one of the institute's top priorities and most innovative aspects of its work.

Marin County/San Francisco Bay Area

San Francisco Bay Area activists established their own community-based research projects several years after the Silent Spring Institute launched its projects. In October 1994, New York State Senator Bella Abzug hosted the Women, Health, and Environment Summit at San Francisco City Hall, with many breast cancer and environmental health activists, as well as concerned citizens, in attendance. During the summit, an unknown person distributed a copy of the *Greater Bay Area Registry Report: A Publication of the Northern California Cancer Center*. Previously, the California Department of Human Health, which contracted the Northern California Cancer Center to conduct the study, had released the report to researchers, public health professionals, and medical providers. It did not make the report readily accessible to the public. As a result of the report's circulation at the summit, activists and other citizens learned that the Bay Area, specifically Marin County, had the highest rates of breast cancer not only in the state but in the world.[72] Before the summit, Bay Area breast cancer activists already suspected that the region had particularly high breast cancer rates. Indeed, this suspicion had motivated activists to found various breast cancer organizations in the early 1990s. The release of the report at the summit served to confirm their suspicions.[73]

The Women, Health, and Environment Summit was a call to action for Marin County residents. Francine Levien and Wendy Tanowitz, two local women with breast cancer who attended the meeting, established Marin Breast Cancer Watch to raise awareness of the county's breast cancer problem. Levien became the group's executive director. Following Levien's death from metastatic breast cancer in 2001, Janice Barlow took over as interim director. Barlow began volunteering for the organization in 2001 after she read in a local newspaper about the organization's research efforts and called up to ask how she could become involved. As a nurse practitioner, Barlow was especially interested in the relationship between radiation and breast cancer. Over the course of the year, she helped to develop materials for various research projects and write grant applications. In 2002, she became the organization's executive director. Given her medical background, and her research and grant-writing experiences while at the organization, she was well suited for the position.[74]

In 2005, the organization changed its name to Zero Breast Cancer as its work increasingly extended beyond Marin County to the San Francisco Bay Area more generally; the group's staff and board members wanted its name to reflect their broadened focus. They also wanted to distinguish the organization from other Marin County groups with similar names, for example, the Marin Breast Cancer Council and Marin Cancer Project. Further, they wanted their name to emphasize the organization's transition from a focus on breast cancer awareness to a focus on environmental factors and disease prevention, especially in conjunction with community-based participatory research. The organization viewed such research as "a process by which members of a community identify a problem, engage outside researchers in a collaborative that promotes co-learning, and achieve a balance between research and action."[75]

Zero Breast Cancer began its scientific work in 1997. While attending the First World Conference on Breast Cancer in Ontario that October, Levien, along with several Marin residents and organization board members, learned that California's Breast Cancer Research Program had recently launched an effort to fund community-based participatory research projects. Zero Breast Cancer decided to pursue a project examining factors in adolescence that increased a woman's risk for developing the disease. To apply for funding, the organization needed an academic partner in California. When the members arrived home, they began cold-calling epidemiologists. None expressed interest. Finally, Margaret Wrensch, an epidemiologist at the University of California San Francisco (UCSF), said yes. Individuals from Zero Breast Cancer and UCSF put together a proposal for the Adolescent Risk Factor Study, comparing adolescent and preadolescent "exposures and experiences," involving three hundred women with breast cancer and three hundred without the disease. Factors to be looked at included physical development, stress, family and social connections, socioeconomic characteristics, passive and active smoking, residency and migration patterns, and established risk factors for the disease.[76] In the end, the Breast Cancer Research Program agreed to fund a pilot project that allowed the research team to develop the main survey and other study materials. Two years later, the team received funding from the Breast Cancer Research Program to conduct the study.

In 1998, Zero Breast Cancer received five hundred thousand dollars from the Marin County Department of Health and Human Services to study possible environmental causes of the county's high breast cancer incidence rates. U.S.

senator Barbara Boxer, along with Representatives Nancy Pelosi and Lynn Woolsey, all of California, worked with the Centers for Disease Control and Prevention to allocate this money to the Marin County department, which then passed it along to Zero Breast Cancer. The organization used the funds to initiate three projects. The first consisted of town forums. Each year, Zero Breast Cancer brings one to two nationally renowned scientists to meet with residents from Marin and its surrounding areas over several days. Speakers have included researchers Ana Soto, Julia Brody, Peggy Reynolds, Tina Clarke, Kirstin Moyish, and Leslie Bernstein. The purpose of these town forums is to create a "three-way flow of information" among researchers, activists, and the community. As Barlow explains, "It was an opportunity for the community to be educated and give input into the research being done, and for researchers to learn about the concerns and interests of community members.[77]

Zero Breast Cancer also used the Centers for Disease Control money to fund two research studies. To help design and carry out these projects, the organization turned to UCSF and the Lawrence Livermore National Laboratory for assistance. The yearlong Breast Cancer and Personal Environmental Risk Factors in Marin County—Pilot Study (PERFS) developed the foundation for a future case control investigation that would examine the relationship between a select group of environmental risk factors and breast cancer. The factors identified in the pilot study included alcohol use; physical activity; birth control pills; hormone replacement therapy; polycyclic aromatic hydrocarbons (PAH) exposure; and exposure to light at night, an occupational risk factor associated with working the night shift. As a companion project to PERFS, researchers developed the Marin Environmental Data Study, a one-year effort to produce a database of environmental exposures that may have contributed to the region's high breast cancer incidence rates. Categories of exposure included air pollution, electromagnetic fields, geology and land use, pesticide use, toxic sites, hazardous waste, leaking underground storage tanks, and water quality. Although Zero Breast Cancer and its collaborators applied for funds from the California Breast Cancer Research program to carry out the full PERFS study, the program turned down their request.[78]

To foster collaboration with scientists, Zero Breast Cancer helped to design and carry out the actual research projects. Janice Barlow served as the lead investigator for the Marin Environmental Data Study and as a co-author of the Adolescent Risk Factor Study publication. Current board members Roni Peskin-Mentzer and Flavia Belli, as well as past board members Ginger Sounders-Mason and Mary Gould, were co-investigators for the Adolescent Risk Factor Study. Along with Margaret Wrensch, Dr. Georgie Farren served as the project's community principal investigator. Meanwhile, the organization's research assistant, Safie Yaghoubi, served as a co-investigator for the Marin Environmental Data Study, while current board member Fern Bellow was a co-investigator for both PERFS and the Marin Environmental Data Study.[79]

The studies also provided opportunities for community participation more generally. As part of the Adolescent Risk Factor Study, for example, Zero Watch staff held focus groups and town hall meetings to solicit feedback on what questions they should include in the study's main survey. Similarly, activists and scientists from the Marin Environmental Data Study collected information from local women about the women's personal environmental exposures. Women provided this information by completing an online questionnaire, answering the survey by telephone, submitting it by e-mail, or attending workshops. Investigators trained Zero Breast Cancer staff and a small group of community members in the use of the geographic information system for data collection and how to identify correlations between particular health problems and toxic exposures. Investigators for PERFS, in turn, considered the environmental concerns raised by community members to determine what types of environmental risk factors to examine in future studies. Community input was obtained through e-mail, by mail, by telephone, and through an open-ended question on the Adolescent Risk Factors Study that asked for women's thoughts on what causes breast cancer. Women had the opportunity to document their past and present environmental exposures by drawing maps of their neighborhoods, the San Francisco Bay Area more generally, and other geographic sites. In all, community members suggested more than fifteen hundred environmental factors to the PERFS investigators.[80]

Currently, Zero Breast Cancer serves as community investigators for two studies, both funded by the NCI. In partnership with the Northern California Kaiser Division of Research, the organization is helping to conduct the Prospective Study of Breast Cancer Survivorship in the Bay Area. This project examines the therapeutic role of lifestyle factors (including diet and physical activity), complementary medicine, and genetic and environmental interactions in "preventing breast cancer recurrences, increasing survival, and enhancing quality of life." The second project, Cancer Clustering for Residential Histories, builds on an earlier study by Zero Breast Cancer and an NCI geographer. This "Phase I" project, completed in May 2008, geo-coded the residential histories that were collected in the Adolescent Risk Factor Study. The study found several statistically significant local clusters of breast cancer that "began in the 1960s, intensified through the 1970s and 1980s, and were observed in the 2000s." The "Phase II" Cancer Clustering project, which Zero Breast Cancer is carrying out with BioMedware, will assess the extent to which established risk factors and possible environmental factors contribute to the formation of the clusters.[81] In addition to serving as community investigator for these studies, Zero Breast Cancer heads the Community Outreach and Translation Core for the Bay Area Breast Cancer and Environmental Research Center, one of four centers across the country funded by the National Institute of Environmental Health Sciences and NCI to study early environmental exposures that may affect the development of breast cancer in adulthood.[82]

The Interpretation of Research Results

The community-based studies on Long Island and Cape Cod and in Marin County represent a small, albeit significant, portion of the total research conducted on environmental causes of breast cancer. Since the late 1980s, scientists from around the world have conducted hundreds of epidemiological, experimental, and ecological studies on the topic. Although activists were not directly involved in all these studies, the attention that they brought to the issue helped to fuel such investigations, especially in the past decade. Given that this research permits improved understanding of the role played by environmental factors in the disease's development, an important ingredient of activists' work is collecting these studies, assessing their results, and presenting them to the public. Along these lines, they regularly present pieces of evidence in their newsletters, fact sheets, print advertisements, e-mail alerts, public presentations, films, meetings, and other social and discursive arenas. Some have also played roles in developing comprehensive analyses of environmental breast cancer research in scientific reports, CDs, and online databases.

Despite the efforts of activists to promote awareness of a link between environmental exposures and breast cancer, the body of evidence on this topic remains inconsistent. Indeed, the inconsistencies emerge even in the community-based studies that activists helped to establish and carry out. To be sure, the Long Island Breast Cancer Study Project found several associations between the development of breast cancer and exposure to certain chemicals. Marilie Gammon and her colleagues found that exposure to PAHs were associated with a modest increase in breast cancer risk.[83] Researcher Erin O'Leary and her team found that women who lived within one mile of hazardous waste sites containing organochlorine pesticides had increased breast cancer risk.[84] Steven Stellman and his colleagues found an association between PCB congener 183 and increased risk of breast cancer and discovered a link between PCBs and increased risk of breast cancer reoccurrence in women with a history of the disease.[85] No other studies, however, found links between breast cancer and organochlorine compounds. Nor did these studies find a connection between electromagnetic fields and the disease.[86] O'Leary and her colleagues observed no relationship between breast cancer and volatile organic compounds, heavy metals, and nitrates found in drinking water. They further determined that living near Toxic Release Inventory sites and hazardous waste sites containing volatile organic compounds and heavy metals did not increase one's risk for the disease.[87]

In keeping with this picture, the Silent Spring Institute's research produced mixed results. On the one hand, the Newton Breast Cancer Study found that traditional risk factors accounted for 5 percent of the difference in breast cancer rates between higher- and lower-incidence areas, whereas possible environmental factors, such as the use of professional lawn services, pesticide applications, and termite treatments, were associated with 14 percent of these differences.[88] The Household Exposure Study found fifty-two toxic compounds in the air of the 120 examined homes, sixty-six compounds in the dust of the homes, and twenty compounds in women's urine.[89] The Breast Cancer and Environment Study found that breast cancer rates were 20 to 80 percent higher among women who lived "in or near areas treated for tree pests in 1948–1995 . . . near cranberry bogs in 1948 to the mid 1970s . . . [and] near agricultural land since the mid 1970s." These findings from the Breast Cancer and Environment Study, however, were not statistically significant. Similarly, researchers found no clear link between breast cancer and the nitrates and endocrine disrupters found in drinking water.[90]

Zero Breast Cancer's studies yielded limited results as well. The Adolescent Risk Factor Study found no association between breast cancer and the use of hormone replacement therapy and birth control pills. In fact, the study found that women with breast cancer were more likely to have never used birth control pills than were women with no history of the disease. The women with breast cancer showed more traditional risk factors, including a higher socioeconomic status before the age of twenty-one, four or more mammograms between 1990 and 1994, giving birth without breastfeeding, and drinking on average two or more alcoholic drinks a day.[91] At the same time, a later study relying on Adolescent Risk Factor Study data found a geographic excess of estrogen-receptor-positive breast cancer among breast cancer cases in Marin County. It is uncertain, however, whether hormones—as opposed to other reproductive, biological, or environmental factors—played a role.[92]

The mixed results of the community-based studies noted above—not to mention the broader body of research on environmental links to breast cancer— lend themselves to what sociologists Trevor Pinch and Wiebe Bijker call "interpretive flexibility."[93] That is, scientists, activists, and other interested parties sometimes rely on different epistemological frameworks for assessing what constitutes a well-designed and properly conducted study, the amount of evidence needed to warrant concern and preventative action, and the types of evidence needed to justify such concern and action. To some extent, the interpretive flexibility associated with the community-based breast cancer projects results from scientific factors. After all, environmental health research in general is fraught with methodological difficulties when it comes to showing that toxic substances cause disease in humans. Endocrine disrupters further complicate the situation for researchers. Yet the ways in which individuals and institutions interpret environmental health evidence is also shaped by their professional, political, and personal vantage points.

Many mainstream scientists and health organizations interpret the inconsistencies within the broader body of research to mean that environmental factors—especially chemicals—do not cause breast cancer. Indeed, critics point to community-based research projects to support this viewpoint. Consider the American Cancer Society's summary of the Long Island Breast Cancer Study Project (LIBCSP). Although the report acknowledged Gammon's findings on PAHs, it goes on to explain why these results are questionable: the increased risk was only modest, the study was based on small population sample, and the measurements did not show increased levels of "PAH in smokers [as compared with] non-smokers among women never diagnosed with cancer."[94] Deborah Winn, a scientist in the Epidemiology and Genetics Research Program at the National Cancer Institute who served as the institute's representative for the LIBCSP, takes a similar stance. Although she acknowledges the evidence that indicates a link between particular toxins and breast cancer, she ultimately concludes that the LIBCSP found environmental factors to be an insignificant cause of the region's high incidence rates. "In short, the reports arising from the LIBCSP have not identified any environmental factors that could be responsible for the high incidence of breast cancer in the area," she writes. "The exceptions among the many negative findings are a report of modest increased in the risk of breast cancer from PAH exposure in the largest of these studies, a risk with proximity to organochlorine-containing hazardous waste sites in one smaller study, and a possible risk of breast cancer recurrence in women who have been exposed to B-hexachlorocyclohexene." Winn also asserts that the findings from the Marin County and Cape Cod studies reaffirm that environmental factors are not associated with breast cancer.[95]

Not surprisingly, activists and their scientist allies take a different approach to interpreting the research on environmental causes of breast cancer.

To be sure, they acknowledge the array of studies that show no association between environmental exposures and the disease, and they recognize the limitations of studies that demonstrate a possible association. They also sometimes disagree among themselves about the meaning and significance of particular bodies of research. Nevertheless, on the whole they conclude that the existing scientific literature suggests that environmental factors play a role in the development of breast cancer. In doing so, they rely on interpretive strategies that sometimes differ from those of their critics.

Emphasizing the Evidence That Does Exist

In contrast to critics who dismiss the environmental breast cancer theory by emphasizing the studies that demonstrate no link between toxic exposures and the disease, proponents of the theory emphasize the evidence that does demonstrate a link. Sometimes they take this approach with respect to individual studies. The Huntington Breast Cancer Action Coalition's description of Susan L. Teitelbaum's 2007 study, "Residential Pesticide Use and Breast Cancer Risk on Long Island, New York," illustrates this strategy. The case control study (which relied on data collected by Teitelbaum, Gammon, and other researchers in 1996 and 1997 as part of the LIBCSP) examined the relationship between breast cancer risk among Long Island residents and self-reported lifetime residential pesticide use. The investigators reported on two main sets of findings. First, over-lifetime resident pesticide use was linked to increased breast cancer risk, even though no dose response was observed. In other words, such pesticide use led to increased breast cancer risk, but greater levels of over-lifetime pesticide use did not lead to greater levels of increased risk. Second, lawn and garden pesticides increased one's risk, whereas pest control products, such as insect repellents and flea medications for pets, did not. In discussing the study's results, the Huntington Breast Cancer Action Coalition highlighted the positive findings rather than the negative ones by ending its report with the following statement: "This study is the first known to suggest that self-reported use of residential pesticides may increase breast cancer risk. Further investigation in other populations is necessary to confirm these findings."[96]

Proponents also take this interpretive approach in discussing the existing body of research as a whole. Rather then emphasizing the body of evidence showing little or no association between environmental factors and breast cancer, they emphasize the body of evidence that does demonstrate an association. As *State of the Evidence: What Is the Connection between the Environment and Breast Cancer*, a scientific report published jointly by the Breast Cancer Fund and Breast Cancer Action, explained in its fourth edition (2006), "Compelling scientific evidence points to some of the 100,000 synthetic chemicals in use today as contributing to the development of breast cancer, either by altering hormone function or gene-expression."[97] The rest of the report discusses individual findings from more than one hundred studies—including those from the LIBCSP and Silent Spring Institute research projects that Winn and others disregarded—to strengthen this general point. Although the report acknowledges that no individual study proves that a particular toxicant causes the disease, it argues that the body of evidence as a whole demonstrates that toxic exposures are likely factors. For example, one section of the report's "Probable Links" discussion examines the evidence surrounding PAHs and breast cancer. After stating that "various studies have shown that PAHs appear to play a role in the development of breast cancer," the report, to support its argument, cites seventeen studies, among them epidemiological research on the impact of smoking (active and passive) and car exhaust on breast cancer risk, studies demonstrating how PAHS damage DNA and disrupt estrogen, and investigations highlighting interactions between genes and PAH exposure. When it comes to the LIBCSP, the report frames the results in positive terms: "One of the several studies from the Long Island Breast Cancer Study Project found that PAHs create a distinctive type of damage on genetic material—referred to as a fingerprint—where the compounds directly bind up with the basic building blocks of DNA into what is known as a DNA adduct. Women with the highest PAH body burdens had a 50 percent increased risk of breast cancer. This Long Island study validated the earlier work of researchers at Columbia University who also found a close relationship between DNA damage from exposure to PAHs in breast tissue and increased risk of breast cancer."[98]

The Limitations of Existing Research

A second set of interpretive tactics highlights the limitations of existing research. Whereas critics of the environmental breast cancer theory use this strategy to highlight flaws in research that demonstrates a link between breast cancer and environmental factors, proponents of the theory rely on it to help explain why researchers have not found more evidence linking the disease to toxic exposures. From this latter perspective, absence of evidence does not necessarily mean absence of harm. One key limitation of research to date is the relative dearth of studies conducted on environmental causes and breast cancer. Although the volume of research conducted on this topic has increased in recent years—in large part because of activists' efforts—many knowledge gaps persist. As the Silent Spring Institute explains in an overview of its project Breast Cancer and Environment: Science Reviews, a comprehensive analysis of existing environmental breast cancer research: "Results demonstrate that much more work needs to be done." The overwhelming majority of chemicals identified as animal mammary carcinogens or hormone disrupting compounds have never been included in a study of breast cancer in women. Further, the vast majority of chemicals we are exposed to have never been tested to see if they cause cancer in an animal study."[99] Such gaps also exist in particular studies. With regard to the LIBCSP's limited findings, for example, Devra Davis argues, "A number of epidemiological studies have identified workplace factors as important causes of breast cancer. This study failed to gather information on women's workplace exposures or their use of household cleaning and personal care products." Janette Sherman, a toxicologist and environmental health writer, further notes that the LIBCSP "did not address adverse effects from exposure to chemicals known to have been used on Long Island [and] did not address radiation exposures."[100]

Another limit of research relates to flaws in study design. Consider *State of the Evidence's* assessment of PCBs, which it lists as having a "probable link" to breast cancer. The report discusses a number of studies linking PCBs to breast cancer in pre-menopausal women and to the recurrence of breast cancer in non-metastatic women. It also presents in vitro studies demonstrating PCBs' xeno-estrogenic effects. At the same time, the report states that the broader body of evidence is divided, with many studies demonstrating no association between PCBs and the disease. Explaining these inconsistencies and negative findings, the report notes that most studies do not distinguish between types of PCBs when examining them: "PCBs are classified in three types based on their effects on cells, but there are more than 200 PCB congeners with perhaps as many different effect mechanisms. One type acts like an estrogen. A second type acts like an anti-estrogen. The third type appears not to be hormonally active, but can stimulate enzyme systems of animals and humans in a manner similar to certain drugs . . . and other toxic chemicals. . . . Unfortunately, most research studies have looked at total PCB levels without identifying individual types." The report then describes three studies to support its argument that different PCBs congeners have different effects. One study linked particular types of PCB congeners to breast cancer cell proliferation, whereas the other two found that women with breast cancer had higher levels of certain PCB types compared with their healthy counterparts.[101]

Yet another limitation of existing research relates to exposure assessment, a particularly important component of study design. Exposure assessment is central to epidemiological research, as it enables scientists to understand the relationship between the type, dose, pathway, and timing of exposure, on the one hand, and disease outcomes, on the other. At the same time, however, exposure assessment—particularly when used in the study of toxic substances—is fraught with difficulties and has the potential to overlook actual environmental risks. Activists and their allied scientists often highlight these assessment difficulties as part of their argument for why many studies might not find links between environmental toxicants and breast cancer. Indeed, they argue that such difficulties are among the more important barriers to accurate research results. For Julia Brody and her Silent Spring colleagues, "Designing meaningful exposure measures is 1 of the most significant challenges in translating mechanistic observations from the laboratory, in which exposure parameters are known and controlled, to epidemiologic studies. . . . Unfortunately, the exposure assessment strategies that underlie current knowledge regarding breast cancer risk are ill suited to studies of environmental pollutants."[102]

Some exposure assessment difficulties relate to the use of self-reporting by human subjects. Self-reporting can be an important way for researchers to learn the types of risk factors that women have experienced during their lifetime. Although this strategy may work when it comes to studying individuals' food consumption, medication usage, and daily living habits, it does not always work as well when it comes to studying their environmental exposures. Many women are not aware of their exposures, particularly ambient ones in the air and water, and they may neither remember nor have knowledge of exposures that took place during critical moments of development such as adolescence and in utero. Another assessment concern revolves around the measurement of multiple exposures. Diseases such as breast cancer are thought to be caused by multiple exposures. Sometimes the effects of these exposures are additive, meaning that they equal the sum of their individual parts. In other cases, the effects of multiple exposures—especially in case of xenoestrogens—are synergistic, meaning that the health impact of each toxin is magnified by its contact with the others. Unfortunately, current assessment methods are generally designed to test one chemical exposure at a time. Thus, it can be difficult to ascertain the health effects of multiple exposures, especially those that act synergistically.[103]

One frequently discussed assessment problem relates to body burden studies, which attempt to find associations between current levels of chemicals in the body and particular disease outcomes. Although body burden studies can sometimes engender useful results, they have significant limitations, especially in studying endocrine disrupters. Individuals are most susceptible to the health effects from these chemicals during "embryonic, fetal and early post-natal development." Consequently, studies that attempt to find a connection between an individual's health problems and that individual's direct exposure to endocrine disrupters may fail because they consider neither individuals' early postnatal exposures nor their parents' exposure levels at the time of conception and during pregnancy.[104] This methodological difficulty is particularly relevant to research on breast cancer, as the disease may be triggered by exposures that take place years—if not decades—before it develops. Thus, a woman's current level of toxic burden may not provide an accurate assessment of the role that chemicals played in the onset of her breast cancer. As the 2002 edition of *State of the Evidence* explains, body burden studies "are unable to show the *timing of exposure* to a chemical, which scientists now know is as critical as the dose of that chemical. The female breast is most vulnerable to chemical insult during prenatal development, adolescence, pregnancy and perimenopause. Thus exposure at age twelve may lead to cancer at age thirty-two or forty-two. Body burden measurement at or near the time of diagnosis will not reflect the levels at the time of exposure."[105]

Rethinking the Value of Certain Types of Evidence

A third set of strategies used to bolster the case that environmental factors increase the risk of breast cancer consists of placing increased epistemological importance on experimental and ecological evidence. When it comes to determining disease causation in humans, scientists, health professionals, and policy makers rely first and foremost on epidemiological research. Epidemiological studies, however, can seldom prove a causal link between particular toxicants and particular diseases. Rather, they typically find correlations between types, levels, and route of exposure, on the one hand, and particular health effects, on the other. To establish proof of harm as defined by the current regulatory system, investigators must support their epidemiological evidence with experimental evidence highlighting the toxicological mechanisms of particular chemicals. In the case of community-based studies, researchers may also rely on ecological evidence that demonstrates correlations between particular disease outcomes and local sources of toxic exposure. To be sure, activists and their scientist allies believe that epidemiological research should play an important role in determining causation. At the same time, the limitations associated with epidemiological research methods often make it difficult to assess accurately the relationship between environmental exposures and disease. Thus, activists believe that increased weight should be given to experimental and ecological evidence in the absence of adequate epidemiological results.

One type of experimental research is animal, or "in vivo" studies. In vivo studies analyze a chemical's possible toxicity. In studies on carcinogens, laboratory animals are exposed to high levels of a chemical in a relatively short period of time. Although these exposure levels are assumed to be higher than those to which most animals—much less most humans—would be exposed at any given point in their daily lives, the results may provide insight into the chemical's potential carcinogenicity at lower, but still potent, exposure levels. Although conducting animal studies is standard practice in toxicology, there are institutions, organizations, and industries—notably, those that downplay environmental causes of cancer—that challenge their relevance to human health. One of their criticisms is that humans and animals have different biologies and consequently may have different responses to the same toxic substance; a finding that certain chemicals cause cancer in animals does not mean that they cause the disease in humans. Individuals, moreover, are not exposed to the high doses of chemicals used in animal studies. Accordingly, such studies may overestimate the risk that these toxins pose to humans. Consider the American Cancer Society's position on the relevance of animal studies to understandings of environmental breast cancer risks among humans: "Although animal studies have demonstrated that prolonged high dose exposure to many industrial chemicals can increase mammary tumors, there are no current methods to determine whether the much lower concentrations of these chemicals that occur—alone or in combination, in air, drinking water, or consumer products—increase the risk of human breast cancer."[106]

Despite these limitations, animal studies are still important when it comes to understanding the relationship between breast cancer and toxic compounds, especially carcinogens. As part of its Breast Cancer and Environment: Science Reviews project, Silent Spring Institute compiled and analyzed data on 216 carcinogens linked to mammary gland tumors in animals, as well as assessed 450 epidemiological studies on breast cancer in humans. In the summary of its findings, the institute explains why animal studies are important to understanding environmental breast cancer risks in humans: "Testing chemicals in animal studies is currently the primary means of identifying chemicals that might cause cancer in humans. . . . Animal studies are a particularly important resource for understanding environmental pollutants and breast cancer, because there are only a limited number of humans studies and those are hampered by difficulties in estimating relevant exposures." The institute also responds to the skepticism surrounding the general relevance of animal studies to human health: "All known human carcinogens that have been tested on animals have been found to cause cancer in animals as well. . . . Sometimes, people question whether the relatively high doses of chemicals are relevant to typical human exposures. Scientists use high doses so they do not need to study a very large number of animals to find chemical risks of public health importance. In addition, research suggests that low levels of exposure to many chemicals can also have negative effects."[107]

When Science Is Not Enough

In the years since activists first helped to establish and carry out the research projects on Long Island, in Massachusetts, and in Marin County, they have participated in numerous other research efforts conducted by federal agencies, state agencies, universities, and private institutions. Whereas some of this research has focused solely on breast cancer, other research has examined the links between particular chemicals and an array of disorders. Among other projects, activists helped to develop—and, later on, uphold—the scientific and procedural guidelines for the EPA's Endocrine Disrupter Screening and Testing Program, which determines whether chemicals are hormonally active and what endocrine processes they disrupt. They also worked to pass bills that mandate "biomonitoring" programs to measure the amount of chemicals in people's bodies. Likewise, they helped to establish a federal research program to understand the environmental exposures faced by girls that put them at risk for breast cancer later in life. This scientific work, however, is not an end in itself. Rather, activists use the knowledge gleaned from such studies to promote their political and public health efforts.

Nevertheless, uncertainty surrounding the relationship between breast cancer and synthetic chemicals endures. Given that regulatory institutions require proof of harm before establishing more stringent environmental policies, such uncertainty has made it difficult for activists to achieve their prevention goals. To be sure, activists believe that more and better research can partly solve this problem. At the same time, science may not be enough. Even under the best research conditions, financial, ethical, political, scientific, and technological barriers that make it difficult to ascertain proof of harm in humans are likely to persist. This is especially true for diseases such as breast cancer that are caused by a complex intermingling of environmental, lifestyle, and genetic factors across a person's lifespan. Consequently, activists began to address the uncertainty problems in the late 1990s by arguing that evidence of harm— rather than proof of harm—should be the basis for taking regulatory and other types of preventative actions.

Chapter 4

"We Should Not Have to Be the Bodies of Evidence"

The Precautionary Principle in Policy, Science, and Daily Life

On May 15, 1999, the Massachusetts Precautionary Principle Project (MPPP) embarked on a three-year campaign, launching it at a well-attended meeting. A partnership between environmental health advocacy, scientific, and academic communities, the MPPP was the first activist campaign in the United States directed exclusively at implementing the precautionary principle in environmental health policymaking. The one-day event, held at Framingham College, a small school fifty miles west of Boston, exemplified the growing importance of the precautionary principle to environmental breast cancer activism and the bourgeoning environmental health movement more generally.

The precautionary principle is a multifaceted framework for conceptualizing and alleviating environmental health risks. It is most commonly understood as an approach to environmental health policy that encourages regulatory action in the face of uncertainty when some evidence of harm exists. The goal of the MPPP was to develop precautionary-based policies in Massachusetts, with the eventual aim of expanding the campaign nationally. During its first year, the MPPP would work with its participants to define its political agenda and develop strategies for action. Its second-year activities would be educating the public about the coalition's plan and the precautionary principle in general, as well as promoting public involvement in the campaign. In its third year, coalition participants would work to effect legislative change. The purpose of the kick-off meeting was to bring participants together to begin the first phase of the MPPP and lay the groundwork for the upcoming year's campaign efforts.

Representatives from an array of environmental health and public health organizations—numbered among them were Health Care Without Harm,

Physicians for Social Responsibility, and the World Wildlife Foundation—attended the meeting, but breast cancer activists and allied scientists from the Greater Boston area played a particularly prominent role. Along with the Clean Water Fund and the Lowell Center for Sustainable Production, the Massachusetts Breast Cancer Coalition co-organized both the meeting and the MPPP campaign. Activists and scientists from the Women's Community Cancer Project and Silent Spring Institute led workshops and facilitated discussions. Devra Davis gave the event's keynote speech, which revolved around her widely presented slide show, titled "The Case for the Precautionary Principle: Better Safe Than Sorry." In her talk, Davis discussed the case of xenoestrogens and breast cancer to bolster her argument for the necessity of the precautionary principle. She also outlined ways to implement the principle as part of a broader breast cancer prevention program.

Environmental breast cancer activists' newfound support for the precautionary principle during the late 1990s went hand in hand with their growing focus on identifying and eliminating suspected environmental causes of breast cancer, especially endocrine disrupters. To be sure, activists responded to the scientific uncertainty surrounding environmental factors by pushing for more and better research that they believed would lead to more definitive answers. At the same time, they came to realize that advocating for increased research without also changing the environmental regulatory system was not enough to protect women's health. Tens of thousands of chemicals were already on the market, and dozens more are developed every year. Obtaining the scientific data necessary to determine proof of harm based on the standards set by regulatory agencies could take decades, if not longer, especially given that so little is currently known about possible health effects. The limitations of conventional scientific methods, particularly in regard to endocrine disrupters, add to the time line. Not only would the research take a great deal of time to complete; scientists would also need to develop new testing paradigms, research methods, technologies, and risk assessment tools—efforts that could take years to complete in and of themselves.

For these reasons, activists embraced the precautionary principle to challenge the established assumption that proof of harm should be the basis for taking regulatory and other preventative actions. Although activists continue to demand more and better research, they also believe that enough evidence exists to take preventative actions to protect women from suspected environmental causes of breast cancer. As Nancy Evans writes in the fourth edition of *State of the Evidence*, "The public's health cannot and should not have to wait for absolute proof that certain chemicals cause breast cancer before moving to reduce the risk of such harm occurring. Too many people will suffer from the disease if we delay action until a 'scientific standard' of proof is met. Such a standard requires a 95 percent certainty of cause and effect. While this strict standard is supported by industry when policy changes under consideration would have an impact on profits, less stringent standards are followed in other settings. . . . What may work for science and industry does not serve, in this case, to protect public health."[1]

Over the past decade, breast cancer activists and their allied scientists have worked to implement the precautionary principle in various ways. Like the bulk of precautionary principle advocacy taking place in the United States and around the world, the efforts by such activists and scientists focus on implementing the principle into environmental health policymaking at the local, state, and federal levels. Just as important, they also approach the principle as an ethic for scientific practice and for everyday life. Understanding how activists have conceptualized and sought to implement the precautionary principle in these multiple ways not only demonstrates the principle's growing importance to the environmental breast cancer movement, but also highlights the many ways in which the movement contributes to the broader development of the precautionary principle.

A Brief History of the Precautionary Principle

The idea for the MPPP emerged in 1998 in the wake of the "Implementing the Precautionary Principle" conference at the Wingspread Retreat Center in Racine, Wisconsin. Thirty-two scientists and activists from the United States, Canada, and Europe attended this event and developed the first international consensus statement to outline the principle and the reasons why "corporations, government entities, organizations, communities, scientists, and other individuals must adopt a precautionary approach to all human endeavors."[2] After learning about the event and its consensus statement, Lee Ketelsen, the New England director of the Clean Water Fund, spoke with conference participant Peter Montague of the Environmental Research Foundation about ways to implement the precautionary principle in Massachusetts. Montague suggested that Ketelsen call Joel Tickner, a fellow conference participant and graduate student at the Lowell Center for Sustainable Production, one of the conference's co-sponsors.[3] The center's involvement in the precautionary principle issues made sense. Lowell, a city with more than one hundred thousand residents, was established in 1826 as a textile manufacturing center in the hills where the Merrimack and Concord rivers meet. Considered the cradle of the Industrial Revolution in the United States, Lowell was the largest city in New England during its heyday in the nineteenth century. The city's industrial power declined after the Great Depression, however, and by the 1970s it had lost much of its economic viability and infrastructure. In 1975, the Lowell Technological Institute merged with Lowell State College to become the University of Lowell (in 1991 renamed the University of Massachusetts at Lowell), with the purpose of catalyzing new technology in the area. By the 1990s, the economy had rebounded as a result of new technology and new service industries.[4] The Lowell Center for Sustainable Production was established in 1995 to ensure that technological and industrial development—both within the Merrimack River area and beyond—would foster not only economic growth but also healthy environments and communities.[5]

Soon after Ketelsen called Tickner, the latter spoke with Amy Pett, the Massachusetts Breast Cancer Coalition's director at the time, about the same idea. Consequently, the three organizations joined forces, procured funds from various foundations interested in environmental health issues, and spearheaded the MPPP. They consulted with Carolyn Raffensperger, an environmental lawyer from North Dakota and the executive director of the Science and Environmental Health Network (SEHN), for guidance on the coalition's kick-off meeting.[6] Established in 1994 by a group of environmental organizations, SEHN became an independent nonprofit in 1999. It currently functions as a "virtual organization" with six staff and nine board members across the country. Intent on promoting the use of science to protect the environment and human health, the organization has been one of the nation's leading proponents of the precautionary principle.[7] Not only did Raffensperger participate in the Wingspread conference; SEHN was one of its co-sponsors. Moreover, Tickner and Raffensperger co-edited *Protecting Public Health and the Environment: Implementing the Precautionary Principle* in 1999.

For its inauguration, MPPP packed many activities into the one-day event. Discussion sessions for the entire group of some one hundred participants were interspersed with the keynote speech, remarks by the event's organizers, small-group workshops and planning sessions, and opportunities for informal intermingling during breaks. Although participants hashed out a number of issues related to the precautionary principle throughout the day, a common discussion topic was how to define the meaning of the principle for the individuals and organizations involved. Most participants viewed the precautionary principle first and foremost as a commitment to taking preventative actions to protect health in the face of scientific uncertainty when some evidence of harm exists, as opposed to waiting for the proof of harm that the current regulatory system demands. Yet participants also pointed to several other important elements of the approach. They discussed the need to require proof from manufacturers that their products were safe, as opposed to not harmful, before they put them on the market. Similarly, they emphasized the importance of placing the burden of proof of safety on manufacturers before products were released rather than on consumers after the products were on the market. Further, participants sought to broaden established notions of risk by considering social and cultural factors in addition to economic ones when conducting environmental risk assessment. Finally, they brought up the need to make the environmental regulatory system more democratic through including the perspectives and interests of lay citizens in decision-making processes that traditionally have been dominated by the interests of politicians, policymakers, and industries.

Participants defined the precautionary principle in ways that reflected what they viewed as the necessary steps for environmental health policy change in Massachusetts and beyond. In crafting their ideas for change, they drew on several decades of precautionary principle advocacy, especially efforts that had occurred in Europe. The principle first emerged as *Vorsorgeprinzip* (the foresight principle) in West Germany in the early 1970s as a policy framework for preventing environmental damage through "forward-thinking" planning. It then entered the international environmental policy arena at the 1984 First International Convention on the Protection of the North Sea, with European governments working to incorporate it into their laws and policies from the mid-1980s into the early 1990s. Although the precautionary principle entered U.S. environmental policy discourses as an explicit concept in the early 1990s, when the U.S. government signed on to the 1992 Rio Declaration on Environmental and Development, it was not until 1998 that scientists, activists, and government researchers from the United States, Canada, and Europe met at the Wingspread Retreat Center in Racine, Wisconsin, to discuss ways to formalize the meaning of the principle and implement it in practice.[8] This meeting, convened by the North Dakota–based Science and Environmental Health Network, ended with the participants' writing and signing on to the Wingspread Statement on the Precautionary Principle.

As public support for the precautionary principle increased in the mid- to late 1990s, proponents pointed to a number of pressing environmental health issues in making the case for its implementation. These included mercury poisoning, arsenic in drinking water, air pollution, problems of children's health, ozone depletion, and global warming. Each of these issues represented serious health problems for which the evidence from the current regulatory perspective was not certain enough to warrant more stringent action. Still, the growing scientific and public concerns about the health effects from endocrine disrupters played a particularly crucial role in fueling precautionary efforts. Many scholars, scientists, policymakers, and activists advocating the precautionary principle discussed the scientific and technical difficulties surrounding the study of endocrine disrupters as a rationale for why the principle was needed.[9] Some of the principle's proponents even presented the specific case of xenoestrogens and breast cancer to bolster their position.[10]

To understand fully the relationship between the precautionary principle and endocrine disrupter theory it is important to recognize how the influence has gone both ways. Not only have the principle's proponents used the endocrine disrupter problem to promote the framework; many individuals have also invoked the principle to strengthen their argument for why increased public protection from these toxins is warranted. One of the earliest links between these two issues appeared in Theo Colborn, Dianne Dumanoski, and John Peterson Myers's *Our Stolen Future*. In response to criticism of the theory's inability to draw definitive links between endocrine disrupters and particular health disorders, the authors pointed to the problem of misapplied and inadequate research methods. They went on to argue that most of this criticism was based on misunderstandings of the theory's scientific principles:

> Just as it is difficult, with current knowledge, to affirm *all* the human health impacts we raise in this book, it is impossible to dismiss biologically plausible theories that hormone-disrupting chemicals may be a factor eroding human health, undermining intelligence, and reducing reproductive capacity. . . . If one detects worrisome trends in a variety of health problems linked to hormone disruption, the pattern may be far more telling than any single trend. It is a profound mistake to view this issue through the narrow lens of a single illness or physical deficiency or to consider human evidence alone. The power of this book's argument rests on the cumulative weight of the evidence and the compelling patterns that emerge when it is considered as a whole.[11]

Like their critics, Colborn, Dumanoski, and Myers acknowledged that definitive links between hormone-disrupting chemicals and most human health disorders did not exist. Yet they stressed that the general theory of endocrine disruption is more an interpretive framework than a scientific fact. Consequently, their purpose in writing the book was not, as some critics suggested, to bring this array of evidence together in order to "prove" that endocrine disrupters caused specific health disorders. Instead, they wished to make the case that despite the scientific uncertainty, enough overall evidence already existed to warrant public concern, further scientific inquiry, and increased regulatory action to protect human health from potential harm. Although they did not discuss the precautionary principle per se, they did emphasize the need for "caution" in the concluding paragraphs of the book's paperback edition: "We raised some daunting questions, knowing at the outset that it is not yet possible to answer all of them. We are pleased that the book and the controversy surrounding it have served to invigorate research. . . . In the meantime, even though the case has not been proven to the satisfaction of all, we urge caution. The possible consequences of widespread hormone disruption are immense and irreversible."[12] Other scientific writings and efforts since the mid-1990s have likewise invoked precautionary language in their warnings about the possible health risks from endocrine disrupters.[13]

Despite growing support for the precautionary principle from the environmental breast cancer and environmental health movements, the approach has been criticized by some scientists, policymakers, and industrialists. Consider *Rethinking Risk and the Precautionary Principle*, a collection of essays edited by Julian Morris, the director of the Environmental and Technology Programme at the Institute of Economic Affairs in London, as a response to the 1998 Wingspread Statement on the Precautionary Principle. In the introduction, Morris laid out some problems with precautionary thinking, claiming, for example, that the precautionary principle is not well defined and that its lack of concrete protocols leaves it too open for interpretation. He views the principle as antiscience and antitechnology, because obtaining proof of safety is epistemologically impossible and requirements to provide it would halt the development of new science and technology. Along these lines, he believes that the principle's impossibly high standards of proof of safety contradict the scientific method and society's emphasis on learning by trial and error. Moreover, the principle may lead to more harm than good, as taking small technological risks often benefits the public at large. Morris goes on to argue that implementing the precautionary principle would be too expensive, as it would require a dramatic expansion of the current regulatory apparatus and of the resources needed to conduct the necessary safety testing. Similarly, he believes that requiring an examination of the full range of safer alternatives to prospective new technologies would prove too costly and would take too long.[14]

Proponents of the precautionary principle counter these charges by emphasizing that its implementation demands more and better science. It will lead to more scientific and technological innovation, as it will require scientists, engineers, and manufacturers to think in creative and novel ways. The precautionary principle will also fuel—rather than hinder—economic growth by reducing the financial costs associated with environmental damage and public health problems that result from the use harmful products, technologies, and practices. To be sure, supporters acknowledge the principle's vagueness when it comes to its lack of concrete protocols. Instead of viewing this characteristic as a weakness, however, they view it as a strength. Given that the precautionary principle is not so much a set of well-defined rules as much as a conceptual framework, a set of general guidelines, and an environmental health ethic, it can be implemented to meet the specific needs of the particular problem at hand.

From this perspective, the principle functions as what sociologists Susan Leigh Star and James Griesemer call a "boundary object."[15] That is, the precautionary principle's meaning is stable enough to attract the support of many differently situated individuals and groups. At the same time, its meaning is flexible enough for them to define it in ways that meet their own particular political and public health needs. On the one hand, the precautionary principle's flexibility plays out across various domains: whereas most proponents tend to construct the principle as an environmental policy ethic, some construct it as an ethic for scientific practice and everyday life. On the other hand, its flexibility is evident in each of these domains, with activists and scientists constructing its policy, scientific, and quotidian dimensions in different ways. The precautionary principle's multiple meanings within—and across—these domains are apparent in the work that activists and their allied scientists do on suspected environmental causes of breast cancer, especially xenoestrogens.

The Precautionary Principle as a Policy Ethic

As the first U.S. campaign of its kind, the MPPP set the stage for a wave of precautionary principle activism during the subsequent decade. Many environmental health organizations, including those focusing on breast cancer, led this wave of policy advocacy and reform. The Alliance for a Healthy Tomorrow (AHT), for example, began in October 2000 to give the MPPP a more permanent existence.[16] Like the MPPP, the AHT takes a statewide approach to implementing the precautionary principle by seeking to "correct fundamental flaws in government policies that *allow harm* to our health and environment." The coalition aims to "create proactive policies to *prevent harm* before the damage is done, and to choose the safest alternatives." To these ends, the coalition promotes a number of "proactive" policies that it believes the state government should take to protect the public's health from environmental dangers. Such policies are based on the core values of the AHT: "choice, progress, and innovation; rigorous science; individual and corporate responsibility; democracy; [and] precautionary action and foresight."[17]

The Massachusetts Breast Cancer Coalition, the Clean Water Fund, and several other members of MPPP started the coalition, which encompasses a diverse group of "citizens, scientists, health professionals, workers, [and] educators seeking preventative action on toxic hazards."[18] The Lowell Center for Sustainable Production provides scientific support for the group.[19] Its members number more than 160 organizations and more than nineteen hundred individual activists and citizens; it has a governing board, a labor committee, and a senior advisory council. Breast cancer activists and their allied scientists play prominent roles in the coalition. The Massachusetts Breast Cancer Coalition and the Women's Community Cancer Project are two of the coalition's organizational board members. Julia Brody, executive directive of the Silent Spring Institute, and Nancy Krieger, associate professor in the Department of Health and Social Behavior at the Harvard School of Public Health, are also members of the coalition's Senior Advisory Council. Additionally, San Francisco's Breast Cancer Action is one of ten national organizations that are coalition members.[20]

In working to reduce exposure to toxic chemicals, the AHT strives to eliminate a range of environmental health problems, including breast cancer. The measures sought by the AHT are geared toward both adults and children. In its 2003 campaign, centered around protecting children's health, the AHT stated: "We need to start by protecting our children. Children are more vulnerable than adults to toxins. Recent research has demonstrated that children—and especially the developing fetus—are uniquely vulnerable to health damage from toxic substances. Children are not little adults. Their organs and physiological processes are still developing. Toxic chemicals can disrupt the development of organs and systems during childhood, causing long-term, irreversible damage. When adults are exposed to some toxins before and during pregnancy, their children can develop lifelong health problems." By making children's health a priority, the coalition not only strives to protect the health of one of the most biologically, socially, politically, and economically vulnerable human populations; it also aims to prevent many disease and disorders (such as breast cancer) afflicting adults believed to be caused by childhood exposure to harmful toxins.[21]

Recently, the AHT called on Massachusetts governor Deval Patrick to support the group's proposed five-pronged approach, intended for the state government to follow, to protect public health and the environment in Massachusetts. The strategies suggested by the AHT included prioritizing "clean economic growth," purchasing nontoxic products and services, banning toxic substances from consumer products, upholding laws and providing resources for state agencies "dedicated to reducing toxic chemicals," and promoting more stringent environmental legislation.[22] The coalition had helped to pass the Mercury Products Bill, which former governor Mitt Romney signed into law on July 28, 2006. One of the most stringent mercury-reduction laws in the country, this bill was framed to "dramatically reduce emissions resulting from the use of mercury-containing products," especially in municipal waste incinerators.[23] Although this effort does not have particular implications for breast cancer, the coalition's other legislative efforts do. In 2007, the AHT lobbied the state legislature on behalf of two other proposed bills: the Safer Alternatives Bill and the Safer Cleaning Products Bill. If passed, the former would build on the Massachusetts Toxics Use Reduction Act (TURA) program by helping to create "a comprehensive program to replace toxic chemicals with safer alternatives in consumer products and other businesses."[24] Similarly, the Safer Cleaning Products Bill "would reduce asthma and other health threats by requiring that only cleaning products approved by the Department of Public Health be used in public schools, hospitals, health care facilities, day care centers and public housing common spaces."[25]

Like the breast cancer activists in Massachusetts, those in the San Francisco Bay Area work to implement the precautionary principle in environmental health policy. For example, Breast Cancer Action, the Women's Cancer Resource Center in Oakland, and other members of the Toxic Links Coalition founded the campaign Stop Where It Starts in 2000. They recognized that more research was needed to find more conclusive links between toxic exposures and cancer, especially breast cancer, but they also believed that "there is also enough evidence now to encourage us to decrease the use and production of environmental pollutants in an effort to stop the increased rates of cancer."[26]

Whereas the AHT focuses on changing statewide policies, Stop Cancer Where It Starts works to pass environmental health resolutions that protect health at the city level. Moreover, the Bay Area campaign focuses not on environmental health issues faced by specific populations but on reducing the incidence of a specific group of diseases—primarily breast cancer and other cancers—among local community members of all ages. Stopping cancer where it starts entails the implementation of prevention strategies at the local sources of environmental contamination to which communities are exposed on a daily basis, often over long periods. By promoting policies to be enacted citywide, activists involved in Stop Cancer Where It Starts strive to eliminate immediate sources of pollution that may pose a greater threat to local residents than more geographically distant contamination sources.

To these same ends, the Toxic Links Coalition worked with the city of Berkeley in October 2000 to pass the "Resolution for the City of Berkeley

Establishing October as 'Stop Cancer Where It Starts' Month." They chose the month of October, National Breast Cancer Awareness Month, to counter the emphasis on early detection that is so prevalent during that month, by highlighting cancer prevention and emphasizing a precautionary approach toward suspected environmental causes. The resolution read, "WHEREAS, health and environmental policies, as well as industrial and other business practices, should be guided by the Precautionary Principle: When an activity raises threats of harm to human health or the environment, precautionary measures should be taken even if some of the cause and effect relationships are not established with absolute scientific certainty. In this context, the proponent of an activity or substance, rather than the public, should bear the burden of proof of harmlessness." Among other things, Berkeley's resolution called for citywide actions that would reduce the local sources of pollution linked to breast cancer and other cancers. One effort, the Healthy Buildings ordinance, eliminated the use of PVC plastic, formaldehyde, and other toxic materials in new construction. Other proposed actions included replacing the pesticides used on city property and land with safer alternatives; eliminating the use of PVC medical products, particularly in hospitals; requiring city institutions to buy chlorine-free paper items; and educating local businesses, hospitals, schools, organizations, and community members about not only the possible dangers associated with commonly used toxic products but also the availability of less harmful alternatives to these products.[27]

Following the passage of Berkeley's resolution, Breast Cancer Action, Women's Cancer Resource Center, and other members of the Toxic Links Coalition helped to pass similar resolutions in the Bay Area cities of San Francisco and Oakland, as well as in nearby Marin County.[28] Breast Cancer Action built on these local successes to promote the campaign nationally. On October 25, 2000, the organization ran a Stop Cancer Where It Starts advertisement in the *New York Times*. The ad, endorsed by eighteen individuals and organizations with ties to cancer and breast cancer activism, critiqued National Breast Cancer Awareness Month's emphasis on early detection over disease prevention, as well as encouraged readers to tackle environmental breast cancer issues in their local communities.

Prevention First: A Coalition of Independent Health Organizations is yet another group of environmental breast cancer activists carrying out precautionary policy work. In 2001, eight breast cancer, women's cancer, women's health, and consumer advocacy groups from the United States and Canada founded the organization (originally named Putting People First) to promote disease prevention, especially in regards to breast cancer and women's health more

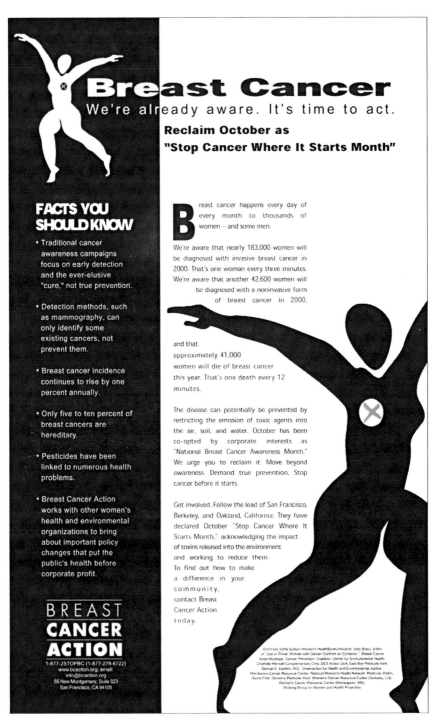

Figure 4.1 The Stop Cancer Where It Starts campaign's advertisement in the *New York Times*, October 25, 2000. Courtesy of Breast Cancer Action (San Francisco).

generally.[29] By the time the coalition officially disbanded in 2007, it consisted of twenty-four nonprofit organizations (and one business) from the United States, Canada, Australia, and Europe. Environmental breast cancer organizations that belonged to the coalition included Breast Cancer Action (San Francisco and Montreal), the Women's Cancer Resource Center in Oakland, the Massachusetts Breast Cancer Coalition, and two Long Island groups: the Babylon Breast Cancer Coalition and the West Islip Breast Cancer Coalition.[30] Unlike the Alliance for a Healthy Tomorrow and Stop Cancer Where It Starts campaigns, Prevention First did not focus on environmental health policy change in a particular geographic region. Rather, the coalition targeted pharmaceutical and biomedical industries, by critiquing the growing trend toward the "medicalization of prevention."[31] That is, it favored "shifting the emphasis in disease prevention away from drugs, medical products, and procedures" and promoted a focus on "true prevention" that eliminates the root causes of diseases, particularly suspected environmental causes.[32] Despite the coalition's dissolution, the organizations affiliated with it continue to work on these issues, on their own and in conjunction with one another.

The precautionary principle structured Prevention First's efforts, especially its central assertion that pharmaceutical companies market so-called prevention pills to bolster their economic profits rather than to protect public health. After all, the use of such pills—many of which the drug companies and the FDA did not adequately judge to be safe before they were marketed to the public—can often cause other health problems. Addressing the precautionary principle in this context, the coalition stated, "The Precautionary Principle is a formal statement of two commonsense ideas about protecting health and the environment. Implementing the principle requires that new drugs and technologies only be introduced into society when we have reasonably good evidence that they are safe, and that those who want to introduce a new drug or technology must first demonstrate that it is safe." The coalition suggested that if companies truly cared about the public's health, they would work to better understand and eliminate the actual causes of disease, especially environmental toxins—rather than develop costly medical interventions as an alternative to "true prevention."[33]

Although Prevention First challenged the marketing of prevention pills in general, it directed much of its efforts toward tamoxifen (Novaldex) and raloxifene (Evista). Both drugs, selective estrogen receptor molecules, reduce the risk of estrogen-receptor positive breast cancers by acting as anti-estrogens.[34] In the late 1970s, the FDA approved tamoxifen for the prevention of reoccurrences of breast cancer in women. In 1992, the National Cancer Institute (NCI) established the five-year Breast Cancer Prevention Trial to examine whether the drug could prevent breast cancer in healthy women (premenopausal and postmenopausal) over the age of thirty-five at increased risk for developing the disease.[35] By 1998, the study had determined that tamoxifen reduced such risk by 49 percent; it also, however, significantly increased the risk of blood clots, endometrial cancer, uterine sarcomas, strokes, and cataracts, especially in women over the age of fifty. Notwithstanding these serious side effects—and despite criticism from many breast cancer and women's health activist groups—the FDA approved the drug for use in healthy women that year. A follow-up study in 2005, however, led researchers to advise that healthy women over the age of sixty should not take the drug because it harms such women more than it helps them.[36]

Also in 2005, the NCI established the Study of Tamoxifen and Raloxifene study to compare the use of raloxifene to that of tamoxifen in healthy postmenopausal women at increased risk for breast cancer. The FDA had approved raloxifene in 1997 for the prevention of osteoporosis in postmenopausal women. Two years later, the agency approved it for the treatment of osteoporosis. That same year, investigators for the Multiple Outcomes of Raloxifene Evaluation study found that postmenopausal women taking the drug for osteoporosis also had fewer invasive breast cancers than participants who took a placebo. In a 2004 follow-up project, the Continuing Outcomes Relevant to Evista, NCI confirmed these findings. Furthermore, the Raloxifene Use for the Heart trial found that raloxifene decreased the incidence of invasive breast cancer in postmenopausal women at increased risk for coronary problems. Building on these earlier findings, the STAR study assessed the safety and efficacy of raloxifene in postmenopausal women at increased risk for breast cancer. Researchers concluded in 2006 that raloxifene prevented invasive breast cancer just as well as tamoxifen. Unlike tamoxifen, however, raloxifene did not decrease the incidence of noninvasive breast cancers. Although the study also found that those taking raloxifene had 36 percent fewer uterine cancers and 29 percent fewer blood clots than those taking tamoxifen, women taking both drugs had the same increased risk for developing strokes. In 2007, the FDA approved raloxifene for postmenopausal women at risk for invasive breast cancer.[37]

As forms of chemoprevention for healthy women at risk for breast cancer, both drugs received much hype within the medical community and the media. Prevention First, however, was not impressed, not only because of the drugs' serious side effects but also because of the ways in which they treat "a risk factor as though it were a disease."[38] "True prevention isn't a shell game," the National Women's Health Network, one of the coalition's founding members, stated. "Instead of women lifting up the shell and finding a prize (less breast cancer), they're just as likely to raise a shell and reveal a stroke, blood clot, or other kind of cancer."[39] Along this line, Prevention First additionally targeted the direct-to-consumer (DTC) ads for chemoprevention drugs. In December 2001, the FDA sent a regulatory letter to tamoxifen's maker, AstraZeneca, stating that the company had violated the agency's DTC advertisement requirements by "making misleading efficacy claims, minimizing health risks, and failing to comply with postmarketing reporting requirements."[40] Prevention First pressured the FDA to make sure that AstraZeneca responded to the agency's charges by improving its ads. The coalition further encouraged other breast cancer groups, women's health groups, and concerned citizens to take action by sending their own letters to the FDA about the tamoxifen ads, challenging the misleading claims made by DTC ads more generally, and working toward "public policy that puts people's health before corporate profit."[41]

The Precautionary Principle as a Scientific Ethic

At the Massachusetts Precautionary Principle Project's second annual coalition meeting in December 2000, participants formed subcommittees, each of which focused on a particular set of precautionary principle issues. One committee addressed the relationship between the precautionary principle and science. The discussions that took place among its members over the subsequent months led its chair, Joel Tickner of Lowell's Center for Sustainable Production, to organize the three-day "International Summit on Science and the Precautionary Principle" at the University of Massachusetts at Lowell. Eighty-five scientists, scholars, and activists from seventeen countries participated in the September 2001 event.

At the conference, participants developed a consensus statement outlining their understanding of the precautionary principle; the reasons why it should structure environmental health policy; and most important, its relevance to scientific practice. On the one hand, the statement outlined the role that science should play within a precautionary policy framework. For instance, it discussed the need to base policy decisions on evidence of harm rather than proof of harm. It asserted the importance of deeming a product safe, as opposed to harmful, before putting it on the market. It also emphasized that the burden of proof should fall on manufacturers and not consumers. On the other hand, the statement highlighted the significance of precautionary thinking for scientific practice. That is, it critiqued the ways in which "normative" science reflected and reinforced the established model of environmental health policymaking that they sought to revamp: "We believe that there are ways in which the current methods of scientific inquiry may . . . retard precautionary action. Unfortunately, limitations in scientific tools and in the ability to quantify causal relationships are often misinterpreted by government decision-makers, scientists, and proponents of hazardous activities as evidence of safety. However, not knowing whether an action is harmful is not the same thing as knowing that it is safe." To these ends, the consensus statement outlined conceptual and practical strategies for conducting research from a precautionary perspective. Among other things, the statement asserted that practicing science from such a perspective demands new research agendas—particularly an increased focus on primary prevention—and new modes of analysis for assessing the relationship between toxic exposures and health. It described how this science requires not only improved and innovative scientific methods and tools but also a greater integration of quantitative and qualitative research. Scientists also need to go beyond established paradigms in order to develop safer and more cost-effective alternatives to harmful products and technologies currently on the market.[42]

More than one hundred scientists, activists, and scholars signed on to the consensus statement. Three—Ana Soto, Carlos Sonnenschein, and Ruthann Rudel—were breast cancer researchers who had participated in the summit. Four other breast cancer scientists and activists—Devra Davis, Nancy Krieger of Harvard University, Joan Reinhardt Reiss of the Breast Cancer Fund, and Mary Lomont Till of the Women's Community Cancer Project—signed the consensus statement at a later date. The fact that these first four scientists endorsed the statement is worth noting, as most of their breast cancer research has both focused on xenoestrogens and been influenced by a commitment to the precautionary principle.[43]

The precautionary principle influences the ways in which breast cancer scientists conceptualize and assess evidence, as exemplified by the slide show that Davis presented at public venues across the country. When making the case for a precautionary approach to breast cancer prevention, Davis did not provide proof that xenoestrogens caused breast cancer in women. Such proof did not and still does not exist. Instead, she discussed evidence that demonstrated the plausibility of the xenoestrogen theory. Some of the evidence, laid out in the slide show, came from experimental research, including studies demonstrating how DDT and other pesticides disrupted normal breast cell communication and how DDT stimulates breast cancer cell growth.[44] Other evidence came from epidemiological studies showing correlations between increased risk of breast cancer and exposure to DDT, as well as between heightened cancer risk in Scandinavian women and their consumption of contaminated fish.[45] Davis highlighted ecological research from Long Island demonstrating that post-menopausal women living near two or more chemical plants had twice the risk of developing breast cancer compared with women who lived in areas with no such facilities.[46]

In taking this precautionary approach, however, Davis not only rethought what constitutes *enough* evidence; she also rethought what constitutes *relevant* evidence. In addition to describing evidence linking xenoestrogens to breast cancer, she highlighted evidence linking xenoestrogens to reproductive health problems in human males. Specifically, she explained studies demonstrating the declining rates of birth for baby boys in the United States, Canada, Denmark, Norway, and other industrialized countries.[47] She pointed to research showing increased rates of undescended testicles and hypospadias in baby boys, as well as increased rates of testicular cancer in men, in various parts of the world.[48] In some of her presentations, Davis also described a 1999 Japanese documentary that examined possible environmental causes, especially exposure to PCBs, for the steady decrease in testicular weight among Japanese men over the past decade. "Now, let me add some recent findings from Tokyo that I am trying to get translated into English," she stated at the Massachusetts Precautionary Principle Project's kick-off event. "The Tokyo medical examiner has conducted studies of the autopsies of Japanese men killed in accidents from 1970 to 1998. Over the years the men's bodies became taller and heavier. Researchers measured their height, their weight, the weight of their brain, the weight of their liver, and the weight of their testes. And in proportion to the weight increases of their other organs and total body mass, their testes did not continue to grow after 1980. I think this is pretty important. I don't know why Japanese men have smaller testicles, and I think it may be of interest to more than just Japanese women. But I think it is pretty important that we find out."[49]

Finally, Davis's presentation included slides linking xenoestrogens to health problems affecting wildlife, evidence that she called "sentinel indicators." She highlighted studies suggesting that endocrine disrupters caused limb malformations and abnormal sex concentrations in frogs in New Hampshire, as well as deformed frogs and declining frog populations in the Midwest.[50] She summarized research that drew connections between the dichofol, DDT, and other pesticides that polluted Lake Apopka, Florida, and the altered sex ratios and deformed penises in the alligator population that lived there.[51] She also discussed evidence demonstrating that exposure to high levels of synthetic estrogens caused sex reversal in snapping turtles.[52]

By rethinking what counts as relevant evidence in regard to the theory that xenoestrogens cause breast cancer, Davis created a new "ecology of risk"—a term that I use to describe the particular ways in which individuals, institutions, and communities conceptualize the relationship between breast cancer risk and the natural or built environment. Conventional ecological understandings of risk consider the unique set of risk factors associated with a particular disease such as breast cancer. By rethinking the notion of relevant evidence, however, Davis constructed an ecology of risk based not so much on the problem of breast cancer per se but on that of breast cancer as it relates to the broader set of risks associated with endocrine disrupters. In particular, Davis based her ecology of risk on a global framework that linked breast cancer on Long Island to human and wildlife disorders found in other parts of the United States, as well as in Japan, Scandinavia, and Canada. Indeed, much of Davis's precautionary approach to breast cancer prevention reflected her perspective that endocrine disrupters are a global problem that needs a global solution. By presenting a slide on how PCBs and other endocrine-disrupting chemicals are found in the fat of polar bears living in the Arctic Circle—a region with little human presence, much less an industrial one—she argued that increased federal regulations, though important, cannot in themselves protect against the transport of these chemicals into the United States or to more remote areas such as the Arctic Circle by way of rain, ocean currents, and wind. Instead, global solutions are also needed to solve this growing environmental health problem.[53]

Other breast cancer activists who construct their own ecologies of risk take a more local approach. In the early 1990s, Lorraine Pace and other concerned women suspected that the inordinately high increase in rates of breast cancer in their Long Island neighborhoods were caused by environmental factors, particularly xenoestrogens. In part, their suspicion arose from their mapping studies indicating that the highest rates of breast cancer in the neighborhoods occurred among women living on cul-de-sacs where "dead-end water mains" contained high amounts of sewage runoff. Yet their suspicion also resulted from their concerns that xenoestrogens caused other health problems in local human and non-human populations. For instance, some activists speculated that the declining clam population in the nearby bay resulted from cadmium contamination. In Rachel's Daughters, Pace explained that local companies had been dumping cadmium into the bay since 1932 and that some residents, herself included, used cadmium as a fungicide for their lawns, which bordered the bay. She went on to observe that cadmium is known to harm shellfish populations and cause mammary tumors in rats. "When I first moved here," Pace stated, "you could practically walk from clam boat to clam boat. That's how many clam boats there were. Now you're lucky if you see one clam boat. Something is killing the clams. Something is killing the fish. So maybe the same thing that is in their fat cells is in our fat cells."[54] Not surprisingly, cadmium made the list of one hundred suspected endocrine disrupters that Long Island activists wanted the EPA to examine as part of the Long Island Breast Cancer Study Project.

The precautionary principle shapes the structure of research projects and the types of research questions that breast cancer scientists ask. For example, it influences the research practices of toxicologist Ruthann Rudel and her colleagues at the Silent Spring Institute. Rudel joined Silent Spring when it first opened after having spent numerous years at an environmental consulting firm. She made the switch because she wanted to work on a more "proactive" environmental health research agenda. The institute was a good fit for her, because the science done at Silent Spring is policy driven, meaning that its scientists seek to conduct research that "helps to increase the imperative to act," according to Rudel. Much of the science revolves around exposure assessment, especially the development of exposure assessment methods.[55] Exploratory research is conducted to identify new avenues of scientific inquiry, as opposed to more "doable" research—that is, the testing of narrow hypotheses in well-developed research areas that can be easily answered.[56] Silent Spring's research, while innovative in many respects, tends not to land big grants from mainstream research organizations, industries, or government agencies that prefer to support studies with well-defined and testable hypotheses. Rudel points to Silent Spring's multidisciplinary research approach (which includes toxicological, epidemiological, and ecological research) and its collaborative relationship with activists and Cape Cod residents as evidence of the institute's precautionary approach to environmental breast cancer science. Democracy and collaboration are central to the precautionary principle, as they provide an alternative to the top-down model of scientific knowledge production.[57]

The Precautionary Principle as an Ethic for Everyday Living

Five months after the Massachusetts Precautionary Principle Project's kick-off meeting in October 1999, the Massachusetts Breast Cancer Coalition (MBCC) organized its own one-day conference, "At the Heart of Primary Prevention: Breast Cancer and the Precautionary Principle." The purpose was to discuss the principle as it specifically pertained to the issue of environmental links to breast cancer. After making her introductory remarks, MBCC director Deborah Forter introduced the conference's keynote speaker: Mary O'Brien, an Oregon-based scientist, breast cancer survivor, and environmental health activist.

In her talk, "Racing towards the Starting Line: The Radical Nature of Precaution," O'Brien discussed the importance of taking a precautionary perspective in efforts to prevent breast cancer. Much of her speech centered on the need to implement the precautionary principle in environmental health policy-making. Yet she also maintained that envisioning the principle solely as a regulatory framework is not enough; the precautionary principle must also become a framework for everyday life. That is, it must guide the ways in which we inhabit our natural and built environments so that we live our lives in ecologically sustainable and health-promoting ways. In particular, she encouraged people and communities to practice simple living. The social movement that revolved around simple living encourages individuals and communities to reduce their dependence on stressful lifestyles and jobs; unnecessary material goods; fuel-based transportation; environmentally harmful practices, products, and technologies; and food that is overly processed, pesticide ridden, and packaged.[58]

Several days later, O'Brien expanded on these themes in a workshop on "alternatives assessment" at the Lowell Center for Sustainable Production. Unlike conventional risk assessment, which focuses on the economic costs and benefits of particular technology and policy decisions, alternatives assessment also considers social, cultural, personal, spiritual, and other less tangible costs and benefits. Most important, it emphasizes the need for citizens, industrialists, activists, and policymakers to develop safer alternatives and creative strategies for addressing environmental health problems.[59] Along this line, much of the workshop was spent on everyday efforts that communities could take to reduce their environmental risks. O'Brien advised that widespread acceptance of such efforts will require shifts in not only personal but also social and cultural values. That is, they require what anthropologist Linda Layne calls a "cultural fix."[60] O'Brien explained, for example, that individuals will begin to rely on bicycles instead of cars for their primary mode of transportation only when cultural perceptions about time, class status, and physical activity change. In addition, communities will need to build more bike trails and design more bike-friendly roads. People will need to live closer to where they work, shop, and play. For their part, city planners and officials will need to construct their communities with these simple living principles in mind.

Like O'Brien's approach, the final section of Davis' slide show—"Precautionary Approaches to Risk Reduction and Prevention"—presented the precautionary principle as an everyday ethic. In addition to encouraging schools and workplaces to offer healthier food choices to their students and employees, she encouraged individuals to exercise more, eat better, and reduce their reliance on hazardous products linked to breast cancer. Further, she spoke about the need to eradicate the socioeconomic barriers that make it difficult for many people to incorporate healthy living strategies into their lives in the first place. In contrast to O'Brien, Davis incorporated an explicitly spiritual dimension into her precautionary ethic that drew from her strong Jewish faith. After advocating prayer and meditation as facets of a broader plan of breast cancer risk reduction, she ended her slide show with four inspirational quotes to encourage people to join others in working to prevent breast cancer. The last of these quotes comes from the Talmud: "It is not for us to complete the task, but we must begin it."

Sharon Koshar also views the precautionary principle in spiritual terms. Koshar served as MBCC's precautionary principle coordinator from 1999 to 2003 and continues educating people about the principle in the social change class that she teaches at Springfield College.[61] In her presentation at MBCC's October 1999 conference, Koshar described her reliance on spiritual ideals in explaining to local residents why they should strive to incorporate the principle into their daily lives. Unlike Davis, Koshar drew not from Judaism but from Deepak Chopra's Ayurvedic approach to holistic health.[62] In this belief system, one's physical, emotional, and spiritual health are intertwined. To be healthy in one of these ways requires health in all of them; one's body cannot be well, for instance, if one is chronically anxious and stressed. Moreover, Ayurveda emphasizes disease prevention over disease treatment, encouraging people to practice health lifestyles so that they do not get sick in the first place. By incorporating Ayurvedic perspectives into her precautionary principle activism, Koshar situated these three facets of individual health within the broader context of environmental health. One must inhabit a healthy environment to live a healthy physical, emotional, and spiritual life—and vice versa.

In 1999, Karen Miller, founder of the Huntington Breast Cancer Action Coalition established the Prevention Is the Cure (PITC) campaign. This initiative promotes the precautionary principle in dealing with the environmental health concerns facing Long Island and beyond. In partnership with other breast cancer and environmental advocacy groups, the campaign espouses everyday living strategies that individuals can use to lower their environmental health risks. For example, PITC, along with Neighborhood Network, developed a chart of twenty-five "Precautionary Alternatives" to "toxic triggers" that are known to cause or are suspected of causing various cancers, endocrine disorders, respiratory problems, Alzheimer's, and other health problems. Such precautionary measures include relying on organic pest control to minimize exposure to pesticides, using glass and stainless steel containers instead of plastic ones, and choosing paint with low levels of volatile organic chemicals (suspected of triggering asthma and reproductive effects).[63] PITC organizes the annual Prevention Is the Cure Week, comprising a series of educational workshops and local events across Long Island that has been held since 2002. In 2008, such events—most of which are free or encourage a voluntary donation—includes classes on safe cosmetics, environmental factors associated with breast cancer and other diseases (and steps to reduce one's risk), nontoxic home care, organic gardening techniques, and the national and international history of the precautionary principle. Running these events are various local breast cancer groups, such as the Huntington Breast Cancer Coalition, the Babylon Breast Cancer Coalition, the Great Neck Breast Cancer Coalition, the Islip Breast Cancer Coalition, and the Brentwood/Bayshore Breast Cancer Coalition.[64]

Viewing the precautionary principle as an ethic for daily life requires activists to direct their efforts toward not only scientists and policymakers but also the general public. Activists grapple with how best to communicate the meaning and importance of the principle to members of the public. During her presentation at the 1999 MBCC conference, Koshar warned that activists should describe the principle in language that most people can understand. She acknowledged that many activists, scientists, and policymakers feel comfortable using the term *precautionary principle* as it pertains to their political, scientific, and regulatory efforts. Many laypeople, however, find the term cold and overly technical, she explained, especially when it is used in campaigns aimed at educating them about the relevance of the principle to their daily lives. After her talk, audience members discussed these rhetorical concerns in relation to their own precautionary principle activism. They brainstormed alternative ways to describe the concept to the general public. In addition to suggesting such familiar phrases such as "Look before you leap," the audience members discussed the politics of describing the precautionary principle as a form of "common sense," a "gut feeling," and an innate "intuition" that all people shared regarding how to maintain a healthy self, community, and environment.

After the MBCC conference, one local group handed out a flier with "HEALTH FIRST!" printed across the top in bright red. The flier highlighted a way in which activists described the precautionary principle in less technical terms. Pictured below the phrase were nine men, women, and children of different ethnicities standing in front of the earth and smiling. Below them, the fact sheet stated in red and blue letters: "USE THE PRECAUTIONARY PRINCIPLE: For people, businesses, and governments—the first thing to consider when using a substance, creating a product or permitting a practice is: Is it healthful? Or harmful? Today there are over 80,000 chemicals in use. Many of them have polluted our earth, water and air, causing widespread contamination of plants, fish, wildlife and people. We need to take better care of our health and that of all living things. HEALTH FIRST: Let's do our part! Grassroots at WORK for a Healthy World." Without describing the technicalities of risk assessment or environmental regulation, this fact sheet promoted the precautionary principle by encouraging people to embrace a consumer, production, and regulatory ethic that puts the health of humans, wildlife, and the earth first. The fact sheet also highlighted that people of all ages and backgrounds can help implement this precautionary ethic in their daily lives and that such efforts are necessary for creating a healthy and sustainable world.

The title of Davis's slide show, "The Precautionary Principle: Better Safe Than Sorry," illustrates yet another rhetorical strategy for describing the precautionary principle in less technical terms. Like the phrase "Health First!"

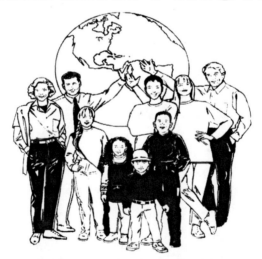

HEALTH FIRST!

USE THE PRECAUTIONARY PRINCIPLE:
For people, businesses, and governments - the first thing to consider when using a substance, creating a product or permitting a practice is: It is healthful? Or harmful?
Today there are over 80,000 chemicals in use. Many of them have polluted our earth, water and air, causing widespread contamination of plants, fish, wildlife, and people.
We need to take better care of our health and that of all living things. HEALTH FIRST: Let's do our part!

Grassroots at Work ✿ for a Healthy World

Figure 4.2 A flier from "At the Heart of Primary Prevention: Breast Cancer and the Precautionary Principle," a conference organized by the Massachusetts Breast Cancer Coalition in October 1999. Courtesy of Lise Beane.

"Better Safe Than Sorry" promotes health over harm by appealing to what Davis and others call "common sense." Davis likes the phrase because is one that people of all ages and backgrounds have heard throughout their lives in relation to many real-life situations, from rechecking whether the coffee pot is turned off to not driving one's car too fast in a snowstorm even if driving slower will make one late for an important event. "In many aspects of our lives, we promote the idea that it's better to be safe than sorry," Davis once explained to me, "So why should the values guiding how we protect public health from environmental dangers be any different?" Long Island's Prevention Is the Cure takes this view, as well: "The science has spoken!" the organization asserts on its Web site. "Harmful environmental toxins are causing disease. Instead of waiting for definitive 'proof' of the toxicity of millions of chemicals and products, we advocate a precautionary health model—one that says it is 'better to be safe than sorry.' "[65]

Davis also likes "Better Safe Than Sorry" because it helps people to understand the importance of erring on the side of caution even when the risk of harm—especially death—is unproven. "We should not have to become the bodies of evidence," declared Davis at many of her public presentations. She borrowed this phrase from Bay Area breast cancer survivor and activist Nancy Evans.[66] Both Davis and Evans use it bring attention to the deaths of women with breast cancer that have occurred when harmful products were deemed "safe" for industry use and public consumption following inadequate safety testing. In addition, they rely on the phrase to highlight how women's breast cancer–ridden bodies have become the evidence of harm within a regulatory system that places the burden of proof on consumers rather than on the manufacturers of toxic products.

Activists' efforts to implement the precautionary principle within the domains of science, policy, and daily life demonstrate its growing relevance to the environmental breast cancer problem, and the principle's flexibility indicates that it will continue to be a useful framework in the future. In the years to come, activists and their allied scientists will identify new chemicals and other toxic substances of concern. They will focus on new geographic, workplace, and other physical sites of exposure. They will better understand not only the toxicological properties of particular chemicals but also the biological, genetic, behavioral, and structural factors that make particular individuals susceptible to environmental health risks. They will develop new research methods and fine-tune older ones. In addition, the changing technoscientific landscape of environmental breast cancer activism will intersect in new ways with the shifting terrain of other health movements. In response to these emerging types of knowledge, issue priorities, technoscientific practices, and kinship opportunities, activists will rethink what strategies count as precautionary and how best to implement them.

Implementing precautionary policies and practices, however, requires more than just the support and compliance of scientists, other activists, industrialists, and policymakers. It also needs support from the public. Activists rely on the public to embrace their objectives and participate in their campaigns as a way to validate their efforts and put pressure on key officials and decision makers. They depend on the money, time, and other resources provided by citizens in carrying out political and public health work. Incorporating precautionary strategies into the daily lives of individuals and communities demands public involvement, as well. Given that breast cancer primarily afflicts women, activists devote much of their outreach efforts to them, often by constructing environmental breast cancer as a women's health issue. Still, the ways in which they construct it as such vary and are subject to debate.

Chapter 5

The Cultural Politics of Sisterhood

In September 1999, the Breast Cancer Fund announced that it would be part of a new coalition, with Susan G. Komen for the Cure and the National Organization for Women (NOW), which would campaign for increased federal research on environmental causes of breast cancer. One of the coalition's first efforts was a two-page letter to President Bill Clinton, copied to presidential candidates Governor George W. Bush of Texas; U.S. senator Bill Bradley of New Jersey; and Vice President Al Gore. Written on Breast Cancer Fund letterhead, the letter called on the president to remedy the nation's failure to address possible environmental causes of the disease and, by extension, breast cancer prevention. The Breast Cancer Fund's decision to send the letter to President Clinton in late October, in the final week of National Breast Cancer Awareness Month, served to sharpen an already existing critique of the dominant breast cancer paradigm. Unlike other activist groups that criticized National Breast Cancer Awareness Month, however, the Breast Cancer Fund did not frame the letter's environmental health demands in relation to critiques of the cancer industry. Instead, the organization conceptualized its environmental health demands and the coalition's broader campaign goals through the lens of the population most affected by breast cancer and by the environmental factors linked the disease: women. In doing so, it took a feminist perspective, situating its demands for more environmental health research within the broader context of women's health politics and activism.

Women's health is arguably one of the most common disease categories in which breast cancer activists situate the breast cancer problem. Thus, it is not surprising that the Breast Cancer Fund's campaign and the environmental breast cancer movement more generally often construct the environmental breast cancer problem through this particular lens. At the same time, the feminist perspective embraced by the campaign reflects only one of the ways in which activists, organizations, and others have constructed the environmental breast cancer problem as a women's health issue. Not only do the gendered elements of environmental breast cancer activism sometimes take place outside a traditional feminist framework; the social, cultural, and political terrain of feminist breast cancer activism, like feminism in general, is also diverse in its own right. Consequently, the various ways in which activists construct the gendered dimensions of the environmental breast cancer issue lead to multiple approaches for addressing the problem. Such differences highlight the array of practices that activists use to inspire women and the broader public to partake in environmental breast cancer activism.

Mapping the Feminist Politics of Environmental Health

The Breast Cancer Fund's 1999 letter to President Clinton outlined four research demands: increasing funding for the National Institute of Environmental Health Sciences (NIEHS), establishing a national registry and inventory of the endocrine-disrupting and carcinogenic chemicals found in our bodies, fully funding the EPA's Endocrine Disrupter Screening Program (EDSP), and establishing a cross-agency committee to oversee government funding for environmental health research. The letter went on to explain how each of these research goals would lead to better understandings of the relationship between breast cancer and toxic exposures. The Breast Cancer Fund argued that increasing the overall NIEHS budget would make more financial and institutional resources available for the study of breast cancer, while increased "biomonitoring" would include a wider range of chemicals as well as the testing of breast milk, which "often contains high levels of carcinogenic and hormone-disrupting chemicals." The letter justifies the EDSP budget by describing how hormone mimickers cause "the rapid growth of cancer cells." Regarding the final demand, the Breast Cancer Fund observed that "recently, a $15 million appropriation earmarked for a study that would have explored environmental factors in regions with high breast cancer incidence was diverted to unrelated projects on genetics and air pollution. A cross-agency oversight committee that includes consumer participation would ensure the correct and wisest placement of new funding."[1]

In making these demands, the coalition did not simply construct breast cancer as an environmental health issue. Rather, it framed the environmental breast cancer problem as a women's health issue. After outlining the four actions that the Breast Cancer Fund wanted President Clinton to take, the letter stated, "We welcome the opportunity to discuss the above in greater detail with you and your staff. Time is of the essence. Women at risk for breast cancer—which is all women—are engaged in a battle to save our bodies and our lives. Until we arm ourselves with new intelligence about the causes of the disease, we will continue to fight blindfolded. On behalf of our mothers, sisters, and daughters, we call on you to vigorously support policy and research that will empower us to fight with both eyes open."[2] The "we" calling on Clinton to take action in this paragraph were the eighty women who signed the letter on behalf of their organizations, businesses, and universities. Although many of the listed parties were representatives from breast cancer organizations such as Breast Cancer Action, the African American Breast Cancer Alliance, and 1 in 9: The Long Island Breast Cancer Action Coalition, they also included representatives from women's cancer organizations, women's health organizations, and other women's groups.

This women's health framework structured the press conference that the Breast Cancer Fund organized on October 27 to discuss the formation of its coalition and the letter that it had sent President Clinton two days prior. Held in the Longwood House of Representatives Office Building on Capitol Hill, the press conference drew several dozen people, including breast cancer activists from East Coast organizations, congressional staffers, and journalists. The event featured speeches by coalition representatives Diane Balma of Susan G. Komen for the Cure, Breast Cancer Fund president Andrea Martin, and NOW president Patricia Ireland. Campaign supporters Wilma Brown of the American Medical Women's Association and Julia Brody, the director of the Silent Spring Institute, among others, also spoke. Both women signed the Breast Cancer Fund's letter on behalf of their organizations. Congresswoman Nancy Pelosi, Democrat of California, and Senator Olympia Snowe, Republican of Maine, longtime proponents of women and women's health issues, expressed their commitment to helping achieve the coalition's demands.[3]

By situating breast cancer within the broader framework of women's health, the Breast Cancer Fund and the campaign's participating organizations formed a disease kinship, linking breast cancer to other health conditions that primarily affect women and to interest organizations working on behalf of women's health. In doing so, the campaign connected activists, affected persons, health care professionals, scientists, concerned citizens, and other individuals who have personal, professional, and political stakes in working together through the broader framework of women's health. The Breast Cancer Fund's focus on environmental health, particularly endocrine disrupters, further helped to construct breast cancer as a women's health issue. Just as xenoestrogens are linked to breast cancer, so too are they implicated in other women's health disorders. Some of these health conditions and their suspected environmental causes are priority issues for many of the organizations that signed the letter. The DES Cancer Network, for example, advocates on behalf of women who have clear-cell adenocarcinoma of the vagina or cervix resulting from in utero exposure to DES. Likewise, the National Women's Health Network takes on environmental causes of breast cancer, endometriosis, and ovarian cancer, while Planned Parenthood works to address the connections between xenoestrogens, reproductive health, and family planning. Indeed, several speakers at the press conference stressed the need to better understand the possible impact of these chemicals on both breast cancer and women's health more generally.[4]

With 99 percent of breast cancer cases occurring in women, it should come as no surprise that the Breast Cancer Fund's 1999 campaign defined the disease as a women's health issue.[5] The environment breast cancer movement—not to mention the broader breast cancer movement—does the same. Women's health is one of the most important disease frameworks used by activists of all kinds to conceptualize and address the breast cancer problem. Yet the Breast Cancer Fund's campaign constructed the category of women's health not simply in biomedical terms but also in feminist terms. That is, it invoked this category to situate its research demands in relation to the social, cultural, political, and economic factors that have historically hindered women's ability to achieve physical and emotional well-being in the United States and beyond.

The majority of those who signed the letter self-identify as feminist. Despite its use of masculine and military metaphors (such as women's "fights" and "battles" against breast cancer) to win the support of Congress, other elected officials, and the public at large, the letter relied on feminist rhetoric in making its case. The letter portrayed women as active participants and key players in scientific and political efforts to eradicate breast cancer. The success of prior campaigns sponsored by the National Breast Cancer Coalition and other organizations to increase federal spending on breast cancer research meant that the Breast Cancer Fund could not justify its demands by simply stating that breast cancer research was underfunded. Thus, it argued that as the federal government increased its environmental health research efforts, it should make sure not to leave women's health issues, particularly breast cancer, behind.

Speakers at the coalition's Capitol Hill press conference made explicit links between feminism, breast cancer, and the need to reform science and policy agendas as they relate to environmental causes of the disease. As Patricia Ireland put it, "Environmentalists and feminists alike share a common interest in research on the impact of environmental degradation on women's health. This concern is reflected in the many women's rights activists who identify themselves as eco-feminists and the many environmental activists who are strong women's rights supporters. Now, we must challenge the scientific research community and policymakers to look for answers to the questions that plague every woman who has ever felt a lump in her breast: Why does this happen? How can we prevent it? And how can we cure it?"[6]

The feminism that structured the Breast Cancer Fund's 1999 campaign shapes the environmental breast cancer movement in broader terms. It fuels activists' arguments that the dominant breast cancer paradigm places blame for breast cancer on women's lifestyle choices rather than the social, political, and economic systems that often hinder women's opportunities to make healthy choices and avoid exposure to toxic substances. It also informs environmental breast cancer activists' engagements with science. Activists point to the historical lack of research on women's health issues, including breast cancer, in their efforts to demand that current and future environmental health research focus on women. They draw on their gender-inflected "embodied knowledge" and "ways of knowing" to make the case for why they should play a role in deciding how much research scientists should conduct, how they should conduct it, and to what politics and policy ends it should be used.[7]

In recent years, scholars, activists, and social critics have written about the environmental breast cancer movement's feminist underpinnings, with many describing how this feminist movement differs from other facets of contemporary breast cancer activism. In particular, some have contrasted environmental breast cancer activism with what feminist, social critic, and breast cancer patient Barbara Ehrenreich calls the "mainstream of breast cancer culture"—a type of activist culture that has come to dominate the social, cultural, and political landscape in the 1990s and early 2000s.[8] Although this mainstream culture emerged in part from the successful efforts of feminist breast cancer activists in raising public awareness about the disease, its critics argue that it is far from feminist.

Ehrenreich's April 2001 *Harper's* article, "Welcome to Cancerland: A Mammogram Leads to a Cult of Pink Kitsch" is a particularly scathing critique of mainstream breast cancer culture. In recounting her ventures into this culture in the wake of her diagnosis with the disease in 2000, she describes it as pink and frilly: "You can dress in pink-beribboned sweatshirts, denim shirts, lingerie, aprons, loungewear, shoelaces, and socks; accessorize with pink rhinestones brooches, angel pins, scarves, caps, earrings, and bracelets; brighten up your home with breast-cancer candles, stained-glass pink-ribbon candleholders, coffee mugs, pendants, wind chimes, and night-lights; pay your bills with special BreastChecks or a separate line of Checks for the Cure."[9] She further notes how mainstream breast cancer culture promotes traditional feminine values through commercialism. Ehrenreich describes the plethora of breast cancer–themed products sold by organizations and businesses—from T-shirts to designer bank checks and teddy bears—in efforts to raise funds for breast cancer research. Such groups also sponsor walks, races, and other fundraising events. For Ehrenreich, this culture embodies a "perkiness" and "cheerfulness" that discourages complaining and getting angry at the disease. The Breast Friends Web site, for instance, offers inspirational quotes and verses, among them "Don't Cry over Anything That Can't Cry over You" and "I Can't Stop the Birds of Sorrow from Circling my Head, but I Can Stop Them from Building a Nest in My Hair."[10] "What does not destroy you," writes Ehrenreich, "to paraphrase Nietzsche, makes you a spunkier, more evolved, sort of person. . . . And in our implacably optimistic breast-cancer culture, the disease offers more than intangible benefits of spiritual upward mobility. You can defy the inevitable disfigurements and come out on the survivor side actually prettier, sexier, more femme."[11]

Ultimately, Ehrenreich claims, the ultrafeminine and infantilizing tendencies of mainstream breast cancer culture perpetuate complacency about the social, political, economic, and environmental policies that she and many others believe are responsible for causing the current breast cancer epidemic. For example, the culture directs women diagnosed with breast cancer to learn makeup techniques so they can look prettier after their treatments, rather than encouraging them to ask what caused their cancer. It promotes the belief that breast cancer is a blessing in disguise and that a cure is just around the corner, instead of cultivating anger at a social system that values financial profit over women's health. It inspires women to become consumers of items decorated with pink ribbons and participants in races that fund research for the ever elusive cure rather than empowering them to become activists who challenge and reform the social, political, and economic system that supports the dominant breast cancer paradigm. The final paragraph of Ehrenreich's article sums up her feelings about mainstream breast cancer culture: "No, this is not my sisterhood. For me at least, breast cancer will never be a source of identity or pride. . . . What it is, along with cancer more generally or any slow and painful way of dying, is an abomination, and to the extent that it's man made, also a crime. This is the one great truth that I bring out of the breast cancer experience, which did not, I can now report, make me prettier or stronger, more feminine or more spiritual—only more deeply angry. What sustained me through the 'treatments' is a purifying rage, a resolve, framed in the sleepless nights of chemotherapy, to see the last polluter, along with, say, the last smug health insurance operative, strangled along with the last pink ribbon."[12]

Ehrenreich's *Harper's* article received considerable public attention and praise. Bloggers, journalists, and others wrote about it in their posts, essays, and editorials. Professors taught it in their women's studies courses. In 2003, the essay was a finalist for a National Magazine Award. It also inspired breast cancer activists. San Francisco's Breast Cancer Action invited Ehrenreich to give the keynote speech at its fifth annual town hall meeting, "Beyond the Pink Ribbon: Challenging the Culture of Breast Cancer," in April 2002. Founded in 1998, this event brings together community members and activists to develop new partnerships and political strategies for addressing the environmental breast cancer problem. Basing the town meeting on Ehrenreich's critique reflected Breast Cancer Action's desire to discuss and dissect what it viewed as the problems with mainstream breast cancer culture.

Accounts such as Ehrenreich's provide important insights into the multiple and often contradictory cultures of action that constitute breast cancer politics and activism. Although the breast cancer movement as a whole often views the breast cancer problem through the lens of women's health, not all facets of the movement necessarily embrace the disease category in the same way. The particular ways in which activists and others conceptualize it carry implications for how they understand the gendered dimensions of living with breast cancer; the impact of gender on the disease's social, cultural, and political dimensions; and the political and public health implications of treating breast cancer as a women's health issue. How activists construct the category of women's health also influences their beliefs and decisions about the best ways to alleviate the breast cancer problem, the specific political actions that they should take, the role that the public (particularly women) should play in this work, and the outreach strategies for getting such individuals involved.

By emphasizing the differences between activist cultures, however, accounts such as Ehrenreich's neglect the heterogeneity that exists within the environmental breast cancer movement. The boundaries between this movement and its mainstream counterpart are not always clear cut. Individuals, organizations, discourses, practices, and political symbols often travel back and forth between these two arenas, embraced by activists and organizations in each. Furthermore, the feminist perspective behind the environmental breast cancer activism is not as unified as the Breast Cancer Fund's 1999 campaign and other accounts such as Ehrenreich's suggest. Rather, the movement is a socially, culturally, and politically diverse terrain when it comes to such perspectives, and downplaying this heterogeneity has the potential to oversimplify the issues of what political and public health efforts best promote women's health in regard to breast cancer prevention, what role feminism should play in these efforts, and what counts as feminist breast cancer activism.

Symbols, Discourses, and Practices

The Breast Cancer Fund's 1999 campaign is a useful springboard for discussing the heterogeneity of feminist environmental breast cancer activism. By signing on to the same letter and set of research demands, the coalition members and the other signatories spoke with a unified activist voice. This form of "strategic essentialism" served an important political purpose: coming together as a unified bloc increased their chances that federal officials would take their demands seriously.[13] In speaking with one voice, however, the Breast Cancer Fund's 1999 campaign erased the differences within the broader environmental breast cancer movement, particularly among the specific groups that signed on to the letter.

In their activist work outside the campaign, these groups have sometimes approached the environmental breast cancer problem in different and even contradictory ways. Such differences, in turn, relate to a wide range of ideological, agenda-setting, practical, organizational, and social factors. One important set of differences relates to the ways in which environmental breast cancer activists define feminist activism and determine what role it should play in their political work. Three issues—the role of corporate support and commercialism, the use of the pink ribbon as a symbol of the breast cancer movement, and the politics of "survivor" identity—exemplify the complexity of feminist breast cancer activism. They also complicate the boundary between mainstream and feminist breast cancer culture.

Corporate Involvement

One facet of mainstream breast cancer culture that Ehrenreich and others critique is corporate involvement in breast cancer advocacy efforts. Since the early 1990s, dozens, if not hundreds, of corporations and businesses have participated in these efforts. Ehrenreich observed, "You can 'shop for the cure' during the week when Saks donates 2 percent of sales to a breast-cancer fund. . . . You can even 'invest for the cure,' in the Kinetics Assets Management's new no-load Medical Fund, which specializes entirely in businesses involved in cancer research. If you can't run, bike, or climb a mountain for the cure—all of which endeavors are routine beneficiaries of corporate sponsorship—you can always purchase one of the many products with a breast cancer theme."[14] Ehrenreich dislikes such corporate sponsorship practices for several reasons. She points out, for example, that a significant portion of the money raised through them goes not to the causes that they supposedly support but to overhead and advertising costs; Avon's Breast Cancer 2-Day Walk spends more than a third of the money it raises on such expenses, while Susan G. Komen's Race for the Cure series "fritter away up to 25 percent of its profits."[15] Further, the money that does go to charity tends to support research to find a cure for breast cancer rather than disease prevention.

Many breast cancer groups share Ehrenreich's concerns. In 2001, ten breast cancer and women's cancer organizations formed a coalition, Follow the Money: An Alliance for Accountability in Breast Cancer, to raise public awareness about the ways in which profits from corporate-sponsored fund-raising events such as Avon's 2-Day Walk and the Susan G. Komen's Race for the Cure series are spent. One member of this coalition, the Massachusetts Breast Cancer Coalition, described the group's mission on its Web site: "We applaud organizations that are committed to raising money to fight the epidemic of breast cancer, and we know that every dollar is critical. The dedication and commitment that participants in fundraising walks, runs, swims, bikes and every other mode of fundraising events show is inspiring. We are concerned with what happened to the money that these walkers, runners, swimmers, and bikers have raised and want to ensure that it is ultimately directed to fighting the breast cancer epidemic." To this end, the coalition lists questions for the public to ask event sponsors before participating in or supporting such events: "What percentage of the events' proceeds will be designated for research? What kind of research will be funded? Will there be funding into environmental links to breast cancer? Will there be local breast cancer advocates involved in the research selection and funding decision process?"[16]

Breast Cancer Action, a member of Follow the Money, established the Think Before You Pink campaign in the wake of its town hall meeting in April 2002. Through brochures, articles, postcards, and other educational materials, Breast Cancer Action seeks to educate the public about the perils of "cause marketing," whereby corporations donate a portion of their sales profits to charitable causes such as breast cancer awareness. The organization maintains that corporations raise little money from these efforts and that they establish such campaigns to gain customers who want to support companies with a social conscience. Think Before You Pink encourages consumers to learn how corporations allocate the profits from their cause marketing campaigns to breast cancer efforts: "How much money from each product sold actually goes toward breast cancer? . . . To what breast cancer organization does the money go, and what types of programs does it support?" Think Before You Pink pushes buyers to consider the ways in which cause marketing campaigns may directly undermine breast cancer prevention, especially as it pertains to potential environmental causes of the disease: "What is the company doing to assure that its products are not contributing to the breast cancer epidemic? . . . Is the promotion a golf tournament on a golf course sprayed with pesticides? Is $1 being given each time you test-drive a polluting car, as in BMW's Ultimate Drive Campaign? Are the products being sold cosmetics containing chemicals linked to breast cancer?"[17]

In October 16, 2002, Breast Cancer Action placed an ad in the *New York Times* illustrating Think Before You Pink's message. In the ad, Breast Cancer Action plays off a cause-marketing campaign promoted by the company Eureka. Eureka (whose name was changed to Electrolux Home Care Products of North America in 2004) is one of the nation's leading producers of vacuum cleaners and their parts. In June 2002, Eureka established its Clean for the Cure campaign. For every Whirlwind LiteSpeed vacuum cleaner purchased, Eureka donated one dollar to research efforts to find a breast cancer cure, with a maximum contribution of $250,000.[18] Breast Cancer Action criticized this and other cause-marketing campaigns—specifically, American Express's Charge for the Cure and BMW's The Ultimate Drive—by suggesting that it is the corporations that "clean up" financially from such campaigns rather than the breast cancer efforts they supposedly benefit. Given that the Whirlwind LiteSpeed vacuums cost $170 each, Eureka donated less than 1 percent of its profits to breast cancer research. Breast Cancer Action's release of its ad in October, National Breast Cancer Awareness Month, is especially appropriate, as many companies promote their cause-marketing efforts at that time, when public sympathy toward breast cancer issues is at its peak. American Express's Charge for the Cure, for instance, took place in 2002 during the month of October.

The fact that many activist groups raise concerns about cause-marketing practices and other corporate fund-raising efforts, however, does not mean that they shun them altogether. Indeed, many groups welcome donations from businesses and corporations that readily extend financial support to environmental breast cancer and prevention fund-raising events. Each year in Cape Cod and in Hopkinton State Park, the Massachusetts Breast Cancer Coalition holds its event Against the Tide, an outdoor fund-raiser involving a one-mile swim, a two-mile kayak ride, and a three-mile walk. Individuals of all ages and skill levels can participate in as many of the events as they want, as long as they raise a minimum of $150 beforehand. Families that want to participate need to raise a minimum of $250. National and local businesses such as Whole Foods Market,

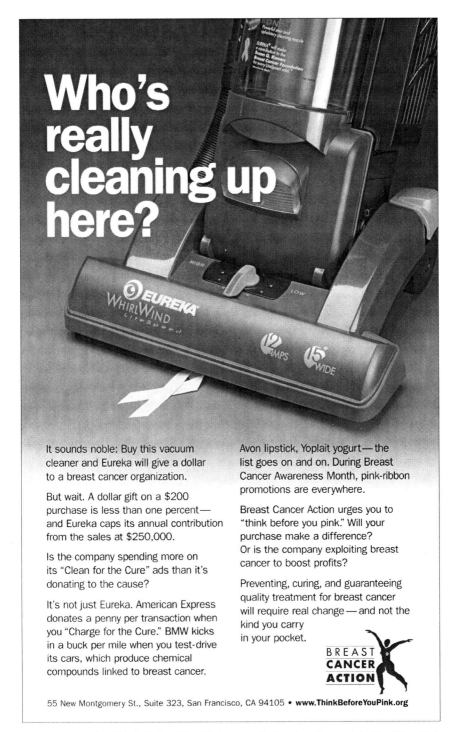

Who's really cleaning up here?

It sounds noble: Buy this vacuum cleaner and Eureka will give a dollar to a breast cancer organization.

But wait. A dollar gift on a $200 purchase is less than one percent— and Eureka caps its annual contribution from the sales at $250,000.

Is the company spending more on its "Clean for the Cure" ads than it's donating to the cause?

It's not just Eureka. American Express donates a penny per transaction when you "Charge for the Cure." BMW kicks in a buck per mile when you test-drive its cars, which produce chemical compounds linked to breast cancer.

Avon lipstick, Yoplait yogurt—the list goes on and on. During Breast Cancer Awareness Month, pink-ribbon promotions are everywhere.

Breast Cancer Action urges you to "think before you pink." Will your purchase make a difference? Or is the company exploiting breast cancer to boost profits?

Preventing, curing, and guaranteeing quality treatment for breast cancer will require real change—and not the kind you carry in your pocket.

BREAST CANCER ACTION

55 New Montgomery St., Suite 323, San Francisco, CA 94105 • www.ThinkBeforeYouPink.org

Figure 5.1 The Think Before You Pink campaign's advertisement in the *New York Times*, October 16, 2002. Courtesy Breast Cancer Action (San Francisco).

Blue Cross/Blue Shield, Dana-Farber Cancer Institute, Edy's Ice Cream, and Quantum Communications of Cape Cod sponsor the event. Net proceeds go not to research efforts to find the cure but to the Silent Spring Institute's research efforts to study environmental links to breast cancer. They have also gone toward the Massachusetts Breast Cancer Coalition's educational and advocacy efforts, the bulk of which focus on environmental breast cancer prevention.[19]

Similarly, the Breast Cancer Fund participates in corporate-sponsored events to raise money for breast cancer prevention and research into environmental causes. Since 1995, it has organized eight mountain expeditions, called Climb Against the Odds, as "collective effort[s] to prevent breast cancer and a personal challenge to beat the disease." Climbing groups have consisted of "breast cancer survivors, supporters and others impacted by the disease." Each climber must raise a minimum of five thousand dollars for research into environmental causes of breast cancer. The expeditions have taken place on Argentina's Mount Aconcagua (1995), Alaska's Mount McKinley (1998), Japan's Mount Fuji (2000), Washington's Mount Rainer (2005), and California's Mount Shasta (2003, 2004, 2006, and 2007). Corporate sponsors of these climbs have included Clif Bar, ISIS, Mountain Hardware, Western Athletic Clubs, and Salomon Sports.[20]

Such corporate-sponsored environmental breast cancer efforts extend beyond public fund-raising events. They also include cause marketing campaigns that support the types of organizations that Barbara Ehrenreich lauds. In October 2002, for instance, *Utne Reader*, a left-leaning monthly magazine focusing on arts, culture, and politics, donated half its new subscription profits to the Breast Cancer Fund.[21] Likewise, the Berkeley-based company Clif Bar donated sales profits from its LUNA bar—an all-natural energy snack marketed to women—to the Breast Cancer Fund's environmental health program in 2003. Since then, the company has identified the organization as the recipient one of several social causes it supports. The company not only raises awareness about the Breast Cancer Fund's environmental breast cancer efforts on the former's product wrappers and Web site, but also sponsors an array of the organization's activities.[22]

Last but not least, some environmental breast cancer groups raise money through online stores. The Breast Cancer Fund sells breast cancer–themed jewelry, clothing, CDs, books, videos, and gifts. The organization's products do not embody the depoliticized "pink kitsch" associated with the marketing practices of mainstream groups. Rather, they promote the feminist values and the preventative efforts that critics of mainstream breast cancer culture espouse. On the Breast Cancer Fund's Web site, one can purchase the documentary *Rachel's*

Daughters: Searching for the Causes of Breast Cancer and *Art.Rage.US: Art and Writing by Women with Breast Cancer*, the latter published by Chronicle Books in 1998. This "powerful juried collection of paintings, drawings, sculpture, poetry, essays, and journals provides a compelling account of the experience of breast cancer and the healing power of art." The art and writings in the book also provide alternatives to the representations of heteronormative white women's bodies and subjectivities that dominate mainstream breast cancer culture. Also on sale are T-shirts that bring attention to environmental health concerns. One top designed for women bears the statement "WARNING: This area contains chemicals known to cause cancer," emblazoned in orange and black across the chest.[23]

The Pink Ribbon

In the past fifteen years, the pink ribbon has become the dominant symbol of the breast cancer movement and breast cancer culture more generally. The use of ribbons during the Iran hostage crisis in 1979 and the AIDS activist movement in the early 1990s led Susan G. Komen for the Cure to devise the pink ribbon, which made its first public appearance at the 1991 New York City's Race for the Cure. Every participant received a ribbon. This massive distribution of pink ribbons at a well-known and highly attended event set the stage for the corporate cooptation that began in 1992, when Alexandra Penney of *Self* magazine collaborated with the Estée Lauder company for that year's National Breast Cancer Awareness Month.[24] Although some businesses have used other symbols to promote breast cancer awareness (such as the blue bull's eye developed by the international fashion industry), the vast majority rely on the pink ribbon. The public at large has embraced the symbol, with many concerned citizens attaching them to lapels, backpacks, cars, and other personal belongings.

To its critics, the pink ribbon symbolizes all that is wrong with mainstream breast cancer culture. Some believe that the pink color—a pastel pink at that—reeks of the femininization and infantilization that belittle women and lead to political complacency.[25] They note that the ribbon is a commodity in its own right, with companies such as Avon selling pink ribbon pens, mugs, and key chains not only to raise money for the breast cancer cause but also to garner profits for themselves.[26] Critics also complain that many businesses and mainstream breast cancer organizations evoke the pink ribbon to promote advocacy focusing on early detection and treatment rather than activism pushing for disease prevention, especially with regard to potential environmental causes.

Environmental breast cancer activists respond to this issue by publicly challenging what they call "pinkwashing." This concept draws on the earlier notion of "greenwashing," a term coined by critics of corporations that constructed themselves as environmentally friendly as a means to bolster their public image at a time of growing public concern about environmental issues. By the same logic, *pinkwashing* refers to the ways in which businesses seek to attract customers by presenting themselves as caring about women's health and wanting to improve it through breast cancer advocacy at a time of rising public concern about breast cancer.[27]

Corporate pinkwashing consists of sponsoring breast cancer fund-raising events such as Komen's Race for the Cure and developing cause-marketing campaigns such as Eureka's Clean for the Cure. It also entails providing breast cancer–related products and information to customers either for free or for a cost. Eureka, for instance, included a postcard in each of its Clean for the Cure Whirlwind LiteSpeed vacuums that explained how to conduct breast self-exams. Given that housework such as vacuuming has historically been construed as women's work, Eureka's decision to design a card geared toward women makes sense.[28] As one component of its Ultimate Drive campaign, BMW developed the Pink Ribbon Collection, a line of pins, watches, T-shirts, teddy bears, photo albums, gym bags, and other products—many of which bear the Ultimate Drive Logo. BMW sells these products at its dealerships, at its Ultimate Drive events, and on its Web site, donating between 22 percent and 55 percent of the profits, depending on the item.[29]

As evidenced by Breast Cancer Action's Think Before You Pink campaign, activists dislike corporate pinkwashing because in their view it benefits the businesses more than the breast cancer efforts the companies supposedly support, by increasing their public visibility and, more important, their profit margins. Corporations focus on breast cancer, as opposed to other diseases such as AIDS (which also had a strong social presence in the early 1990s to mid-1990s) because it is a politically safe disease. Breast cancer, unlike AIDS, is not connected to socially stigmatized populations such as gay men and IV drug users.[30] Similarly, breast cancer is relatively safe in comparison to more controversial women's health issues. As Barbara Ehrenreich asks, "Where were [these companies] ... when the Women's Health Movement was fighting for abortion rights and against involuntary sterilization?"[31]

Given the pink ribbon's problematic meanings, some groups have chosen a different symbol to represent their activist work. In 1996, Breast Cancer Action embraced a design created by one of its interns, Catherine Bullock Theuriet (now Catherine Freeman), that it believes reflects women's collective spirit and power in a way that the pink ribbon does not. Barbara Brenner, the organization's president, explained, "The symbol is an artistic interpretation of a coil

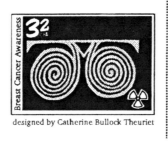

designed by Catherine Bullock Theuriet

Figure 5.2   Breast Cancer Action's alternative to the 1996 United States Postal Service breast cancer postage stamp. Courtesy of Breast Cancer Action (San Francisco) and Catherine Bullock Freeman.

that symbolized the full moon to an ancient Maltese matriarchal society. That culture believed that the lunar cycle was a cycle of rejuvenation, and its women warriors carried the symbol of the moon on breast plates that they wore into battle. I wear that symbol now—embossed in gold color on a deep purple background—as part of the battle I wage everyday against breast cancer. So I don't wear pink ribbons. . . . I don't have time for empty symbols."[32]

Breast Cancer Action put its symbol on its prayer flag pins, sold to the public for five dollars each. The organization also placed the symbol on its alternative to the U.S. Postal Service's original Breast Cancer Awareness stamp, adding in a corner of the stamp a three-sided toxic hazards sign, to link breast cancer to environmental contamination. The stamp, issued in 1996 in conjunction with the Washington, D.C., leg of the Susan G. Komen Race for the Cure, depicts a young, attractive white woman's naked back, with a pink ribbon in the lower right-hand corner and the words "Breast Cancer Awareness" running up the left edge. "I guess it would be too radical to portray an actual women's breast on a postage stamp, and certainly stamps glorifying empty symbols is nothing new," said Brennan, "but I find this stamp particularly offensive in the way it combines a clichéd image of an unclothed woman with the pink ribbon symbol that does nothing to bring attention to what is really needed to end the breast cancer epidemic."[33]

Another strategy organizations take to distance themselves from the pink ribbon is to associate themselves with alternative colors. Zero Breast Cancer, for example, uses the color green in order to emphasize the organization's focus on environmental issues.[34] The Massachusetts Breast Cancer Coalition (MBCC) takes a similar approach. When the organization first opened in the early 1990s, it chose pink and black as its official colors. In 2003, however, it decided to dissociate itself from the colors because of the pink ribbon's increasing exploitation by health organizations, corporations, and other institutions for their own economic gain. MBCC wanted to make its growing focus on environmental issues more explicit. To these ends, MBCC chose green and blue for its new colors. Green is the traditional color of the environmental movement, while blue evokes the sky and water, both of which are polluted spaces of concern to breast cancer and other environmental health activists. Moreover, blue evokes the coastal area of Cape Cod, a region that has inspired as well as served as a political and scientific focus of MBCC's environmental efforts over the years.[35]

Not all environmental breast cancer groups, however, reject the pink ribbon. Some "radicalize" it, as Zillah Eisenstein puts it, by transforming it into a symbol of feminist and environmental breast cancer activism.[36] Long Island's Babylon Breast Cancer Coalition (BBCC) uses the symbol in this way. As shown by its participation in the Follow the Money campaign, the group understands the problems associated with mainstream breast cancer culture, including the pink ribbon commercialization and advocacy that is part of it. Still, the organization continues to use the ribbon as a logo on its Web site and in its newsletters and other campaign materials. Debbie Basile, who has served as BBCC's president since its founding in 1993, explains that the organization has gone beyond its initial focus on breast cancer to emphasize environmental health issues more generally. In this regard, the pink ribbon signifies the organization's breast cancer origins. Moreover, BBCC runs various outreach services geared primarily toward women with breast cancer and their families. Thus, Basile believes that the organization's use of the pink ribbon serves as a "great visual"—that is, a highly recognizable symbol—to raise public awareness about the availability of these services.[37] BBCC's Lend a Helping Hand program provides women with breast cancer (and other gynecological cancers) free housecleaning services, helps them purchase prostheses, and arranges transportation for medical appointments, among other services.[38] Its SOS program provides financial assistance to the families of women who died of the disease to help them pay for funeral costs, housecleaning services, child care, and mental health counseling.[39]

Although MBCC had valid reasons for discontinuing its reliance on pink, its previous use of this color also challenged and complicated the pink ribbon's hegemonic representations in significant ways. Consider the organization's September 2001 newsletter. The pastel pink column that ran up and down the left hand side of the front page proclaimed the organization's mission statement: "Through activism, advocacy and education, our goal is the cure, prevention, and ultimate eradication of breast cancer." It also contained the newsletter's table of contents, which listed articles about a recent Against the Tide event, a research update on environmental links to breast cancer, and Prevention First's efforts to challenge AstraZeneca's marketing practices for tamoxifen. The pastel pink box on the back page listed the dates of upcoming events, among them future Against the Tide fund-raisers, a stage production about Rachel Carson's life called *A Sense of Wonder*, and a public forum on the precautionary principle sponsored by the Massachusetts Precautionary Principle Project.[40] Moreover, the black that accompanied the pink reminded people that breast cancer is not something to celebrate. MBCC's use of black resonates with Breast Cancer Action Ottawa's current logo, a pink ribbon turned upside down to represent "the tears shed at diagnosis" and "lined with black to remember women who have died" from the disease.[41]

The Identity Politics of Breast Cancer "Survivors"

Another contested issue among feminist activists is the breast cancer "survivor" identity. The term *survivor*, prevalent in many activist and public discourses about breast cancer, refers to women who experienced breast cancer, and presumably, overcame the disease. The term manifests itself socially and materially. In June 2001, I participated in the Washington, D.C., leg of Susan G. Komen Race for the Cure. Several weeks before my race, I filled out the application for the event. Besides requesting my name, age, gender, and other personal information, the application required me to check off whether I was a breast cancer survivor (I checked no). At the time, I assumed that Komen wanted this information solely for statistical purposes. On race day, however, I realized that the organization collected the information to determine which colored T-shirt to give to event participants; women with a history of breast cancer received pink T-shirt, while everyone else received a white one. Standing among a sea of pink at the race's starting line helped me experience firsthand the extent of the breast cancer problem.

Despite the term's popularity, some environmental breast cancer activists and social critics dislike it. They believe that it perpetuates the cheerful perkiness of mainstream breast cancer culture and leads to political complacency among women afflicted by the disease. The survivor culture of Komen's Race for the Cure reinforces this point: it equates living with breast cancer with running the race. If you just run hard enough and grit your teeth through the pain, you can finish the race; you can survive it—just as you can survive breast cancer or at least keep yourself alive long enough until a cure is found. In this context, being a breast cancer survivor is all about possessing enough individual strength, courage, and determination to get through the ordeal. It is also about remaining hopeful that a cure—which works on an individual, not collective, level—will be found. Although many women with breast cancer run the race together and cheer one another on, this collective support empowers women to continue running their individual races and to continue fighting their individual diseases. It does not encourage them to band together and change the social, political, and economic conditions that have caused their diseases in the first place. The fact that the event is a race, which by its very nature has individual winners and losers, further perpetuates this social Darwinian rhetoric. As with breast cancer, some will make it, some will not.

For those who reject the survivor identity, this individualizing rhetoric disrespects the dead and dying, especially by erasing the social, political, and economic factors such as access to effective early detection and treatment that make it easier for some people to "survive" breast cancer than others. Barbara Ehrenreich asks, "Did we who live 'fight' harder than those who've died? Can we claim to be 'braver,' better, people than the dead? And why is there no room in this cult for some gracious acceptance of death, when the time comes, which it surely will, through cancer or some other misfortune?"[42] Feminist cancer activist Sandra Steingraber feels that the term "divides [women with cancer] in half and at the same time denies the uncertainty of our prognosis."[43] Similarly, Barbara Brennan chooses not to refer to herself as a survivor because "the term suggests to the world—wrongly—that breast cancer is curable . . . the term survivor also carried a notion that I am not dead of breast cancer because I am somehow better or different from the hundreds of thousands of women who have died of the disease."[44]

For all these reasons, some activists have chosen alternative terms. In the early 1990s, Cambridge's Women's Community Cancer Project replaced the term *survivor* with the phrase "women with cancer and cancer histories."[45] Around the same time, Judy Brady espoused the term *victim*, noting that women with cancer are "victims of a social crime, the crime of poisoning our environment."[46] A decade later, Ehrenreich also used the word, in reference to herself. When discussing the problems with mainstream breast cancer culture at Breast Cancer Action's 2002 town meeting, she asked, "Is there any other disease that has been so warmly embraced by its victims? (And yes, I use the word 'victim'—that's another part of the perkiness—the failure to acknowledge that some of us are in fact victims of a hideous disease)."[47] Currently, Breast Cancer Action employs the phrase "women living with breast cancer" in its materials.[48] Still, Brenner grapples with this term. On the one hand, she likes it because it "tells others that it is possible to live with the disease, while acknowledging implicitly that not all of us are so lucky. It also communicates in a small way that the diagnosis is a life-transforming event." On the other hand, she finds the phrase problematic because "it suggests . . . that the person referred to is currently in treatment or in need of treatment. And, because of the common use of the term 'living with AIDS,' it implies that women with breast cancer will die of the disease, unless something else kills them first."[49]

Other activists do not reject the term *survivor*, instead constructing it in ways that resonate with their feminist and environmental health agendas. The Breast Cancer Fund uses the term "breast cancer survivor" to describe some of the participants in its Climb Against the Odds series. In these mountain treks, breast cancer survivors are women whose fight against breast cancer is equated with climbing a mountain. Some may make it, others may not. Unlike Komen's Race for the Cure, the climb is not just about mobilizing one's physical, technical, and mental strengths; it is also about successfully negotiating the mountain's steep, rocky, snowy, cold, and sometimes unpredictable environment. Moreover, the Climb Against the Odds treks are not races with winner and losers; they are physical, emotional, and spiritual challenges that women take on both individually and collectively. Although individual strength and courage are necessary for women to finish the climbs, reaching the peak of a mountain is truly a team effort. Women help one another up steep inclines, share responsibilities for food and tent preparation, and take turns carrying equipment. In contrast to the Race for Cure—in which it is possible for some individual women to finish with no outside assistance—it is only through collective efforts that individual women can complete these mountain climbs. Thus, individual survival and group survival are intertwined.

When viewed from this perspective, breast cancer survivors are women who have overcome not only their individual diseases but also the harsh environment that may have caused their breast cancers to occur in the first place. To survive their environment, then, women can choose strategies other than finding a cure for their disease; they can also work to clean up their environment so that it no longer poses a threat to their health. It makes sense, then, that the climbing series raises money for the Breast Cancer Fund's efforts to promote research on potential environmental causes of breast cancer and disease prevention policies. Further, women with breast cancer cannot take on their environment alone if they want to succeed at these efforts; although individuals can make a difference, comprehensive social and structural change requires people to work together over the long haul. More broadly, the collective approach embodied by the Climb Against the Odds challenges popular representations of environmental health activism. Although representations of such activism in popular culture often depict determined, strong-willed individuals who fight lone battles against the polluters (such as Jan Schlichtmann, the lawyer depicted by John Travolta in the 1998 movie *A Civil Action*, who tirelessly pursued legal action against polluters in Woburn, Massachusetts), in reality these efforts require the work and cooperation of many other individuals, such as lawyers, activists, community members, scientists, public health officials, government representatives, and journalists.

In offering examples that complicate the division between mainstream and feminist breast cancer cultures, I am not suggesting that such distinctions are meaningless. Rather, my counterexamples demonstrate how political values, practices, and symbols do not necessarily have inherent meanings, feminist or not. Instead, such values, practices, and symbols generate meaning from the social, material, and discursive contexts in which they are used by activists and others. Thus, they carry different meanings depending on how breast cancer activists assemble them in relation to their political objectives. In some circumstances, corporate advocacy can perpetuate a culture of action that detracts attention from environmental causes of breast cancer. In other circumstances, corporate advocacy can foster such attention. Although survivor rhetoric can place the burden of health on individual women, it can also place responsibility on the social institutions and policies that expose women to harmful environmental toxicants. The pink ribbon may symbolize political and environmental complacency in some contexts, but in others it symbolizes political and environmental radicalism.

My counterexamples also highlight some of the differences that exist within the feminist environmental breast cancer movement. It is true that many feminist groups share the same goal, to prevent breast cancer, especially by addressing environmental causes of the disease, and often work together to help achieve this goal (an in the Breast Cancer Fund's campaign to increase federal research on environmental causes of breast cancer). At the same time, activists have their differences. Some are practical; for example, the Breast Cancer Fund tends to spearhead state and national legislative efforts, whereas WomenCARE in Santa Cruz tends to conduct local outreach. Others are discursive and ideological, as with the pink ribbon and survivor rhetoric. In either case, such differences demonstrate that activists can assemble the feminist politics of environmental breast cancer issues in multiple ways. Moreover, such differences demonstrate that the boundary between the so-called feminist and mainstream breast cancer cultures is not as well defined as some critics suggest. This blurring is particularly evident in the work of Susan G. Komen for the Cure.

The Multiple Facets of Komen

In many respects, Susan G. Komen for the Cure epitomizes the mainstream of breast cancer culture. Nancy Brinker established the Texas-based organization—then known as the Susan G. Komen Foundation—in 1982 following the death of her sister, Susan Komen, from breast cancer at the age of thirty-six.[50] By the early 2000s, Komen had become the largest and arguably best-known breast cancer group in the United States. In 2007, the organization celebrated its twenty-five-year anniversary by redefining its focus and changing its name. Although Komen still works to promote education, early detection, and effective treatments, it makes "energiz[ing] science to find the cure" its top priority.[51]

To accomplish its goals, Komen runs a grants and awards program to fund promising biomedical and health research. Since 1982, the group has spent $400 million to fund eleven hundred such projects, most of which focus on basic, clinical, and translational breast cancer research. It also provides financial support for research in the areas of breast cancer education, screening, and treatment.[52] In addition, Komen works on public policy. It educates congressional members about breast cancer issues and encourages them to increase federal funding for breast cancer research, improve mammography equipment standards, and mandate better access to early detection and quality treatment for disadvantaged women. To complement this policy work, the organization established the Komen Champions for a Cure program in 2006, which allows citizens to join forces with their local Komen affiliate to talk with their state and federal representatives about breast cancer issues, especially the importance of finding a cure for the disease.[53]

Along with its research and policy activities, Komen educates the public about breast cancer issues such as early detection, health care options for those with the disease, and ways to support efforts to find a cure. The organization conducts much of this outreach through its 125 affiliates, which work in local communities across the nation and in several foreign countries. It also conducts outreach through public awareness campaigns and fund-raising events. The Race for the Cure series is one of Komen's most popular events. The first race took place in Dallas in 1983. Over the following two decades, the Race for the Cure grew into the largest five-kilometer running/walking series in the world, with more than one hundred events held across the United States, Italy, and Germany each year. Since 2005, more than a million people have participated in the series.[54] In addition to running, walking, or simply watching the event, participants add to their knowledge of breast cancer by meeting other racers affected by the disease; listening to keynote speakers; perusing the information booths set up by Komen and liked-minded health organizations, pharmaceutical companies, and businesses; and reading the free literature provided to racers and their supporters by these institutions. Passionately Pink for the Cure is another Komen awareness campaign. Founded in 2006, the program asks individuals to wear pink during the month of October and encourage their friends, family members, and colleagues to show their support by also wearing pink, as well as by contributing money to the organization's breast cancer programs.[55]

In keeping with this pink theme, Komen further encourages individuals to raise awareness by purchasing the pink-ribbon-themed products (coffee mugs, necklaces, holiday ornaments, socks, shoelaces, and T-shirts) that it sells in its online Promise Shop. In April 2008, Komen offered fifty-six such items for sale.[56] The group relies on celebrity spokespeople to bring attention to breast cancer issues and the work that the organization does to address them and to encourage participation in Komen's fund-raising campaigns and events. Charlie Sheen, for instance, encouraged the public to participate in the ninth annual Lee Jeans for Lee National Denim Day, held on October 8, 2004, which Komen touted as the "world's largest single day fund-raiser for breast cancer." For the event, employees at more than twenty-five thousand companies wore denim to work and donated five dollars each to the organization.[57] The following year, *Desperate Housewives* stars James Denton and Richard Chavira served as spokespeople for the event.[58]

In fiscal year 2005–2006, Komen amassed a $268 million budget for its activities. While the organization generated almost $15 million of this budget through "other public support and revenue," it garnered almost $120 million from the Race for Cure series. It is contributions, however, that represent the largest portion of Komen's budget, at $133 million.[59] Although individuals donated a significant portion of this sum, the bulk of it came from businesses and corporations. As of 2007, Komen had identified fifty-one donor businesses and corporations as "corporate partners," meaning that they raise money for the foundation's research efforts through cause-marketing campaigns. The organization's corporate partners include Boston Market, Dell, LPGA, the Kellogg Company, and Einstein Bros.[60] Komen counts twenty-two of these corporate partners as members of its Million Dollar Council. Each of these selected businesses—among them BMW of North America, Yoplait USA, and American Airlines—has raised more than a million dollars for Komen's research efforts and found "new and innovative ways to spread two important messages: early detection saves lives and only though research can we find a cure."[61]

Despite the ways in which Susan G. Komen for the Cure embodies mainstream breast cancer culture, the organization has taken up numerous efforts since the late 1990s to address the environmental breast cancer problem. In particular, the national organization participated in the Breast Cancer Fund's 1999 campaign to increase federal research on environmental causes of breast cancer. In this campaign, Komen did not merely sign on to the group letter; along with the Breast Cancer Fund and NOW, it was a member of the campaign's founding coalition. More recently, Komen supported the Breast Cancer and Environmental Research Act, which led to the establishment of four national research centers devoted to the study of childhood environmental risk factors that predispose women to the disease. The organization also funded the Silent Spring Institute's Breast Cancer and Environment: Science Reviews project. Indeed, the organization states on its Web site that it "supports the establishment of grant programs to expand biomedical, epidemiological, and behavioral research related to the etiology of breast cancer and the role of the environment" and "ask[s] Congress to devote the necessary resources to fund meaningful research on the potential links between the environment and breast cancer."[62]

Komen's regional affiliates have ties to environmental breast cancer activism as well. Consider the organization's North Jersey affiliate, about which I first learned while working at the World Resources Institute with Devra Davis. Given my prior assumptions about Komen, I was surprised when Davis told me that she had been working closely with the affiliate for the past year on environmental breast cancer issues. Indeed, the organization provided several small grants for Davis's public outreach work. The affiliate also hosted "Exposure: Environmental Links to Breast Cancer," a conference on environmental causes of breast cancer held in October 1999 at Temple B'nai Jeshurun in Livingston, New Jersey. Steven Adubato, an Emmy Award–winning Public Broadcasting Service anchor, moderated the panel discussion. Other participants included Deborah Axelrod, chief of the Comprehensive Breast Cancer Center of the St. Vincent's Comprehensive Cancer Center in New York City; Michael Gallo, director of the National Institute of Environmental Health Sciences Center of Excellence at Robert Wood Johnson Medical School and associate director of Cancer Prevention, Control and Population Sciences at the Cancer Institute of New Jersey; Cheryl Osimo, a co-founder of the Silent Spring Institute and coordinator of its Cape Cod environmental breast cancer study; Annie J. Sasco, a researcher at the International Agency for Research on Cancer and Institut National de la Santé et la Recherche Médicale in Lyon, France; and Shawna C. Willey, chief of breast surgery at the George Washington University Medical Center in Washington, D.C. Barbara Waters, the affiliate's outreach coordinator, also traveled to Washington, D.C., on various occasions to discuss her organization's possible involvement in several environmental breast cancer projects that Davis wanted to develop.

I had the opportunity to work with Waters at other public events. In January 2001, Rutgers University invited me to give a talk about environmental causes of breast cancer following a screening of the 1997 documentary *Rachel's Daughters: Searching for the Causes of Breast Cancer*. Given Rutgers's geographic proximity to Komen's North Jersey affiliate, I encouraged the university's student event coordinator to ask Waters whether the organization would co-sponsor the event. The student called, and Waters agreed. Several months after the Rutgers event, Waters asked me to participate in a panel discussion on environmental causes of breast cancer that she co-organized at nearby Drew University. As with the Rutgers event, a panel discussion followed a public screening of *Rachel's Daughters*. The panel's other two speakers were Deborah Axelrod and Lisa Rodriquez, a twenty-nine-year-old woman with breast cancer who worked at Komen on issues pertaining to young women with the disease.[63]

Lately, Komen's North Jersey affiliate has been working on other environmental projects. In 2007, it developed *Reduce Your Risk*, a twelve-page booklet outlining ten steps women can take to reduce their risk of breast cancer. Lisa Rubin of the North Jersey affiliate wrote the booklet, and Devra Davis and Deborah Axelrod edited it. The booklet encourages women to buy local produce, which is less likely to be treated with pesticides and other preservatives, and to avoid cleaning products, personal care items, and home goods that contain phthalates, parabens, and other xenoestrogens. It also encourages women to avoid certain types of plastics and eliminate the use of outdoor pesticides. The booklet presents alternatives to toxic products and practices, such as natural cleaning recipes and alternative strategies for reducing garden pests. Finally, it lists various organizations to which women can turn for further information, among them the Environmental Working Group, Silent Spring Institute, and the Green Guide.[64]

To be sure, Komen's forays into environmental breast cancer activism account for only a small part of the organization's activities. Even so, recognizing their presence within the group's broader mainstream framework is important, as they help to highlight Komen's multidimensional existence. Although the many dimensions of Komen function as integral parts of the organization's overarching social, discursive, material, and institutional infrastructure, they also possess their own individual identities and ways of being. First, Komen is not a monolithic organization. Rather, it consists of many branches, with each focusing on a particular area of breast cancer activism—scientific and biomedical research, policy, outreach and education, fund-raising, and public relations, among others.

Second, Komen is a multi-sited institution, with offices in not only this country but also abroad. With national headquarters in Dallas, Texas, it has 125 affiliates, found in every state except Alaska and North Dakota, as well as in Puerto Rico, Germany, and Italy. Although the affiliates are overseen by headquarters, they also have a degree of geographic, material, and social autonomy. Each has its own staff, board members, funding sources, goals, practices, and organizational culture. Each has roots in the local community, which influences how it defines its mission and approaches its work.

Third, Komen constitutes what anthropologist James Clifford calls a "regional/national/global nexus" of breast cancer activism.[65] That is, Komen conducts its work at the community, state, national, and international levels. The organization initially took a community-based approach. Over the following two decades, it expanded its focus to include state and national issues as well. In the early 2000s, the organization began to reposition itself from a national organization to an international one. It funded more than $14.8 million in breast cancer research taking place outside of the United States and more than $5.5 million in overseas community education and early detection efforts. Another international project that the organization runs is the Susan G. Komen for the Cure Global Initiative. Founded in 2007, this program "aims to create a dynamic global network of dedicated activists with the skills, knowledge and vision to play a strategic role in shaping their country's response to the breast cancer crisis."[66]

Finally, Komen's existence has multiple temporal dimensions as well as spatial ones. Although it retains a general level of organizational stability, Komen's identity, infrastructure, and everyday practices are constantly in flux: staff members come and go, board members change, and volunteers help out on some projects but not others. Additionally, Komen revamps its policies and campaigns on a regular basis, gains funding sources at the same time that it loses older ones, and provides grant money to a new set of research projects each year.

In the end, we cannot fully understand how each particular facet of Komen functions within—and perhaps apart from—the broader organization without also considering the local webs of people, places, institutions, policies, practices, communities, and cultures in which it is embedded.[67] It is not surprising that the North Jersey Komen affiliate is environmentally active; it is located near Long Island, one of the nation's epicenters of environmental breast cancer activism and community-based environmental breast cancer research. The North Jersey area is also home to its own share of toxic sites. Additionally, Deborah Axelrod's involvement in the organization—first as a member of its board of trustees and then as a member of its Medical Advisory Board—has shaped its environmental efforts. Axelrod devotes some of her professional work to the environmental breast cancer problem, including co-writing several articles with Devra Davis on the subject. Moreover, her relationship with Davis led the latter to become involved with the North Jersey organization. Furthermore, Barbara Water's personal initiative has driven much of the North Jersey Affiliate's environmental focus. Soon after her breast cancer diagnosis at age forty-six, she began working at the organization. She believed that environmental factors contribute to breast cancer—it's "common sense" she told me—even before she began her environmental work at the organization.[68]

Komen is not the only mainstream cancer organization to have multiple existences in regards to environmental issues. So, too, does the American Cancer Society (ACS). Although the institution as a whole, led by its national headquarters, tends to dismiss environmental theories of breast cancer causation, facets of it have acknowledged their possible validity. For example, Breast Cancer Action met with the California division in 1993 to encourage it to give more attention to possible environmental causes of breast cancer and other cancers. This meeting led the San Francisco ACS chapter to organize—with the cooperation of Breast Cancer Action and other local groups—a November 2004 program examining the possible role of agricultural chemicals, exercise, and nutrition in the development of breast cancer. Although Nancy Evans, Breast Cancer Action's president at the time, criticized ACS national headquarters for dismissing environmental factors, she called this regional conference a "baby step forward" for the cancer organization.[69] In 2007, *Cancer,* the ACS's scientific journal, published the review articles that the Silent Spring Institute wrote as part of its Breast Cancer and Environment: Science Reviews database project.[70]

Viewing Komen and other mainstream organizations through the lens of their multiple existences allows us to understand the complex and sometimes contradictory relationships that they have formed with different environmental breast cancer groups. This perspective helps to explain, for instance, how Breast Cancer Action teamed with Komen's national headquarters for the Breast Cancer Fund's 1999 environmental health research campaign but protested Komen's San Francisco affiliate a year later by chanting, "You can run for the cure but you can't run from the cause" at the San Francisco Race for the Cure.[71] It offers insight into a similar set of dynamics between Komen and the Massachusetts Breast Cancer Coalition. On the one hand, Komen's Boston affiliate donated money from its Race for the Cure funds to help pay for the production of the coalition's May 2001 "Beyond the Headlines," a paper that discussed the formation of Prevention First and its campaign to challenge the FDA's regulation of direct-to-consumer ads, particularly those created by AstraZeneca to market tamoxifen to healthy women. The focus on AstraZeneca's ads was part of Prevention First's broader campaign against the prescribing of tamoxifen to such women and the National Cancer Institute's "chemoprevention research" more generally.[72] On the other hand, Komen's national organization supported this research and the use of tamoxifen in healthy women.[73]

Examining Komen's environmental efforts complicates what counts as environmental breast cancer activism and its long-standing feminist culture. After all, the fact that Komen's North Jersey affiliate helped to organize—among other things—the environmental breast cancer events at Rutgers and Drew universities does not mean that it completely lost its mainstream identity. On the contrary, the written materials that lined the tables at these events focused on early detection and treatment issues, the free Komen pens were pastel pink, and the Komen film that Barbara Waters showed at the start of each event left the audience feeling hopeful that a cure was just around the corner. Waters brought enough pink ribbons for everyone who wanted one. Yet the seeming disjuncture between Komen's being situated in the mainstream and the environmental breast cancer activism that it espouses may signify not so much an ideological contradiction as an alternative way to assemble the social and cultural terrain of this body of activism. Moreover, the social and political significance of Komen's particular type of environmental breast cancer activism should not be overlooked, as it may appeal to some facets of the public in ways that more radical types of feminist activism may not.

Women Living Their Environmental Health Politics

When I registered for the 2001 Washington, D.C., Race for the Cure, I sought to glean from the experience ethnographic insight into its cultural politics. I wanted to observe how many people attended this race, who walked it, and who ran it. I wanted to understand the ways in which the breast cancer problem was depicted on the T-shirts that people wore, the signs that people carried, and the materials that one could pick up from the organizations and businesses that ran booths near the race's finish line. In sum, I wanted to learn more about the event's culture of action. Given my prior knowledge of Komen and its Race for the Cure series, I entered the event expecting to be saturated by mainstream breast cancer culture. In many ways, I was not surprised by what I saw: lots of pink this and that; white people; survivor rhetoric; and written materials addressing early detection, treatments, and research on a cure. I did not hear a single statement about prevention or environmental links to breast cancer, nor did any of the written materials I gathered mention these subjects. Washington, D.C.–based feminist women's health groups such as NOW, National Women's Health Network, and the Mautner Foundation for Lesbians with Cancer did not attend the event, as far as I could tell.

What I did not anticipate was the emotional reaction that I had halfway through the race. Going into the event, I had taken for granted the criticisms of the race—it is not feminist enough, not political enough, and therefore not good enough. As I looked around at the people jogging in place and stretching before the gun went off, I wondered what they really thought of Komen and whether they knew about the organization's general lack of attention to environmental health issues and prevention. As I began walking the course and then, several minutes later, running it, my perspective on the race started to change.

Despite my initial criticisms of Komen's Race for the Cure, I wound up feeling moved by the event: so many women with breast cancer histories banding together and cheering each other on, so many people wearing T-shirts with pictures of their mothers, wives, partners, and daughters who had died of breast cancer. At times, I was close to tears, not only because I was reminded of the impact—both negative and positive—that breast cancer has had on people's lives, but also because the collective spirit and energy generated by the racers and their supporters on the sidelines motivated me to run the entire five kilometers. Before the race, I did not think that this would be possible, because a series of prior athletic injuries had left me unable to run for more than five minutes without pain. Running the race gave me a firsthand appreciation for the event's ability to inspire and empower women—an appreciation that I would not have experienced had I based my analysis solely on Komen's promotional materials and other people's written accounts of the event.

I know that critics of mainstream breast cancer culture would probably tell me that my emotional response was exactly what Komen and its corporate sponsors wanted—a reaction that kept me focused on my positive feelings rather than on the fact that Komen's races do nothing to address breast cancer's possible environmental links. To be sure, I do not completely disagree with this perspective. I do, however, find it limiting. Perhaps the event did not empower affected women to track down their local water polluters, but maybe it motivated them to get through another round of chemotherapy. Perhaps it did not lead affected family members to join Breast Cancer Action or stop buying breast cancer stamps, but maybe it made them feel more connected to the mothers, daughters, and sisters whom they had lost to the disease. If the event provided affected women with crucial psychological, spiritual, or even physical healing that they would not have received otherwise; if it made them feel more confident about their athletic potential and their ability to take on physical challenges; if it made them feel more connected to and supported by other women with breast cancer who ran the race, then who am I to say that their experience at this event was not feminist enough?

I am not the only feminist to hold mixed feelings about the critiques of mainstream breast cancer culture. Describing her experiences with her own and her sister's breast cancer, Zillah Eisenstein writes, "I wear the [pink ribbon] pin to connect my individual self to a larger collectivity of women living with breast cancer. I like the fact that wearing the pin does not mean that I, personally, have breast cancer. My cancer is not just about my own body but involves women as a group more broadly. This collective identity that I wear publicly is more than simply personal." At the same time, Eisenstein recognizes how this symbol is used to boost corporate profits and support breast cancer action paradigms that she finds problematic. "Once again," Eisenstein observes, "there is no simple inside and outside in this instance."[74] Similarly, Jennifer Keck, a Canadian woman living with breast cancer who concurs with negative critiques of the cancer industry and the commercialization of breast cancer, explains how her experiences in a breast cancer support group led her to question blanket criticism of mainstream breast cancer culture: "Sometime I look around the room and try to imagine how we would have come together without the curious tie of a disease. We certainly do not all share a common political worldview. But the women who call with messages of support, who are there when my world is collapsing and who want to help other women get through the worst part of the disease form an important part of my life. These women are my sisters."[75]

The fact that I could see some good in Komen's Race for the Cure but still recognize its political downsides makes me wonder whether the women who like aspects of mainstream breast cancer culture—that is, women who may like the cheery pink teddy bears and T-shirts, who may want to learn makeup techniques that can hide the damaging effects of chemotherapy, and who may feel more comfortable participating in Komen's Race for the Cure than in Breast Cancer Action's protest of it—might also support breast cancer prevention and increased attention to environmental factors. After all, personal worldviews are often multifaceted and sometimes contradictory; they do not always fit into the clear ideological categories constructed by media, cultural, and other public narratives.[76]

The complex relationship between the feminist breast cancer culture and its mainstream counterpart was in evidence at a talk about environmental breast cancer activism that I gave to members of a local New Jersey chapter of the Daughters of the American Revolution (DAR) at their monthly luncheon in May 2002. Although I do not know these women's opinion of feminism, I do know that their organization was built on a notion of "sisterhood" that promotes the patriotic values of their American forefathers more than the political values of their second-wave feminist foremothers. At one meeting the previous year, for instance, the guest speaker discussed the history of the American Revolution and afterward had members stand up and sing patriotic songs. My mother, a DAR member, who had invited me to speak to the group, told me that when she had raised the subject of my talk to the organization's board several months beforehand, one of its members expressed a worry that it would be "too negative and depressing."

I found the luncheon's setting quite appropriate—in an ironic sort of way—given the topic of my talk. The restaurant where I gave my talk was in a converted row house in an older working-class neighborhood of a postindustrial town near Trenton. Across the street from the restaurant was a large deteriorating industrial lot, which, according to the sign attached to the six-foot-high chain-link fence surrounding the property, happened to be an EPA Superfund site. That said, the scene in the restaurant's dining room did little to challenge the culture of conservatism that is associated with the organization. The twenty or so women who attended were white, and most were middle-aged or older. Some wore American flag pins or other red, white, and blue paraphernalia on their shirts and jackets. Even the gift package from DAR that each woman, including myself, received for attending this meeting reflected traditional gender values: it contained a small box holding several spools of thread, needles, and a black comb.

Given my initial reading of this group of women, I was unsure what they would think of my presentation, in which I gave an overview of environmental breast cancer activism and its links to the broader breast cancer and women's health movements, explained endocrine disrupters and other suspected environmental causes, and described strategies the women could take to reduce their risks. As I glanced around the room during my talk, it seemed that some of the women were nodding off. When I asked whether any of them had questions, however, it was apparent that most had paid attention. One woman asked me to give more details about pesticides and the benefits of organic food. Another wanted to know what I thought about a recent study that found some brands of bottled water to be just as contaminated as tap water. Some wanted me to explain why it was bad to microwave food in plastic containers (the heat causes the xenoestrogens in the plastic to leach into the food). Several women expressed their belief that environmental toxins caused their loved ones' cancers. I also had an in-depth exchange with a woman who worked in the environmental health division of New Jersey's Health and Human Services about the problems with science-based regulation and the need for the precautionary principle, during which other women chimed in to ask us questions about the topic at hand. After the discussion period ended and I was getting ready to leave, a woman who looked about eighty years old and who sported more than a dozen DAR and other patriotic pins on her jacket came over and, in a whisper, proudly told me how she had refused to take hormone replacement therapy even though her doctors had recommended it for years. "I don't like the idea of putting all those hormones in my body," she said. "I went through menopause the natural way, hot flashes and everything."

Certainly, environmental breast cancer activism entails research, policy, and public education campaigns run by bona fide activists. As this account suggests, however, it also involves common actions that all women may take to protect their health and that of their families and communities. The women who take these ordinary actions may not necessarily align themselves with the feminist culture that undergirds much of the environmental breast cancer movement. Instead, they may assemble the issue of environmental causes of breast cancer in ways that resonate with their own beliefs and lived experiences. Further, the multiple ways in which activists and other women incorporate the environmental breast cancer issue into their political work and daily lives is especially evident with regard to the race and class dimensions of the environmental breast cancer movement.

Chapter 6

Toxic Tours Move Indoors

Race, Class, and Breast Cancer Prevention

Around the same time that the Breast Cancer Fund held its press conference on Capitol Hill urging Congress to devote more funds to environmental health research, the U.S. Navy was working to clean up Parcel A—a large tract of land in Hunters Point Shipyard (HPS), an EPA Superfund site. Located next to the Bayview Hunters Point neighborhood in southeast San Francisco, the shipyard was established in 1869 as the Pacific Coast's first commercial dry dock. In 1940, the U.S. Navy bought the 936-acre property for its shipbuilding and repair efforts. After World War II, the navy used the shipyard for submarine service and testing, as well as nuclear weapons research. By 1976, it had ceased its operations and leased the bulk of HPS to Triple A Machine Shop, a privately owned ship repair firm, which subleased select buildings to other businesses. In 1986, Triple A Machine Shop faced allegations of improper waste disposal, which led the navy to shut the industry down, reoccupy the property, and assess the extent of toxic contamination at the site. The investigation found PCBs, solvents, pesticides, petroleum hydrocarbons, metals, and low-level radiation at various locations throughout the shipyard. Researchers attributed the pollution not only to Triple A but also to other businesses that had occupied the site and to the navy's long-term activities there. The federal government declared HPS to be one of the nation's worst Superfund sites and demanded that the navy remove the toxins from the property. In April 1999, the navy finally declared that it had completed the cleanup for Parcel A and that the land was ready for commercial development.[1]

The cleanup of Parcel A marked a significant step toward the cleanup of HPS, as it represented one of the largest sections of the site. That said, some residents received the news with skepticism. It had taken years of fighting to push the navy to complete its work, and the navy seemed to be dragging its feet on other cleanup projects. Then, officials did not alert residents to an August 16, 2000, landfill fire on Parcel E that emitted assorted chemicals and toxic gases into the air—at least not until residents began calling officials about the strange respiratory ailments and skin rashes that they were experiencing.[2] Ultimately, HPS was only one source of toxic pollution in the community. Bayview Hunters Point is home to one of the heaviest concentrations of industry—and consequently, pollution—in San Francisco. Local activists have long believed that the community carries the burden of such industrial problems because its residents are mostly low-income people of color. These activists also suspect that the disproportionately high rates of various diseases within the community result from its heavy toxic load.

One disease of particular concern is breast cancer, which is associated with various toxins found at HPS. Several studies conducted over the past fifteen years have found that breast cancer incidence rates in Bayview Hunters Point (BVHP) are equal to or greater than those in other parts of the region. One of the most notable studies was among the earliest. In 1995, the San Francisco Department of Health released a study finding that between 1988 and 1992 women under the age of fifty in BVHP suffered twice the rate of breast cancer incidence as that of women in the rest of the city. The study also noted that overall incidence rates of breast cancer in this neighborhood almost equaled those in Marin County.[3] Like their Marin counterparts, BVHP residents have mobilized to address possible environmental causes of the disease in the community. Yet the breast cancer problem in BVHP has arguably garnered less public attention and action than has the problem in Marin, and media outlets in the San Francisco Bay Area, throughout the state, and across the nation have covered BVHP's breast cancer problem less frequently than they have the situation in Marin.[4]

In certain respects, the case of environmental breast cancer in BVHP reflects broader dynamics that play out in the environmental breast cancer movement as a whole. Despite the best intentions of many activists, assorted factors have led the movement to orient much of its environmental breast cancer work toward white, middle-class women. Activists' increasing efforts to integrate the needs of socially and economically marginalized women into the environmental breast cancer movement have not only broadened the movement's demographic base, however, but also highlight the ways in which gender, race, and class shape understandings of the environmental breast cancer problem, the strategies for addressing it, and disease prevention efforts more generally.

The Race and Class Dimensions of Environmental Breast Cancer Activism

Breast cancer affects one in seven women, but it does not affect all women in the same way. Significant racial differences and disparities exist with regard to the disease. Health professionals and researchers have identified various factors based on established understandings of and approaches to the disease that may help to explain why white women suffer higher overall incidence rates than women of color. Because of their higher socioeconomic status, white women are more likely than members of other racial groups to have fewer children and to delay childbirth, both of which are breast cancer risk factors.[5] In addition, white women are more likely than their nonwhite counterparts, especially African Americans, to use hormone replacement therapy. African American women's incidence rates did not drop after it was announced that hormone replacement therapy increased breast cancer risk, even as overall rates declined. Lower incidence rates among women of color may also reflect the fact that they receive regular mammography and other forms of screening less frequently than do white women.[6]

At the same time, explanations have been advanced to account for why women of color, especially African American women, die from breast cancer more frequently than white women. Lack of health insurance; lower levels of personal income; and disparities in health care resulting from racism, classism, and language and other cultural barriers contribute to a situation in which women of color receive diagnoses at later stages of the disease. The later a woman's breast cancer is diagnosed, the less likely she is to survive it. The same mitigating factors also leave women of color with less access to quality breast cancer treatment and care. The presence of multiple health conditions may contribute to higher breast cancer mortality rates among women of color, as well.[7]

Another lamentable fact is that African American women, especially younger women, develop a particularly aggressive form of breast cancer more frequently than do women in other racial groups. This "triple negative" cancer grows quickly and is not fueled by estrogen, progesterone, or human epidermal growth factor receptor 2 (HER2) and thus responds less well to hormone and immune therapies than most other types of breast cancer; it also recurs more frequently. For these reasons, it tends to be more deadly than other forms of breast cancer.[8]

For their part, environmental breast cancer activists and allied scientists strive to understand and address the racial dimensions of breast cancer, especially with regard to potential environmental risks and disease prevention.

Women of color face many of the same types of toxic exposures that white women face, but they sometimes encounter particular types of community, workplace, and personal exposures that many white women—especially more affluent ones—may not. Moreover, the disproportionately high, and increasing, rates of breast cancer incidence among young African American women suggest that women of color may face exposures that put them at greater risk for developing the disease than those of white women. Similarly, women of color, especially African Americans, sometimes face particular types of community and workplace exposures that may contribute to their high rates of breast cancer mortality.

The environmental breast cancer movement's attention to issues of race and class goes back to its early roots in women's cancer and environmental justice activism. These early efforts helped to spark the kinds of political work that the movement embraced over the years: supporting industrial and governmental policies to protect the health of disadvantaged communities, partnering with environmental justice activists, raising general awareness about environmental justice issues, and more recently, promoting research initiatives to better understand the environmental risks faced by socially and economically marginalized communities. Still, the movement as a whole has not viewed the environmental breast cancer problem through the lens of race and class, and its default approach to the problem tends to reflect a white and arguably middle-class perspective.

In many ways, this tendency is not unique to the environmental breast cancer movement; mainstream breast cancer culture embodies a similar perspective. Images of white women's bodies tend to prevail on the covers of magazines, in articles about the disease, in public service announcements, and on postage stamps. Most of the famous women who have publicly announced and received extensive media coverage of their breast cancer diagnosis are white women—some notable examples being Happy Rockefeller, Betty Ford, and Sheryl Crowe. Such popular slogans as "Early detection is your best protection" and "Get a mammogram now" assume that the only barrier to early detection facing women is a forgetful mind or a busy schedule, as opposed to inadequate health insurance. The white and middle-class construction of mainstream breast cancer culture is even evident in this culture's consumerist and hyperfeminine mindset. Encouraging women to help fund a cure by purchasing vacuum cleaners, test-driving BMWs, and buying high-end makeup from Avon and Estée Lauder presumes that they possess a high level of financial stability, and the "pink kitsch," as Barbara Ehrenreich call is it, that many breast cancer groups and companies sell reflects a hyperfemininity associated with white, middle-class culture.

It is also the case that most environmental breast cancer activists, like most breast cancer activists in general, are white, middle-class women. Just as such women run many of the nation's largest, most powerful, and best-known mainstream breast cancer organizations, they run many of the most prominent environmental breast cancer groups, and the public health goals and political strategies embraced by both sorts of groups tend to reflect these women's particular needs, values, and perspectives.[9] These circumstances are not surprising. After all, white middle-class women suffer the highest incidence rates in the nation and account for the largest number of deaths from this disease. With regard to environmental breast cancer groups, the most extensive, established, and influential networks of activism emerged in regions with some of the highest breast cancer incidence rates in the country—regions that also happened to be predominantly white and relatively well-off communities in the San Francisco Bay Area, in Greater Boston, and on Long Island. Yet the demographics of breast cancer only partly account for the environmental breast cancer movement's tendency to embody a white, middle-class perspective. More extensive social and cultural factors also play a role.

One set of factors relates to resources. As white, middle-class women, environmental breast cancer activists—many of whom are lawyers, businesswomen, and educators or have personal and professional relationship with such persons—tend to possess time, money, education, social capital, professional experiences, and political connections to bring to their activist efforts. Such resources have advanced their efforts to gain public credibility; procure grants; develop and disseminate educational materials to the public; form coalitions with other activists; garner media attention; develop scientific research studies; and implement regulations at the local, state, and federal level. In other words, these activists have the ability to "work from the inside out" because they already are, in many respects, on the inside socially, culturally, politically, and economically.[10]

Consider Lorraine Pace's efforts on Long Island. "Connections, media attention," she explained, "that's how everything got started." A West Islip resident for more than fifty years, Pace had personal connections that allowed her to carry out the West Islip Mapping Project. She went to high school with the owner of the dry cleaner business who agreed to pin the project's surveys to the plastic bags that covered customers' clean clothes. She relied on her local priest to encourage his congregants to participate in the study. Her husband, John, was friends with Lou Grasso, the editor of the regional newspaper, *Suffolk Life*, who agreed to run the survey on the front page of the edition that went to West Islip residents. Her husband is a lawyer, and he worked pro bono to help establish the West Islip Breast Cancer Coalition. He used his professional ties with local businesses and elected officials to procure funding and donations for the organization's work. Pace's brother-in-law, Anthony Pace, was a prominent Republican leader who had participated in Senator Alphonse D'Amato's election campaign. D'Amato worked with Lorraine Pace and other activists to develop the legislation that mandated the Long Island Breast Cancer Study Project. Pace also credits the media for bringing attention to the region's breast cancer problem. She has collected several hundred newspaper and magazine articles and records of television interviews related to the mapping project and possible environmental causes of breast cancer. Indeed, coverage by the *New York Times*, CNN, and other major media outlets brought national and even global attention to the problem.[11]

Contrast Pace's experience to that of environmental justice and breast cancer groups working on behalf of low-income communities and communities of color. Such organizations often have access to fewer social and economic resources than do their white, middle-class counterparts. Some groups lack the resources needed to develop and maintain an informative Web site (assuming they have a Web site at all). One group, for example, does not have its own office, e-mail address, or phone number. Instead, its Web site lists the personal phone numbers of its co-coordinators for its contact information. The problem of inadequate resources may be exacerbated for organizations, such as the Bayview Hunters Point Community Advocates, that work on multiple issues facing their communities. Communities of color and low-income communities may also experience social and political marginalization with regard to their environmental justice and breast cancer work. One African American breast cancer activist with whom I spoke believes that state officials do not take her town's environmental health concerns seriously. Although these officials have held public forums to discuss such concerns, they have done little to remedy them. She also notes that her organization has little contact with some of the more prominent and affluent breast cancer groups in the area.[12] Moreover, race and class biases within the news media often contribute to inadequate coverage of the social and health issues affecting communities of color, especially if they are also low income.[13] This problem may be especially marked in the case of breast cancer, given that the particular issues facing such communities tend to exist outside the mainstream breast cancer culture that dominates public discourses, discussions, and understanding of the disease.

Another set of factors relates to the construction of risk. The ways in which individuals and groups perceive risk depends partly on their personal, cultural, social, and economic vantage points. Such vantage points influence not only what they consider a risk but also how they prioritize certain risks over others.[14] Disadvantaged women sometimes experience environmental breast cancer risk differently when compared with their white and middle-class counterparts. Given that low-income women and women of color, particularly African Americans, suffer disproportionately high breast cancer mortality rates, the bulk of efforts directed at these women emphasize enhancing the survival of those already affected by the disease, rather than preventing a disease that may not occur until decades later, if at all. Such efforts include educating women of color about the importance of obtaining regular breast cancer screenings and of seeking medical care for any suspected incidence of cancer as soon as possible; providing mammography to poor and disadvantaged women for free or at low cost; creating support services to meet the emotional and psychosocial needs of women of color with the disease and their families; and educating health professionals about cultural issues, language barriers, and racism that may arise in their interactions with women of color in therapeutic settings or that may prevent women of color from seeking medical care in the first place.

Consider Sisters of Greater Long Island, which is an organization run for and by African American women with breast cancer in Suffolk County. The group devotes some of its efforts to educating its African American constituents about environmental risks and strategies to minimize them. Given that the organization is located in a region known not only for its environmental health and breast cancer issues but also its strong networks of environmental breast cancer activism, such efforts are not surprising. At the same time, environmental breast cancer issues are not the organization's main focus; rather, its mission is to "remove the fear of cancer and its treatments from the minds of African-American women and men in the Long Island community." The organization offers support groups for "newly diagnosed and long term survivors," financial assistance for patients struggling to pay for their medical care, information about the importance of early detection, and strategies for addressing the health care disparities that its clients may face.[15] In fact, the medical disparities and financial barriers experienced by women of color and low-income women inspired Breast Cancer Action, Women's Community Cancer Project, 1 in 9, and several other environmental breast cancer groups to work toward achieving universal health care coverage so that all women have access to the care that they need.[16]

The construction of breast cancer risk in disadvantaged communities is shaped by additional environmental health concerns. Such communities are often disproportionately burdened by various types of toxic exposures. Bayview

Hunters Point (BVHP), besides being in close proximity to the Hunters Point Shipyard, is home to the Hunter's Point Power Plant, which operated for seventy-seven years before closing in 2006, emitting high levels of particulate matter and other air pollutants. Bayview's Southeast Water Pollution Control Plant treats 80 percent of the city's sewage. Cement production and the storage of city buses also take place nearby. In addition to enduring industrial pollution, low-income communities such as BVHP face high levels of indoor pollution from smoking, poor ventilation, mold, dust mites, and cockroach infestations.[17]

As a result of these varied exposures, low-income communities often experience high rates of multiple diseases, some of which may take public health precedence over breast cancer. Of particular note in BVHP is the community's asthma problem, which health officials attribute to both indoor and outdoor sources of pollution. Nationwide, 6.9 percent of African Americans and 5.6 percent of the general population have the disease. In contrast, 10 percent of BVHP's total population has asthma, including 15.5 percent of its children. BVHP has a far higher asthma hospitalization rate (24.9 per 100,000) than does San Francisco as a whole (9.7 per 100,000). With proper medical management, asthma is a controllable condition. When treated improperly or not at all, however, a severe asthma attack can kill. Given that so many BVHP residents (especially children) have this life-threatening disease but lack adequate health care coverage, both public health officials and residents view asthma as one of the community's most serious health problems and are working to eliminate the factors that cause the disease and to provide better access to appropriate medical care.[18]

It is also important to recognize that disadvantaged communities often have health concerns that go beyond environmental health. In 2000 and 2001, the BVHP Health and Environmental Assessment Task Force conducted a survey asking residents about their community health concerns. About 45 percent of respondents ranked crime and violence as their number-one concern, followed by drugs and alcohol, AIDS, unemployment, pollution, cancer, and poverty.[19] At times, basic health needs may take precedence over breast cancer prevention. As Barbara Waters of Susan G. Komen for the Cure's North Jersey affiliate explained, many of the poor women with whom the organization works are in "survival mode," worrying not about whether they are eating enough vegetables (much less organic ones), but about whether they can put enough food of any kind on the table.[20]

Finally, organizations, especially those located in predominantly white communities, may face social and cultural barriers when trying to reach out to women of color. The Huntington Breast Cancer Action Coalition (HBCAC) faced this situation when carrying out its mapping project in the mid-1990s. HBCAC wished to encourage the participation of the town's African American and Latino residents, and to aid the latter, it published its survey in both English and Spanish. Staff and volunteers met with potential participants in person about the project. Despite these efforts, HBCAC noticed that minority residents responded at a lower rate than that of Caucasian residents. To address this situation, two HBCAC volunteers representing the Latino and African American communities partnered to enhance the organization's presence in these communities. The coalition's goal was to provide health information and outreach with cultural sensitivity. Both women agreed to do this work at churches, beauty salons, and other community gathering places. Along with Karen Miller, founder and president of HBCAC, the women hosted a breast health awareness segment on a local radio show. The outreach project ended several years later, unfortunately, when one of the women passed away.[21]

Obviously, many activists are cognizant of and concerned about the environmental breast cancer movement's orientation toward white, middle-class women, as well as the factors that have contributed to it. Over the years, they have increasingly strived to integrate the needs, experiences, and perspectives of low-income women and women of color into their efforts and the movement more generally. Doing so, however, has led them not only to expand the movement's demographics; it has also led them—and, in some cases their allied scientists—to broaden their understandings of the environmental breast cancer problem and their strategies for addressing it.

Broadening the Scope of Scientific Research

Science is an arena in which the environmental breast cancer movement's race and class dynamics play out. Who conducts science can determine how it is done. For example, the historical predominance of white men in science has contributed to, and reflected, gender and racial biases in the research questions asked, the methods used to conduct research, the interpretation of results, scientific language and discourse, and the application of scientific knowledge to daily life. Increasing the number of women and people of color who work in science has helped to counter such gender and racial biases by providing alternative perspectives about the research process.[22] Likewise, the growing participation of activists and lay citizens in environmental breast cancer research has influenced this science in important and innovative ways. At the same time, the fact that these activists are, for the most part, white and middle-class women has its own implications for the research that they pursue.

The impact of the race and class backgrounds of activists on the research process is evident in the community-based studies that they pursued in the 1990s. Despite efforts to include residents of color in such studies, racial diversity was sometimes difficult to achieve. For example, the mapping projects that took place in communities across Nassau and Suffolk countries tended to focus on white and middle-class households. As evidenced by the HBCAC's mapping efforts, social and cultural factors may have contributed to this tendency. More significant, however, is that many of the ZIP codes that identified the study areas had relatively few residents of color. At the time of when HBCAC conducted its mapping project, 90 percent of the town's residents identified as white, 4 percent as African American, another 4 percent as Hispanic, and 2 percent as Asian.[23]

Several recent environmental breast cancer studies reflect intensified efforts to include communities of color in the research process. Such efforts include increasing representation of citizens of color on the advisory boards and committees that oversee the design and conduct of particular studies, as well as in the interpretation and public dissemination of study results. They also include the development of studies examining environmental breast cancer issues facing women of color. Increasing the participation of communities of color in these areas of the research process not only contributes to the democratization of science, but also has the potential to provide new insights and perspectives into the environmental causes of breast cancer and the best ways to study them.

One important study in this regard relates to the Breast Cancer Fund, Susan G. Komen for the Cure, and NOW's 1999 campaign to increase federal research on environmental causes of breast cancer. This campaign, in conjunction with the subsequent advocacy efforts by many other breast cancer activists and organizations, prompted Congresswoman Nita Lowey (Democrat of New York) and Senator Lincoln Chaffee (Republican of Rhode Island) to introduce the Breast Cancer and Environmental Research Act, a bill to "authorize $30 million a year for Fiscal Years 2000–2005 for the NIEHS [National Institute of Environmental Health Sciences] to establish up to eight multi-disciplinary research centers to study environmental factors related to the etiology of breast cancer."[24] The passage of this bill in 2001 led to the establishment of the Breast Cancer and Environment Research Centers the following year. Funded by the NIEHS and the National Cancer Institute, the seven-year project allots $5 million annually for the identification and assessment of the prenatal, infant, and adolescent exposures that raise women's risk of developing breast cancer. The research takes place at four centers across the country and is directed by the University of California at San Francisco, Michigan State University, the Fox Chase Cancer Center in Philadelphia, and the University of Cincinnati.[25]

The working group that overseas the broader research program includes representatives from various breast cancer organizations, including Silent Spring Institute's Julia Brody and Ruthann Rudel, Karen Miller of HBCAC, Maria Caroline Hinestrosa of the National Breast Cancer Coalition, and Wendy Mason of Susan G. Komen for the Cure.[26] Breast cancer groups also participate in the activities of each regional center. In the case of the Bay Area Breast Cancer and the Environment Research Center, Zero Breast Cancer serves as a center collaborator along with the California Department of Public Health, Kaiser Permanente of Northern California, Lawrence Berkeley National Laboratory, Marin County Department of Health and Human Services, Roswell Park Cancer Center, and the University of Michigan. Also involved are the Breast Cancer Fund, the Bay Area Breast Cancer SPORE Advocacy Group, and the Bayview Hunters Point Environmental Assessment Task Force.[27] Zero Breast Cancer runs the center's Community Outreach and Translation Core, facilitating communication between scientists and the community. Karen Goodson-Pierce of Bayview Hunters Point Health and Environmental Assessment Task Force and several other advocates also participate in this effort.[28]

The Breast Cancer and Environmental Research Centers run two projects. The first, Environmental Effects on the Molecular Architecture and Function of the Mammary Gland across the Lifespan, conducts experiments with animal and cell culture models to study the molecular development of the mammary gland across the lifespan and the impact that environmental exposures may have on such development. The second, Environmental and Genetic Determinants of Puberty, tracks cohorts of young girls over time to determine how "hormonal changes, obesity, diet, family history, psychosocial stressors, environmental exposures, and genetic polymorphisms, among other factors, may interact to control mammary gland development and other landmarks of puberty." The latter study has significant representation of girls of color. Researchers at the Fox Chase Cancer Center are examining six hundred seven- and eight-year-old girls from East Harlem, with Latinas constituting 60 percent of the study population and African Americans constituting 40 percent. University of Cincinnati scientists are studying four hundred six- and seven-year-old girls from the greater Cincinnati area. Sixty-five percent of these girls are white, and 30 percent are African American. The study population for the San Francisco Bay Area part of the project is four hundred seven-year-old girls, of whom 18 percent are Asian, 9 percent are Pacific Islander, 19 percent are African American, 20 percent are Latino, and 35 percent are white.[29]

Substantial inclusion of girls of color may provide important insights into the early exposures that increase the risk of breast cancer, especially among young African American women. A particularly compelling set of factors that the Breast Cancer and Environment Research Centers addresses relates to the "falling age of puberty." In 1900, the average age at which girls in the United States began menarche was 14.2 years. By 1970, the average was 12.8. Since then, it has dropped by several more months. Currently, the mean age for menarche is 12.6 among white girls, 12.2 among African American girls, and 12.1 among Mexican American girls. The decline among the last two groups has been quicker than that among white girls.[30] The onset of thelarche and pubarche (the development of breasts and pubic hair, respectively) has also dropped over the past century. In the 1960s, girls began to develop breasts at an average age of 11.2 years. Today, 50 percent of girls demonstrate signs of breast development by age 10. Fourteen percent show signs of such development between the ages of 8 and 9. African American girls show the first signs of puberty a year earlier than their white counterparts (at 9 years of age compared with 10).[31]

Among the possible causes of the declining age of puberty are low birth weight, premature birth, weight gain and obesity, formula feeding, physical inactivity, psychosocial stressors, use of television and other media, and environmental exposures to such elements as endocrine disrupters and tobacco smoke. Some of these factors may also help to explain the racial disparities surrounding early puberty. African American girls are more likely than their white counterparts to have experienced many of these possible causes. Moreover, researchers have implicated the use of hair products containing endocrine-disrupting compounds to early puberty in this racial group.[32] These products, which are aimed primarily at African Americans, contain placenta and other hormonal agents. Such products have the potential to affect the health of not only the girls and women who use them but also the children of users. One study found that the female toddlers of women who used the hair products began to develop breasts. When their mothers stopped using these products, the toddlers' emerging breasts dissipated.[33]

The decreasing age of puberty increases the risk of health problems. Girls who go through early puberty are more likely to develop psychological problems such as anxiety, depression, eating disorders, and suicidal tendencies. They are more susceptible to cigarette smoking and the abuse of drugs and alcohol. They become sexually active at younger ages, increasing their risk for teen pregnancy. They have higher rates of delinquency, conduct disorders, and criminal histories, as well as lower levels of academic education. Of particular note, researchers have linked early puberty to polycystic ovary syndrome and breast cancer, because of the increased lifetime exposure to hormones.[34]

Indeed, the fact that African American girls are disproportionately afflicted with early puberty may help to explain why young black women now have the highest incidence rates of breast cancer in the United States.

Beyond the research on early exposures, a second trajectory focuses on daily exposures faced by low-income communities and communities of color that may increase the risk of breast cancer and other illnesses. In 2006, Silent Spring Institute teamed with Communities for a Better Environment (CBE) and Brown University to conduct a study titled "Breast Cancer and Environmental Justice." After completing their Household Exposure Study on Cape Cod, Silent Spring researchers sought to determine whether the chemicals they found in homes were present in the residences of individuals from different socioeconomic backgrounds and geographic regions. For help in conducting the study, the investigators contacted Rachel Morello-Frosh, a professor at Brown University who studies environmental health issues facing disadvantaged communities. A breast cancer survivor who participated in *Rachel's Daughters* as a lay investigator, she expressed interest in participating in the project and recommended that they also team with CBE, with whom she had an existing relationship.[35] CBE addresses the environmental justice issues faced by low-income African American, Latino, and other minority communities in Northern and Southern California. Such communities experience high rates of asthma, cancer, respiratory illnesses, and miscarriages, which some activists and health professionals suspect are caused partly by their close proximity to power plants, freeways, oil refineries, seaports, and other hazardous sites. The organization helps residents identify and develop strategies for addressing the health problems and social injustices that they face. In particular, its staff—organizers, lawyers, policy analysts, and scientists—provide assistance with organizing, research, policy initiatives, and legal efforts.[36]

Funded by the National Institute of Environmental Health Sciences, the study conducted an exposure assessment of household pollutants, specifically endocrine disrupters, associated with various health problems, including breast cancer. The three groups decided to focus on Richmond, California, as CBE already had ties to the environmental justice groups there. A large number of people of color who reside in this town live near an oil refinery and other industrial sites. CBE sought to compare Richmond to another California town, one that was geographically and demographically different, so they added Bolinas, a rural coastal community, to the study.[37] Fifty California homes were included in the project, forty from Richmond and ten from Bolinas. Sampling from inside and outside the homes centered on consumer products. Chemicals of concern include pesticides, phthalates (plastics and vinyl in toys and cosmetics), flame retardants (clothing, bedding, carpet, and electronic equipment), PCBs (older electrical equipment and building materials), PAHs (combustion from fireplaces, smoke, outdoor air pollution, and heaters), alkyphenols (detergents, plastics, and pesticides), other phenols (plastics, disinfectants, and fungicides), parabens (cosmetics and skin lotions), metals (emissions and cigarette smoke), particulate matter (engines, frying food, dust, and cigarette smoke), and ammonia (emissions, fertilizers, cleaning products, and natural processes). The study also assessed the presence of ambient pollution in and around the homes.[38]

Broadening the scope of environmental breast cancer research to emphasize disadvantaged groups has occasionally led activists to rethink their approaches, as evidenced by the Breast Cancer and Environmental Justice study. Overall, the collaboration between Silent Spring and CBE went well. Both groups agreed on a project design that met the needs of researchers and residents from both communities. Silent Spring sent research equipment to CBE and taught the organization's staff how to collect home samples. Residents of Richmond and Bolinas attended community meetings for the project and participated in the study at the same rate as that of Cape Cod residents. Still, the CBE investigators confronted problems during the data collection process that the Silent Spring researchers did not face in their part of the project. The homes tested by Silent Spring on Cape Cod tended to be owned by older, financially secure, retired women, many of whom had flexible schedules. Nor did the residents have many qualms about participating in the study. Consequently, researchers found it relatively easy to arrange to come to their houses and collect samples. In contrast, the CBE investigators faced obstacles in scheduling their home visits, especially in Richmond. Given that many of the town's residents had low incomes, they tended to work long hours and have erratic schedules. Many of the residents whom investigators contacted to participate in the study rented their apartments or houses, and they expressed concern about being evicted if the researchers found evidence of toxic exposures. Finally, many residents were undocumented workers who worried that participating in the project would expose their immigration status.[39]

Science is only one arena in which environmental breast cancer activists, and their allied scientists, rework their strategies when reaching out to low-income communities and communities of color. Breast cancer prevention efforts is another. The movement's increased focus on chemicals, especially those found in personal care products and other household items, provides a compelling case for examining the ways in which activists grapple with race and class issues in their efforts to reduce exposures to harmful substances.

Constructing Risk Factors and Prevention

Breast cancer risk factors are not only biological constructs, but also social and cultural ones. That is, the race and class roots that shape the environmental breast cancer movement as a whole also influence the particular ways in which activists construct risk factors and prevention strategies. To understand the social construction of breast cancer risk, it is important to understand the "riskscapes" that women inhabit on a daily basis. Such riskscapes are shaped by the complex interplay between "geographies of exposure" and "geographies of susceptibility." The term *geographies of exposure* refers to the spaces—communities, homes, and workplaces—in which women encounter toxic exposures, such as air pollution from local industries, occupational hazards, and the pesticides that landlords spray on the grass of their rental properties. *Geographies of susceptibility* refers to the social, cultural, developmental, psychological, and economic conditions that influence the extent to which women are vulnerable to such exposures. For example, low-income women may have little choice but to live in toxic communities, as these may be the only places where they can afford to live. For certain women of color, the psychosocial stress from living daily with racism can also increase the risk of developing breast cancer.[40]

One way in which race and class shape the construction of environmental risk factors relates to the types of toxic exposure with which women are concerned. Donna Jurasits, executive director of the Babylon Breast Cancer Coalition, explains how her organization works with women in Suffolk County, Long Island, who come from various socioeconomic backgrounds. One of the coalition's programs, Time for a Change, educates such women about environmental health risks facing themselves and their families. The program also provides protective strategies that they can take. According to Jurasits, women across the socioeconomic spectrum express concern about the health impact of everyday chemicals. Their concerns, however, sometimes differ. For example, wealthy women have asked Jurasits whether the chlorine in their home pools is safe to use and whether organic home landscapers do quality work. In contrast, many of the poorer women with whom the coalition works do not have lawns, much less swimming pools. Their questions revolve around whether the local schools spray chemicals on the school fields and whether the home products the women buy from the dollar store are safe.[41]

Race and class may shape how organizations construct environmental breast cancer risk factors. In *Pathways for Prevention: Eight Practical Steps—from the Personal to the Political—towards Reducing the Risk of Breast Cancer*, Nancy Evans and Andrea Ravinett Martin of the Breast Cancer Fund discuss strategies that women can use to reduce their risk of breast cancer: exercising regularly; eating ample fruits, vegetables, and other healthy foods (especially organic); avoiding unnecessary mammograms and other X-rays; limiting the use of birth control pills; relying on natural alternatives to hormone replacement therapy; using nontoxic pest management and household cleaning products; learning which canned food manufacturers do not use plastic lining and buying cans from these companies instead of cans lined with plastic; installing filters on faucets for drinking and bathing; and participating in environmental health and public health campaigns.[42]

Without a doubt, such risk reduction measures are important tools. In the spirit of the feminist health movement, they empower women to take control of their health, particularly in the absence of adequate regulatory protections and the presence of other breast cancer risk factors—such as genetic inheritance or reproductive history—that they cannot control. Unlike local or state-based policy reforms, which form the bulk of environmental health protections passed by activists, personal risk reduction strategies have the potential to help women across a wide range of geographic regions. Moreover, the focus on personal risk reduction serves as an effective introduction to the environmental health movement for lay citizens. Sharon Koshar, the Massachusetts Breast Cancer Coalition's former precautionary principle coordinator, maintains that it provides people with a "way in," a means of connecting environmental health issues to their own lives and the lives of their family and friends. Once they make this connection, they (ideally) begin to understand the importance of protecting human health through environmental policy change and other types of structural and societal reform.[43]

However, the risk reduction measures as cited in *Pathways for Prevention* assume a white and economically advantaged readership. Advising women to limit their use of mammography assumes that women have basic access to health care and health insurance. The primary users of birth control pills and hormone replacement therapy are not disadvantaged women but white, middle-class women who have access to health care and health insurance that will cover the procedures. Other risk reduction strategies assume that women not only have the financial means to pay for organic and nontoxic products, which often cost more than the conventional items, but also have access to them. Many disadvantaged communities, especially those in urban areas, have no natural food stores, farmers markets, or general grocery stores that may stock organic products. In fact, some urban areas have no access to fresh produce of any kind because they lack supermarkets. In such communities, residents often rely on fast food restaurants and neighborhood convenience stores that sell primarily prepackaged and processed goods.[44]

Such barriers highlight the limitations of risk reduction strategies that Evans and Martin call "pocketbook activism." Certainly, the impact—both positive and negative—of consumer activism should not be dismissed, as economic pressure can lead to significant political and public health reform. Indeed, this approach reflects a growing trend in recent decades toward a consumer-based activism that encourages individuals to express their political views and work for social change not through voting or direct action but through their purchasing decisions. "The more we use our power as consumers to indicate our preference for non-toxic products through our purchases," Evans and Martin write, "the more industry will have reason to create better, more affordable products free of dangerous chemicals."[45] The promotion of pocketbook activism is evident not only in the environmental breast cancer movement's risk reduction tips but also in its corporate-related campaigns. Some of these campaigns (such as that created through the Breast Cancer Fund's partnership with Clif Bar) encourage individuals to support companies that donate profits to environmental breast cancer efforts, while others (such as the Think Before You Pink campaign) discourage consumers from supporting businesses that have ideological and financial stakes in promoting the dominant cancer paradigm. Still, such activism tends to be geared toward economically advantaged individuals who have the opportunity to pick and choose what they want to buy even if it means purchasing more expensive items or products they would not normally buy.

Given all this, activists increasingly view personal risk reduction through the lens of racial and class disparities. Breast Cancer Action, for example, publishes *Saber es Poder*, a Spanish-language newsletter. Appearing several times a year since 1999, the newsletter discusses a wide range of breast cancer issues of relevance to Latina women. Issue 19, published in late 2007, focused on environmental causes of breast cancer. Besides discussing the latest research linking toxic chemicals to the disease, it suggested low-cost strategies for avoiding such chemicals. Rather than simply declaring that women should buy organic produce, however, it listed which types of produce had less pesticide contamination (such as broccoli and mango) and which had more (such as spinach and nectarines). Women on limited budgets could thus judge which foods to buy and which to avoid. The newsletter also provided directions for making nontoxic cleaning products using basic ingredients such as baking soda, castile soap, vinegar, and water. Finally, the newsletter discussed the formation of a cooperative called Natural Home Cleaning and its importance from a public health and social justice standpoint.[46]

Other groups take similar approaches. At a monthly cooking class in 2007, the Women's Cancer Resource Center in Oakland discussed strategies for buying organic on a budget. Among other things, the organization encouraged women to compare the cost of conventional and organic produce, as sometimes the prices are similar. Participants learned about the "pesticide free" option. Some produce is grown without pesticides but is not labeled organic because the farm from which it came did not meet requirements pertaining to certain factors such as soil quality. Pesticide-free produce can be cheaper than fully organic. The presenters encouraged women to shop at farmers markets, which often sell organic produce at a cheaper price than do supermarkets. They also told women to compare the prices at the markets (some markets in town are more expensive than others) and suggested that they shop at them right before they close, as farmers may offer to sell the produce at a cheaper price to get rid of it before they pack up and leave for the day.[47] The Babylon Breast Cancer Coalition suggests that low-income women volunteer at local organic farms if possible, as volunteers often receive discounts on the food that they have a part in growing.[48] Using a different strategy, 1 in 9 encourages women to shop together at Costco and other wholesale stores where they can purchase safer products at a discount by buying them in bulk and dividing up their purchases.[49]

Social justice strategies can work through policy reform. Many recent initiatives have focused on banning dangerous chemicals from consumer products such as toys, cosmetics, and other household goods, with a number of groups seeking to pass regulations requiring companies to identify harmful chemicals in their products and packaging. Such reforms have the potential to benefit large numbers of people, as individuals from many racial and class backgrounds buy these products. In the case of labeling policies, however, the focus on consumer safety assumes that individuals have the opportunity to buy less toxic alternatives if they so choose. It also downplays the harmful exposures to the chemicals that workers face on the job. Indeed, workplace exposures disproportionately affect people of color. Although African Americans number one in eight Americans, they make up one in three housekeepers, one in three blue-collar workers, and one in two sanitation workers.[50] Latinos make up only 11 percent of the U.S. population, but 41 percent of "private household cleaners and servants," 27 percent of "non-private household cleaning and building services," and 30 percent of "laundering and dry cleaning machine operators."[51]

To address workplace disparities such as these, breast cancer activists increasingly seek legislation to protect the health of workers in addition to the health of consumers. In October 2005, Governor Arnold Schwarzenegger of California signed Senate Bill 484, the Safe Cosmetics Bill, into law. Breast Cancer Action, the Breast Cancer Fund, the and National Environmental Trust spearheaded the campaign to pass the bill. In addition to protecting consumers by requiring companies to disclose the latter's use of toxic chemicals in cosmetic products, the bill gives CalOSHA, California's Division of Occupational Safety and Health, the authority to regulate the use of harmful products in nail and beauty salons to protect salon workers.[52] Cosmetologists face twice the risk of breast cancer as that of other women, as well as some of the highest levels of toxic exposures. The majority of workers whom such regulations would protect are women of color, many of them recent immigrants. In the case of nail salons, 93 percent of workers are women and 80 percent are of Vietnamese descent.[53] Similarly, the Safer Alternatives and Safer Cleaning Products bills that the Alliance for a Healthy Tomorrow, a coalition that includes breast cancer and environmental justice groups, aims to pass in Massachusetts would protect workers, among other vulnerable populations, by requiring businesses, public schools, hospitals, public housing facilities, and other institutions to reduce their use of toxic chemicals and products.[54]

Another way in which activists address workers' health is by reforming local business practices. Breast Cancer Action and the Breast Cancer Fund are members of the California Healthy Nail Salon Collaborative, formed in 2005 "out of growing concern for the health and safety of nail salon and other cosmetology workers, owners, and consumers." Asian Health Services in Oakland manages the collaborative. In addition to pushing for laws and policies to protect the nail salon community, the group encourages the use of safer products and practices in nail salons owned by Asian Americans and in hair salons owned by African Americans. The group meets with workers and salon owners to identify "issues of concern and [develop] solutions to benefit the nail salon workforce, their families, and small businesses." It also holds community forums and conducts outreach activities to raise awareness about the "environmental health concerns facing nail salon workers and about toxins found in nail, beauty and personal care products."[55] These efforts come on the heels of other Bay Area attempts to protect the health of workers, particularly workers of color. WAGES (Women's Action to Gain Economic Security) helps low-income Latina women open their own ecofriendly housecleaning cooperatives, such as Natural Home Cleaning.[56] Founded in 2003, this cooperative is run by fourteen women and serves San Francisco's East Bay communities.

The women's mission is "to support our families and be economically self-sufficient while providing our clients with high-quality service. By using least toxic cleaning products, we protect the health of our clients, our own health, and the health of our planet."[57] WAGES helps in starting up other ecofriendly cooperative businesses, among them Eco-Bay Landscaping in Oakland.[58]

Of course, campaigns advocating for the health of workers are not new. Since the 1990s, breast cancer activists across the country have helped to protect the health of farm workers, teachers, dry cleaning staff, and health care professionals, among others, from toxins at occupational sites and from the diseases linked to these harmful chemicals. Still, the bulk of breast cancer activism over the years has focused more on consumers than on workers. This tendency is especially apparent in the movement's growing concentration on personal care products, cosmetics, toys, baby items, and other home items. Viewed from this perspective, recent efforts to frame the dangers posed by such products as occupational health problems signify an important political and public health strategy.

Rethinking the Environment, Rethinking Environmental Justice

Efforts by environmental breast cancer activists to address the needs of socially and economically marginalized groups illuminate the ideological tensions that sometimes exist between the environmental justice and environmental health movements. Certainly, both movements emerged in response to some common social, political, and public health concerns, and both embrace the notion that the people have a right to healthy bodies, communities, and environments. The boundaries between the two fields are blurred and are arguably becoming more so, especially given that activists in these fields recognize that both are needed to address the full scope of the health problems on which they work. That said, significant differences between the two movements exist.

Breast Cancer Action, an organization that strives to integrate environmental justice and environmental health approaches in its work, provides a particularly useful model for conceptualizing their differences. According to the group, an environmental justice framework emphasizes grassroots, community-based efforts to challenge the practices, policies, and malfeasance of local industries, and sometimes governments, that contribute to the disproportionate health problems faced by low-income communities, particularly those of color. It also strives to eradicate the systemic racism, classism, and other inequities that contribute to the environmental health problems affecting such communities. In doing so, an environmental justice framework seeks to empower disenfranchised communities by demanding that they play a role in the decision-making processes of relevance to the health of their residents and their environment. In contrast, an environmental health approach identifies "the human and/or environment exposure to toxins as the core problem." To these ends, it advocates for increased scientific research; access to safer products and healthier environments; increased information about the health risks from toxic substances; local, state, national, and international laws to limit the production and use of such substances; and public involvement in scientific and policy decision making. It does not, however, "address the disproportionate exposures for different populations, or the root causes of these disparities."[59]

One way in which these ideological tensions play out in the context of environmental breast cancer activism relates to the movement's increasing focus on the dangers from household good and products. In many respects, the environment is what anthropologist Melissa Checker calls a "flexible narrative," its meaning changing over time.[60] During the 1980s, activists working on behalf of disadvantaged communities helped to redefine notions of the environment by insisting that so-called built environments, especially urban areas, deserved the same environmental protections as the wilderness, forests, and waterways that the Sierra Club and other groups spent decades trying to preserve.[61] Over the following decade, environmental justice, breast cancer, and other activists expanded this concept by defining the environment to mean an array of "outside" sources of pollution such as air pollution, contaminated drinking water, and agricultural pesticides to which many individuals and communities are exposed. More recently, breast cancer activists and their environmental health counterparts further broadened the scope of the environment to include "inside" sources of contamination, particularly those found in the home.

Many types of indoor exposure fit into a traditional environmental justice framework. For example, many low-income residents live in houses and apartments with cockroach infestation, mold growth, and lead paint exposure. Often, these living conditions result from landlords' taking advantage of their tenants' socioeconomic situation by neglecting to maintain the properties. The fact that low-income individuals have few choices in the first place when it comes to housing reflects the racism, classism, and poverty embedded in the country's socioeconomic structure. Indoor pollution can also result from outdoor pollution sources, such as car emissions and factories and other industrial sites that are located in or near communities of color. The indoor exposures—personal care products, household items, and other consumer goods—on which the environmental breast cancer movement tends to focus, however, fall outside the traditional scope of environmental justice, as they do not relate to pollution and toxic exposures forced into the home by malfeasance on the part of industries, local governments, or landlords but rather are connected with the common, and seemingly benign, products that individuals bring into the home as a result of their own consumer purchases and choices. The makers of harmful products are most likely located not in the residents' communities but in other parts of the state; the country; or, in the age of globalization, the world.

This is not to say that personal care and home products are irrelevant to the traditional environmental justice concerns. After all, women of color constitute a significant portion of cleaning and salon staff who must work with such products daily. Companies market to African Americans hair care products that are especially high in estrogenic compounds. Because of poverty and racism, women of color and low-income women often have less access to safer products than do their economically advantaged counterparts. Still, the emphasis on consumer products, personal risk reduction, and purchasing habits—while important—complicates the traditional environmental justice focus on the structural causes of disproportionate exposure, on collective grassroots action, and on community participation in local environmental decision making. The Massachusetts Breast Cancer Coalition's educational campaign Toxic Tours of Your Bathroom, designed to encourage individuals to learn which of their products contain harmful chemicals, exemplifies this complication.[62]

The ideological tensions between environmental justice and environmental health also play out in the context of science. Across the nation, environmental justice activists and the residents they represent increasingly play a prominent role in community-based participatory research on health issues affecting their communities.[63] Yet some activists and residents are skeptical of efforts to study the relationship between toxic exposures and human health, as they view the institution of science as part of the social, political, and economic system that contributes to their marginalization. For one thing, conventional environmental risk assessment often discounts the experiences of low-income communities and communities of color, especially by excluding "tacit" and other forms of local knowledge from this scientific process.[64] Skepticism is especially strong when it comes to research examining the interactions between genes and the environment, as some environmental justice activists and residents worry that scientists and policymakers will hold individuals' genetic makeup, rather than industry malfeasance, responsible for their communities' health problems. They worry that science will function as a strategy for delaying political action and industrial reform.[65] Activists also condemn researchers who rely on residents' participation when conducting their studies but do not use their studies' findings to help the community.[66] Further, low-income communities and communities of color often lack the money, time, social capital, and infrastructure to carry out research projects successfully.[67]

Such tensions are evident in the Breast Cancer and Environmental Justice Project conducted by Silent Spring, Communities for a Better Environment, and Brown University. One set of tensions revolved around the types of exposures on which the project focused. Given Silent Spring's desire to extend its Cape Cod Household Study, its scientists wanted the Richmond and Bolinas study to focus on indoor exposures. Communities for a Better Environment (CBE), however, wanted the study to examine outdoor exposures, to build on the community's long-standing efforts to challenge the local refineries and other sources of industrial pollution. In the end, individuals from both organizations agreed that the study would focus on a combination of indoor and outdoor exposures. As the study progressed, CBE raised concerns that Silent Spring researchers would declare that the indoor sources of contamination put residents in more danger than the outdoor exposures. The organization worried that such a position would invalidate the community's fight against local polluters.[68]

Another set of issues revolved around the process of choosing participants. For the Cape Cod study, Silent Spring had chosen participants in a traditionally scientific manner, systematically and randomly selecting people's names from the phone book. They then mailed letters asking the selected households to participate in the study and followed the letters up with phone calls. After the researchers completed the study, they sent the results to participants by mail. Given the success of this approach, the Silent Spring researchers wanted to use it for the Richmond and Bolinas study. CBE staff, however, had other ideas. First, they wanted to recruit participants by encouraging individuals to volunteer for the study. Although this approach was not scientific in the traditional sense, it embodied environmental justice values by empowering community members to become involved and by reducing the possibility of coercion. Moreover, CBE wanted to conduct the participant outreach in person. In the end, the two organizations compromised. Half of the study's participants were selected randomly, while the other half volunteered. Moreover, the investigators for the Richmond study decided to go door to door asking members of the community to participate in the study. They also used this in-person approach to provide participants with the study results.[69]

Negotiating Differences

Integrating the needs and perspectives of women of color and low-income women into the environmental breast cancer movement continues to be a vital goal, as it has the potential to benefit the health not only of these particular women but of women in general. At the same time, efforts to do so demonstrate how the push for breast cancer prevention—particularly in regard to environmental factors—is, in many respects, a mark of privilege. That is, having social, cultural, and economic access to health insurance, state-of-the-art treatment, early detection, basic medical care, and ample (if not organic) produce allows women to devote their energies and efforts to preventing the disease. If the environmental breast cancer movement strives to make breast cancer prevention more accessible to women who are socially and economically marginalized, it should continue to address the underlying barriers that make it difficult for such women to make prevention a greater priority.

Viewing the emphasis on breast cancer prevention as a reflection of privilege complicates the environmental breast cancer movement's criticism of mainstream breast cancer culture. What implications does challenging the dominant breast cancer paradigm have for disadvantaged women whose immediate need for improved access to early detection and proper treatment may be greater than their longer-term need for prevention? What significance do critiques of the pink ribbon hold for activists of color who find that handing out the ribbons to women in their community is a useful strategy for encouraging them to get a mammogram?[70] In discussing these complexities, I am not suggesting that the charges against mainstream breast cancer culture are irrelevant to the lives of disadvantaged women. After all, downplaying the causes of prevention of breast cancer benefits no one, and challenges to the cancer industry guide the work of many environmental justice groups. Nevertheless, critiques of mainstream breast cancer culture warrant more nuanced analyses when considering the priorities and needs of women of color and low-income women.

Examining the tensions that can arise between environmental justice and environmental health approaches raises the question of how to address the environmental breast cancer problem in socially and economically marginalized communities. It also highlights the ways in which the two approaches shape one another. The participation of marginalized communities in local research efforts, for example, leads to the "resistance and reconstruction," as sociologist Jennifer Fishman puts it, of conventional scientific and risk assessment practices.[71] Similarly, the growing political and public health emphasis on household products and consumer goods complicates the environmental justice movement's ideological focus and boundaries. Underlying this all is the broader issue of what constitutes the environment—a concept that has evolved and will likely evolve even further over time. Thus, the discussions and debates over the definition of environmental health and environmental justice and how they can best come together will go on.

The politics of race and class is not the only arena in which environmental breast cancer activists grapple with the movement's tendency to privilege certain populations over others. These tendencies also play out in the connections that activists make between breast cancer in women and diseases and disorders afflicting other populations, such as children, men, and wildlife. Not surprisingly, such connections have significant implications for how activists situate their breast cancer work in relation to the broader environmental health movement.

Chapter 7

Beyond Breast Cancer, Beyond Women's Health

In February 2000, the American Association for the Advancement of Science (AAAS) held its annual meeting in Washington, D.C. One of its sessions was an all-day workshop titled "Environment and Fertility." Organized by the National Audubon Society, Population International, Natural Resources Defense Council, National Family Planning and Reproductive Health Association, and Planned Parenthood Federation of America, this session brought together more than thirty representatives from the environmental, population, public health, women's health, children's health, and learning disabilities communities. The purpose of the meeting was to assess the status of existing evidence linking endocrine disrupters to human reproductive health concerns, especially in the areas of fertility and population health. Participants discussed the work they did to address these issues and the ways in which they could work together in the future. "Within the environmental community," the program agenda explained, "several campaigns and projects are tackling aspects of the issue (for example, Health Care Without Harm, the Citizen's Dioxin Report, and the international Persistent Organic Pollutants [POPs] Campaign). The children's health, women's health, birth defects and learning disabilities communities are also addressing the impacts of these chemicals on human health and the environment. At this time, however, no coalition or alliance of organizations has come together to take on the specific and complex set of issues related to population growth, fertility and environmental contamination."

During the first part of the meeting, participants focused on why scientists and policymakers had not adequately addressed the human health impacts of endocrine disrupters. In addition to noting the profit motives of those with economic stakes in the production and use of toxins, participants discussed the failure of epidemiological, toxicological, and risk assessment methods for effectively assessing the specific biological mechanisms and health risks of endocrine disrupters. They listed the strengths and the weaknesses of the EPA's newly created Endocrine Disrupter Screening and Testing Program. Participants shared information about Web sites and newsletters devoted to endocrine disrupter issues. In short, workshop participants highlighted how the very category of endocrine disrupters led to social, material, and discursive restructuring in the arenas of science, policy, and advocacy, especially in regard to reproductive health.

In the meeting's second half, participants discussed plans to form a new coalition of groups that would focus on endocrine disrupters and reproductive health. They generated a contact list of names and numbers. They made lists of issues that the coalition could address, political actions and outreach strategies that they could take, and points of connection and disconnection among the groups. They then brainstormed possible names for the group. Most interestingly, the planning session demonstrated how endocrine disrupter theory could facilitate alliances between organizations that previously seemed to have little in common. A representative from Planned Parenthood stood up to say how her organization had only recently seen the connection between environmental contamination and the local and global issues related to reproductive health, fertility, and population. Indeed, the organization's newfound awareness led it to co-organize this meeting.

Sociologists Sheryl Ruzek, Virginia Olesen, and Adele Clarke maintain that women's health is embedded in communities; women's physical, psychological, and emotional well-being go hand in hand with the health of their families, their social networks, and societal institutions. "Without creating and maintaining social relationships and institutions that actually produce health," they write, "efforts to reduce the burdens of disease and the costs of biomedicine will remain unrealized."[1] Similarly, the AAAS meeting illustrates how the health of women is dependent on the environmental health of their communities, particularly the indoor and outdoor spaces in which they live, work, and play. Just as important, the meeting highlights the ways in which the environmental health of women is connected to the environmental health of other populations.

Not surprisingly, environmental breast cancer activists take this approach by constructing disease kinships between breast cancer in women and disorders afflicting humans and other living beings. They construct kinships between environmental breast cancer groups and the organizations working on other diseases and affected populations. The context of endocrine disrupter theory provides a compelling case for examining the significance of such kinships for environmental breast cancer activism and its relationship to the bourgeoning environmental health movement. Although the theory enables environmental breast cancer groups to promote the health of human and nonhuman populations, activists' approaches to these populations tend to differ. Contrasts of this sort reflect factors with which activists must negotiate when developing agendas, campaigns, and action strategies that best meet their political and public health needs.

From Women's Health to Children's Health

Participants at the AAAS Environmental and Fertility workshop spent considerable time discussing children's health. They expressed concern about the impact of prenatal and postnatal exposure to endocrine disrupters on children's physical, cognitive, emotional, and neurological development and noted the risk that such chemicals might pose to both women's and men's ability to have children in the first place. Given this focus, it was not surprising that representatives from children's health organizations, including the Learning Disabilities Association, Advocates for Youth, and Children's Health and Environment Coalition, attended the meeting. Nor was it surprising when representatives from other environmental health and public health organizations such as the World Resources Institutes, the Environmental Working Group, and the Center for Science in the Public Interest, explained the ways in which their organizations addressed children's environmental health issues; this last group distributed materials related to their work on endocrine disrupters and birth defects.

Breast cancer activists began to prioritize children's health during the mid- to late 1990s, particularly in conjunction with their work on endocrine disrupters. In addition to supporting campaigns spearheaded by other organizations, they take on the issue as one of their own. Activists' interest in children's health is especially evident in the 1997 documentary *Rachel's Daughters: Searching for the Causes of Breast Cancer*. As its title suggests, the film initially invokes the image of children to present breast cancer as an issue of particular concern to younger generations of women. Playing the roles of Rachel's daughters, the seven breast cancer activists who conducted the investigation into environmental causes of breast cancer took up where Rachel Carson left off. The investigators were, in a sense, Carson's offspring, the next generation of activist kin. It is little wonder that Nancy Evans and Andrea Martin of the Breast Cancer Fund dedicated their 2000 booklet, *Pathways to Prevention: Eight Practical Steps—from the Personal to the Political—toward Reducing the Risk of Breast Cancer*, to Carson, the "mother of the modern day environmental health movement," as they described her.[2]

The generational perspective embodied in the film's title helps to foreground two of the main questions that framed the activist investigation and motivated Irving Saraf, Allie Light, and Evans to produce the documentary: Why does it seem that so many younger women are dying of breast cancer? Why are so many mothers burying their daughters? To highlight increasing incidence rates among younger women, the documentary begins with footage of a funeral procession for thirty-two-year-old Jennifer Mendoza—one of the investigators who died during the making of the film—slowly making its way across the Northern California foothills. The procession then cuts to Mendoza's burial, with friends, family, and the other investigators tearfully placing flowers on her casket and embracing her aging mother.

The voiceover that narrates Mendoza's funeral procession illuminates how the focus on endocrine disrupters fueled the film's generational understanding of breast cancer: "We are the generation who was born and came of adult age during the most toxic and environmentally unregulated decade ever known, whose baby food was contaminated with traces of DDT, PCBs, and DES. Our neighborhoods were sprayed with pesticides and filled with toxic waste. Most of these chemicals did not exist before World War II. We are the generation whose early idealism opened up the original generation gap. We didn't know that this gap would come to mean premature and early death in our thirties, forties, and fifties. We didn't know that the 'in' generation was destined to become the cancer generation. We didn't know that so many of our mothers would bury us."[3]

The voiceover establishes the connection between the health of this younger generation of women and the health of infants and young children, especially girls. Recent studies have found that infants, children in general, and adolescent girls are more biologically vulnerable to the harmful effects from toxic chemicals—especially endocrine disrupters—than are adult women. Although the mothers of these younger generations of women were also exposed to such chemicals after World War II, the fact that they were first exposed to them as adults may have provided them with a form of protection that their daughters—and now the daughters of these daughters—did not receive. Because the cells and tissues of fetuses and children undergo a state of rapid growth and development, exposure to toxic substances can cause longer-lasting and more powerful damage. Compared with adults, children breathe in more air and drink more water proportional to their body weight and cannot metabolize chemicals as effectively.[4] In a later section of the documentary, Jennifer Mendoza describes firsthand the dangers of this early exposure. As the daughter of Mexican migrant farmworkers, she spent her childhood playing in the streams that flowed by the pesticide-sprayed fields in which her parents worked.

Nancy Evans's involvement with *Rachel's Daughters* was not the first activist work that she had done to promote children's health. "The Persistence of Pesticides: Women and Children First," an article she wrote for the October 1993 issue of Breast Cancer Action's monthly newsletter, described a Breast Cancer Action meeting at which Dr. Marion Moses, the director of the Pesticide Education Center in San Francisco, spoke about the health impacts of DDT and other xenoestrogenic pesticides. The article highlighted how the timing of exposure to a toxin directly relates to the type of health effect that it may trigger. "The same toxic exposure that causes miscarriages early in pregnancy could cause stillbirth if the exposure occurred later in pregnancy," Evans wrote. "Occurring in adolescence when the female breast is developing, that same toxic insult might sow the seeds of breast cancer."[5] Although breast cancer primarily affects adult women, Evans argues that their susceptibility to the disease may have developed when they were children.

In *Rachel's Daughters*, Evans used this knowledge to encourage breast cancer risk reduction among girls and teenage women. When two of the film's investigators ask Devra Davis at her Washington, D.C., office how DDT and other xenoestrogens cause breast cancer, Davis explains how the breast tissue of adolescent girls is particularly susceptible to the damaging impact of endocrine disrupters. After she asserts that breast cancer risk increases as one's lifetime exposure to natural and synthetic estrogens increases, the film cuts to a shot of teenaged girls doing jumping jacks on a field during a gym class. While Davis states in a voiceover how exercise helps to reduce one's total burden of estrogen, one of the exercising girls says, "I do a hundred every night."

Evans also urged breast cancer prevention through pesticide regulation that would protect children's health. At the end of "The Persistence of Pesticides," she mentioned the U.S. Senate hearings on the repeal of the Delaney Clause, a 1958 amendment that barred "even tiny amounts" of known carcinogens from processed foods. She then encouraged readers to contact their congressional representatives to tell them to oppose this repeal—a policy change that Evans argued would benefit only the multibillion-dollar industry that profits from the development of pesticides, insecticides, and herbicides and their use in agricultural and other food products.[6] Although Congress ultimately repealed the Delaney Clause in 1995, many breast cancer groups worked hard to make sure that its replacement, the Food Quality and Protection Act of 1996, included specific regulations to protect the health of children from pesticides.

Breast cancer activists worked to pass other pesticide reforms geared toward children. In its August 2001 newsletter, Breast Cancer Action published an action alert about the Schools Environment Protection Act of 2001, a federal bill to "provide basic level of protection to students and school staff from the use of pesticides on public school buildings and on school grounds." Breast Cancer Action urged readers to contact their congressional representatives to raise concerns about pesticides in schools and ask them to sign one of two "Dear Colleague" letters in support of the act that were circulating on Capitol Hill. The organization provided a sample letter to congressional representatives for readers wanting guidance.[7] Breast cancer groups helped to pass similar legislation at the state and local levels. Breast Cancer Action, the Women's Cancer Resource Center in Oakland, and the Breast Cancer Fund worked to pass California's Healthy Schools Act of 2000, which prevented the use of pesticides on or near the properties of California public schools. As a member of the Toxic Links Coalition, the Women's Cancer Resource Center successfully pressured the Oakland Unified School District in 2001 to implement an integrated pest management plan to eliminate the need for pesticide treatments by preventing pest problems from occurring in the first place.[8] Similarly, Breast Cancer Action informed its constituents about Healthy Schools Trainings. Held in Los Angeles and Oakland, these Pesticide Watch sessions taught parents and community members who supported the implementation of California's Healthy Schools Act of 2002 how to help phase out the use of pesticides in their local school districts.[9]

To some extent, the pesticide reforms promoted by various breast cancer activist groups reinforce their primary focus on breast cancer. Although these efforts target children, they do so with the goal of preventing breast cancer by reducing its risk at the points in women's lives when their bodies are most vulnerable to the impact of endocrine-disrupting chemicals: infancy and early adolescence. At the same time, these regulatory efforts to reduce childhood exposure to pesticides also protect children from other potential cancerous and noncancerous health problems, demonstrating how breast cancer activists' concerns about children's health sometimes go beyond women's health and breast cancer. The focus on children's health for its own sake is particularly evident in activist efforts to pass legislation protecting children from chemicals that have no direct ties to the disease. Consider the efforts of breast cancer groups to reduce the presence of arsenic in the environment. This chemical, a known bladder and kidney carcinogen and a suspected endocrine disrupter that is often used in playground equipment, decks, and other structures, has not been linked to breast cancer in either humans or animals.[10] Nevertheless, breast cancer activists worked to ban its use. Breast Cancer Action sent out a November 15, 2001, action alert urging its members to attend a public meeting held by the San Francisco Commission on the Environment about possible legislation to ban the use of arsenic-treated wood throughout the city.[11] Then, the Breast Cancer Fund sent out an e-mail action alert, headed "Keep Arsenic Out of Our Playgrounds," in January 2002, urging constituents to submit a letter to the EPA's director, Christine Todd Whitman, asking her to ban the use of arsenic-treated wood.[12]

The children's health framework also shapes activists' scientific interventions. In October 2002, various activists, as well as their allied scientists and health professionals, spoke at the "Joint Informational Hearing on Breast Cancer and the Environment" held by the California Senate Health and Human Services Committee and Assembly Health Committee. The purpose of the meeting was to motivate the California Assembly to develop programs that would lead to a better understanding of the causes of breast cancer in California women and help to prevent it. Many speakers addressed the need to develop a statewide, community-based biomonitoring program that would, among other things, track the presence of chemicals in the body. Although the Centers for Disease Control and Prevention (CDC) conducts various biomonitoring projects, it does not focus on the local dimensions of body burden exposures that a regional program could address. Ultimately, such state-based tracking could help researchers construct a community-based ecology of risk by providing clues about the chemicals to which women and other residents are regularly exposed.

To be sure, speakers mentioned that a state-based biomonitoring program would measure the levels of toxins found in bodily substances such as urine, blood, and hair. Even so, they expressed particular concern about assessing the levels of contaminants in breast milk. As Dr. Felix Aguilar, president of the Los Angeles chapter of Physicians for Social Responsibility, explained, "A comprehensive, community-based biomonitoring program using breast milk is a useful approach to measuring community health because it can zero in on toxic hot spots."[13] Once researchers have identified geographies of risk, they can initiate plans to eliminate contaminants. Constructing breast milk as a nonhuman "actant," the executive director of the Breast Cancer Fund, Jeanne Rizzo, asserted, "Conducting biomonitoring using breast milk can be a powerful tool for measuring community-health because when breast milk speaks, people listen."[14] In line with the hearing's purpose, some speakers noted that a statewide biomonitoring project could offer insights into the impact of environmental exposures on the development of breast cancer. Still other speakers discussed what breast milk could reveal about the health of infants and children.

Through breastfeeding, breast milk transfers the chemicals in women's breasts to the bodies of nursing infants, where they can settle in a child's blood, tissues, and body fat for days, months, and even years. Such chemicals include dry cleaning fluids, flame retardants, deodorizers, fungicides, and gasoline vapors. Of particular concern are PCBs and DDT—two banned xenoestrogens linked to breast cancer. Breast milk is one of the most PCB-contaminated foods on the planet, whereas DDT remains the most prevalent contaminant in the breast milk of mothers living in industrialized nations. Toxic accumulation is greater in species high on the food chain. Given that humans rank among the highest species on the food chain, their breast milk is one of the most contaminated substances that infants can imbibe. When compared with their parents, breastfed infants from industrialized countries consume up to fifty times more PCBs per pound of body weight.[15] For these reasons, the case of breast milk contamination provides another lens through which to conceptualize disease kinships and biological relatedness: just as mothers share genes and blood with their children, they share endocrine-disrupting and other toxic chemicals. The case also highlights another way to conceptualize ecologies of risk: endocrine disrupters and other chemicals not only travel across local and global spaces but also through familial lines, from one generation to the next.[16]

In the wake of the 2002 California Assembly hearing, breast cancer activists worked to develop legislation to establish a biomonitoring program in the state. In 2005, they had their first glimmer of success. State senator Deborah Ortiz and Senate president pro tem Don Perata—along with the Breast Cancer Fund and Commonweal—sponsored Senate Bill 600, the Healthy Californians Biomonitoring Program. Inevitably, when promoting the bill, activists discussed its relevance to children health. The Breast Cancer Fund developed a fact sheet devoted to the topic, highlighting the impact that toxic exposures exert on the development of asthma, cancer, birth defects, and disabilities among this population. Another fact sheet explained why contaminated breast milk is still better for infants than formula. Many of the fifty-five organizations and fifty-two scientists and health care professionals who endorsed the bill were devoted to children's health issues. The bill passed the Senate, but Governor Arnold Schwarzenegger vetoed it.[17] The following year, the Breast Cancer Fund and Commonweal tried again. Along with lead authors Perata and Ortiz, they co-sponsored Senate Bill 1379, a revised version of Senate Bill 600. After passing the Senate in August 2006, the bill was signed into law by Governor Schwarzenegger, on September 29. The CDC promised to provide $1.7 million to support development of the project, which is currently the only state-based biomonitoring program in the country.[18]

As shown by the Alliance for a Healthy Tomorrow's efforts to pass more stringent environmental health legislation in Massachusetts, activists use children's health as a justification for implementing the precautionary principle. Also consider Long Island's Prevention Is the Cure campaign. As part of its 2008 Prevention Is The Cure Week, the group organized classes on organic snacks that teens can make at home and steps parents can take to protect their children from toxic exposures.[19] The group also asked individuals to protect children's health by demanding that the New York State Department of Environmental Conservation strengthen its plan to reduce the emission of mercury from the state's power plants. Mercury exposure in utero and during early children can cause memory and vision problems, impaired fine-motor coordination, and attention disorders.[20]

As part of their breast cancer and environmental health efforts, activists sometimes go beyond the issue of children's health to address issues facing men. Their efforts to promote men's health, however, are not as comprehensive as their work on behalf of children, despite the fact that men are at risk for reproductive health disorders thought to be caused by the same endocrine-disrupting chemicals that are linked to breast cancer.

Saving the Males

During the AAAS workshop's coalition-building session, Devra Davis gave a short talk about the research linking breast cancer to xenoestrogens. She described the evidence linking endocrine disrupters to male reproductive health problems such as decreased sex ratio (fewer male births than female), undescended testicles, and decreased sperm count. She offered this information not only to bolster her argument that xenoestrogens might cause breast cancer but also to encourage participants to consider directing some of their future efforts toward male reproductive health. Somewhat tongue in cheek, she proposed, a "save the males" campaign. Although many in the audience chuckled at this suggestion, they also nodded approvingly. Throughout the rest of the workshop, participants referred back to the idea of this campaign.

Davis had called for her Save the Males campaign in other venues, among them the Massachusetts Precautionary Principle Project kick-off meeting that had taken place the previous year. Then, she had said, "Now let me go over a little bit of human evidence that we have. I want to talk about what is happening in men in industrial countries. We need to create a 'save the males' campaign. There are increases in testicular cancer in every industrial country. There are increases in defects of the penis of baby boys, hypospadias, increases in undescended testes of baby boys, and infertility, possibly reduced sex-ratios. These pieces don't really fit together except that they are all examples of things that reflect some disturbance in the hypothalamo-gonado-pituitary axis, in the way the body regulates itself hormonally." She urged meeting participants to pay more attention to the role of paternal exposure to toxins in the formation of birth defects. "The father's role in producing healthy babies and defects in babies has been underestimated,"

Davis declared. "There shouldn't be any surprises here. People have been reluctant to accept the reality: it takes two parents to make a baby."[21]

By promoting her campaign, Davis sought to inspire breast cancer and other environmental health activists to broaden their political scope to address disorders affecting men, particularly those linked to the same types of hormone disrupters associated with breast cancer in women. To some extent, breast cancer activists had already begun embracing this broader focus by the time that Davis made these calls to action. As part of their efforts to build the case that endocrine disrupters cause breast cancer, they sometimes invoked the evidence linking these chemicals to various male reproductive health disorders. From time to time, they mentioned men's health issues in their policy and research updates. In May 2000, for instance, the Breast Cancer Fund sent its constituents a follow-up letter to its October 1999 campaign pushing for increased federal research on environmental causes of breast cancer. In the section describing the outcomes from the campaign, the letter stated that President Bill Clinton's new budget for 2001 allocated increased funding for the CDC's Environmental Health Labs to explore "the largely unknown environmental causes of disease, like breast and prostate cancer."[22] In general, however, the movement's engagement with male reproductive health is somewhat tenuous.

This dynamic became especially apparent several years after Davis's call to action at the AAAS meeting. In June 2002, CDC researchers published a study linking phthalates in cosmetics, shampoo, nail polish, deodorants, and other personal care products used by women to increased rates of testicular sterility and damage in their male children.[23] Six months later, Harvard researchers discovered that phthalates damaged the sperm of adult men.[24] A study in December that year, by Swedish researchers, found a link between a mother's exposure to organochlorine chemicals and an increased risk that her son would develop testicular cancer later on in life.[25] Health groups also conducted their own studies around this time. In July 2002, the Environmental Working Group, Health Care Without Harm, and Coming Clean released the report *Not Too Pretty: Phthalates, Beauty Products, and the FDA*, which discussed the results of a study contracted by various environmental health and public health organizations two months earlier to assess the presence of phthalates in seventy-two personal care products used primarily by women, including fragrances, hair gels, deodorants, body lotions, hairsprays, and nail polish. The researchers not only found phthalates in fifty-two of the products but also noted that none of the products listed these chemicals in their ingredients. The researchers went on to argue that the male reproductive system was especially susceptible to the effects of phthalates. Thus, women who use these products may put their male offspring at risk.[26] Four months later, Health

Care Without Harm teamed up with the European organizations Women's Environmental Network and the Swedish Society for Nature Conservation to publish *Pretty Nasty: Phthalates in European Cosmetics*, which described results similar to those discussed in *Not Too Pretty*.[27]

In conjunction with the release of the *Not Too Pretty* report, U.S. and European groups founded the Not Too Pretty campaign. This organization worked to raise public awareness about the health dangers from cosmetics, put pressure on cosmetic companies to stop using phthalates and other toxic chemicals in their products, and lobby the European Union and U.S. governments to ban the use of phthalates and other toxic chemicals in cosmetics. This organization also printed two lengthy articles about the June and December 2002 studies on its Web site and provided readers with outlets for taking political action.[28] Women's Voices for the Earth, a group that addresses environmental health issues affecting women and children, added to the efforts by publishing the article "Are Her Cosmetics Hurting His Testicles?" on its Web site, posting a link to Not Too Pretty's site, and providing readers with an online letter they could e-mail to their congressional representatives about phthalates.[29]

When I first learned about these anti-phthalates efforts, I assumed that environmental breast cancer activists would get involved. Even before the studies on phthalates appeared, some groups had expressed concern with the chemicals because of their xenoestrogenic qualities. Many activists already targeted cosmetics in their arguments that mainstream culture detracts attention from environmental causes of the disease. These targets included the American Cancer Society's Look Good ... Feel Better program and companies such as Avon and Estée Lauder that promote the dominant breast cancer paradigm over disease prevention through their support for events such as National Breast Cancer Awareness Month and Komen's Race for the Cure series. Last, but not least, the campaigns' attention to the reproductive health of male children seemed to resonate with environmental breast cancer activist efforts' on behalf of children's environmental health.

In some ways, my assumption was correct. In the wake of the June and December 2002 phthalate studies, for example, several breast cancer organizations, including Breast Cancer Action and the Breast Cancer Fund, printed brief summaries about the results in their newsletters and e-mail action alerts, and Breast Cancer Action published the URL for Not Too Pretty's Web site in their newsletter. A few breast cancer groups also became politically involved. For example, the Breast Cancer Fund and Breast Cancer Action were members of Health Care Without Harm and Coming Clean—two of the organizations that produced the Not Too Pretty report. In 2003, the Breast Cancer Fund, along with the Alliance for a Healthy Tomorrow, the Clean Water Fund, Commonweal, the Environmental Working Group, Friends of the Earth, the Massachusetts Breast Cancer Coalition, the National Black Environmental Justice Network, the National Environmental Trust, and Women's Voices for the Earth transformed the Not Too Pretty campaign into the Campaign for Safe Cosmetics.[30] Since its inception, the campaign has supported state and federal legislation that would protect consumers from the toxic chemicals found in beauty and personal care products.[31] In 2004, it created the Compact for Safe Cosmetics, which urges U.S. companies to eliminate the use of toxic chemicals in personal care products.[32] The group encourages consumers to take action in their own lives, and its Web site allows them to search Skin Deep, a database developed by the Environmental Working Group that includes information about the safety of almost twenty-five thousand personal care products.[33]

Although the Campaign for Safe Cosmetics targets a broad range of chemicals, health issues, and affected populations, men's health—particularly male reproductive health—plays a role in the coalition. With their emphasis on the reproductive health of men and boys, the 2002 *Not Too Pretty* and *Pretty Nasty* reports, not to mention the Not Too Pretty campaign, served as catalysts for the Campaign for Safe Cosmetic's development. The organization continues to work on men's health issues. In summer 2007, the organization established Get the Lead Out, an online campaign to eliminate the use of lead acetate in Grecian Formula, a hair dye for men made by Combe Incorporated. Lead acetate is not only a carcinogen but also a neurotoxin and reproductive toxin. "We think gray is distinguished," the article reads, "but if he still wants to dye his hair, refer him to the Skin Deep database, where he can find safer alternatives to Grecian Formula." The article encourages readers to demand, via phone and e-mail, that Combe Incorporated stop using lead acetate in its product.[34] The campaign's Web site links to the *Not Too Pretty* and *Pretty Nasty* reports, as well as to various scientific studies on phthalates and male reproductive health.

Despite the participation of some breast cancer groups in the Campaign for Safe Cosmetics, the broader movement's efforts to promote male reproductive health are limited in several ways. Most important, not all breast cancer groups participate in political campaigns to promote the health of men and boys. Nor do all of them write about such issues in their organizational materials—even when these issues (such as phthalates) overlap with environmental breast cancer concerns. Even the groups that are involved in efforts to address male reproductive health do not deal with the subject in substantial terms through their own organizational materials. Consider their coverage of the reports and scientific studies published in 2002 about phthalates in women's personal care products.

Breast Cancer Action's August 2002 e-mail alert about the *Not Too Pretty* report, for example, states that phthalates can impede healthy "development of the male reproductive health system," among other biological organs and processes, but does not describe the specific impacts of the chemicals on this system.[35] Breast Cancer Action's December 2002 newsletter merely states that phthalates "may lead to dangerous levels of exposure for pregnant women and other vulnerable groups," while the Breast Cancer Fund's December 2002 e-mail alert announces, "Recent findings have shown that levels of phthalates in women surpass government safety standards, and the chemicals have been known to damage the liver, kidney and reproductive health systems, and disrupt hormonal processes that could affect breast cancer risk."[36]

The relative lack of attention to male reproductive health extends to breast cancer groups' coverage of the Campaign for Safe Cosmetics, including the materials written by the breast cancer organizations that belong to the coalition. On the Breast Cancer Fund's Web site, the organization describes the campaign, the issues it addresses, and the political work it has done and continues to do. A section outlining some of the campaign's targeted chemicals is the only place in which the organization mentions male reproductive health issues: "Dibutyl Phthalate—a reproductive toxin used in perfumes, hair spray and deodorant— impairs fertility and causes developmental toxicity in male offspring."[37] In its own organizational materials, the Massachusetts Breast Cancer Coalition (MBCC) presents the issue of male reproductive health within the broader context of children's health, reproductive health, and other general categories. Its Web page for the campaign states: "Many of these chemicals have gotten into our bodies, our breast milk and our children. Some of these chemicals are linked to cancer, birth defects and other health problems that are on the rise in the human population. Some chemicals found in a variety of cosmetics—including phthalates, acrylamide, formaldehyde and ethylene oxide—are listed by the EPA and the state of California as carcinogens or reproductive toxins."[38]

A particularly interesting effort by breast cancer activists to raise awareness about male reproductive health issues that I have come across relates to Prevention Is the Cure's endorsement of the Mount Sinai Medical School Center for Children's Health and the Environment's 2002 ad campaign. One of the seven ads in the series focuses on the impact of pesticides, phthalates, PCBs, dioxin, and other synthetics on male reproductive health problems such as declining sperm count, decreased sex ratio, and increased incidence of undescended testicles. The ad's headline reads, "Pesticides Could Become the Ultimate Male Contraceptive. Why?" Below is a photograph of a seated shirtless man staring pensively into space. Behind him, a woman lies sleeping in (presumably) their bed. The ad ends with a call to action: "Though not the sole cause, it's clear that exposures to endocrine disruptors can be contributors to reproductive problems in both animals and humans. . . . Wouldn't we all be better off if chemicals had to be tested for safety before they were out on the market? Certainly males would be better off." Viewers can download this and other ads in the series.[39]

In many ways, the limited attention paid by breast cancer activists to male reproductive health contrasts with their comprehensive efforts promoting children's environmental health. To address the latter issue, activists not only join coalitions and support the work of other groups; they also promote children's environmental health through their own organizational efforts, including legislation, research, and public awareness. They write extensively about such issues in their newsletters and on their Web sites. The difference between their commitment to children's health and that to male reproductive health highlights how they seem to privilege the former over the latter, and it suggests that breast cancer activists are more likely to take on children's health issues when the health of female children is at stake.

During the time in which activists began to address children's health and male reproductive problems, some of them also began to highlight the environmental health issues facing wildlife. Their efforts on behalf of nonhuman populations, however, are even sparser than those directed toward men and male children.

A Total Ecology Approach

In her keynote speech at the MBCC's 1999 conference, "At the Heart of Primary Prevention: Breast Cancer and the Precautionary Principle," the environmental health activist and breast cancer survivor Mary O'Brien declared that breast cancer activists needed to take a "total ecology" approach in order to eradicate the disease. According to O'Brien, solving the problem of breast cancer requires attention to the health problems affecting the entire ecosystem. Although she encouraged activists to work on other human health issues, especially those affecting children, she stressed the importance of resolving the health issues affecting wildlife and the earth's natural resources. In front of some one hundred activists, scientists, and community members, she said:

> Our breasts are simply ONE marvelous part in Earth's systems. As a scientist, I do not think we are going to be able to stop the breast cancer epidemic until we make sure ALL the Earth's embryos and longest-living individuals are clean. . . . If we're going to put our bodies and our breasts

back together, if we're going to restore functioning of OUR hormone systems, we're going to have to restore the hormone systems of the frogs. We're going to have to allow peregrine falcon eggs to get thicker. We're going to have to put estuaries and streams and grasslands and the winds and the ozone layer back together. We're going to have to reconstruct our transportation systems so we don't mine the Artic National Wildlife refuge for oil and kill each other with exhaust pipes every time we go to the grocery store. We're going to have to reconstruct our agriculture so that farms are not hazardous chemical sites, but instead are safe habitats for wildlife and farmworkers and farm owners' embryos. We're going to have to consider what it means to know and care for children, to avoid forcing them into a world that has no room for anything but humans.

She went on to encourage MBCC and other breast cancer groups to form partnerships with environmental and conservation groups such as "the Sierra Club, the Isaac Walton League, hunters' organizations, the Nature Conservancy, Planned Parenthood, and Republicans for Environmental Protection of America."[40]

O'Brien constructed these kinships because many of the health problems affecting humans, wildlife, and the earth itself are linked to the same types of toxic substances, especially endocrine disrupters. She also did so because she believes that preventing breast cancer—not to mention other environmental health problems—requires a new local and global precautionary ethic that encourages individuals, institutions, and communities to interact with their natural and built environments in healthy and ecologically sustainable ways. For these reasons, she urged breast cancer activists to collaborate with organizations that focus on wildlife and ecological health, as well as with groups that address human health.

By the time of O'Brien's speech, some breast cancer groups were already thinking beyond breast cancer and human health more generally, especially in relation to their work on endocrine disrupters. In addition to incorporating wildlife evidence into their environmental breast cancer efforts, they linked their Web sites to the World Wildlife Foundation and related organizations. Breast cancer activists forged alliances with groups that focused on wildlife and conservation issues to promote their public health agendas. For example, MBCC and the Lowell Center for Sustainable Production teamed with Clean Water Action to form the Massachusetts Precautionary Principle Project. Other breast cancer groups (for instance, Women's Community Cancer Project and Silent Spring Institute), wildlife groups (among them World Wildlife Foundation) and conservation organizations (including the Sierra Club and the Nature

Conservancy) also took part in the project. The National Audubon Society, in turn, helped to organize the 2000 AAAS workshop on endocrine disrupters and fertility. Although the meeting agenda stated that human health was the focus, it argued that wildlife issues were relevant to the meeting because evidence from wildlife presented the strongest case that endocrine-disrupting chemicals compromised the health of living beings.

Despite their collaborations with wildlife and conservation groups in promoting human health, breast cancer groups have done less to promote the health of wildlife itself. To be sure, such groups occasionally promote actions to prevent breast cancer that would also protect the health of animals. The Huntington Breast Cancer Action Coalition runs the "I Am Fed Naturally" lawn flag program, which encourages residents to avoid the use of pesticides on their lawn, in their gardens, and in other areas. Participants in the program can stake a pink flag in their yard declaring that their lawn is chemical free. Ultimately, the purpose is to teach community members organic landscaping techniques so that they can "approach their partnership with the ecosystem in a more natural way. . . . Eliminating the use of toxic pesticides, you can protect your health, children, pets, and wildlife."[41] Such efforts, however, to protect the health of wildlife are the exception rather than the rule.

Consider the Breast Cancer Fund's e-mail action alerts. In 2002, the organization sent such alerts to its constituents asking them to support more stringent policies related to radioactive waste storage, clean air standards, global warming, climate change, clean water, and the production and usage of energy—some of the same ecological issues that O'Brien discussed in her call-to-action speech at the MBCC's 1999 conference.[42] Many alerts discussed the impact of environmental policies on human heath disorders. Its October 2002 action alert, "Demand a Responsible Energy Policy," states, "As we continue to see a rise in diseases linked to environmental toxins, including breast cancer, asthma, and birth defects, it's critical that our government act now to reduce pollution." Other alerts tended to focus on the health of the earth for its own sake. The "Demand a Responsible Energy Policy" alert claims that "the current proposed [energy] bill fails to promote clean energy alternatives, threatens conservation efforts and weakens consumer protections against corporations."[43] Similarly, the November 2002 action alert "Preserve the Clean Water Act," explains, "The Bush Administration has proposed redefining and narrowing the waters that are protected under the law. This change will remove critical waterways and wetlands from federal protection, giving polluters free license to fill, dredge and dump waste into these waters—and their polluted runoff will threaten our water quality."[44] For the most part, however, the Breast Cancer Fund's action alerts have neglected to highlight the relevance of these local, state, and federal efforts to protect the earth's natural resources for wildlife health.

Such inattention from environmental breast cancer organizations is striking, given that wildlife groups embraced some of the aforementioned causes when working to protect the health of nonhuman species. The National Audubon Society has promoted clean water for years, particularly in wetlands, since healthy wetlands are critical to the well-being of the birds and other wildlife that live in them. Most recently, the organization supported the Clean Water Restoration Act of 2007 (H.R. 2421), which would restore not only provisions stripped from the 1972 Clean Water Act in 2001 and 2006 but also the EPA's authority to enforce these provisions.[45] The National Audubon Society sits on the steering committee of the Clean Water Network, a coalition of more than one thousand environmental, conservation, and public health organizations founded in 2000 to promote clean and healthy waterways through new legislation, increased funding for clean water programs, and the enforcement of clean water regulations and laws. The coalition seeks to restore the full scope of the 1972 Clean Water Act, especially through the passage of the 2007 Clean Water Restoration Act.[46] The organization also works to eliminate global warming, in part by developing fact sheets examining its impact on wildlife.[47]

Nor have environmental breast cancer activists participated in campaigns organized by wildlife and conservation groups to address the specific impact of environmental exposures on the health of wildlife. This is true even when the chemicals at hand have ties to breast cancer. Again the case of the National Audubon Society is instructive. Since 2001, the society has sought to block a series of bills in Congress that would open up Alaska's Arctic Wildlife Refuge for oil drilling and has worked to pass legislation to prohibit oil drilling on the reserve. The organization opposes this drilling partly because of the health dangers that oil spills and chemical emissions would likely have on the birds and other wildlife that live in the reserve. The society bases these concerns on the toxic legacy left by the oil drilling at Kenai National Wildlife Refuge, which began in the 1960s. Scientists believe that release of PCBs, benzene, antifreeze, xylene, solvents, and other chemicals from this drilling project into the local environment has led to birth defects and developmental problems among frogs, toads, and salamanders. Such pollution also threatens the habitats of birds and other wildlife that live in the area.[48] Despite all this, I have not seen any newsletter articles or e-mail action alerts written by environmental breast cancer organizations about these wildlife issues.

Although many environmental breast cancer activists seem to share Mary O'Brien's total-ecology approach in theory, few, if any, have truly implemented it in practice. The few groups that take on wildlife issues do so in limited ways. As with their narrow attention to male reproductive health, breast cancer activists' small gestures to the health of wildlife only affirm the privileged status of children's health among activists over other affected populations. At a more fundamental level, the contrast between how breast cancer activists approach the health of children and how they approach the health of wildlife and natural resources demonstrates how such activists privilege the health of humans over that of nonhumans.

The Social Context and Significance of Kinship Building

The fact that activists privilege children's health over men's health and human health over wildlife health is no accident. These kinship decisions reflect the multiple institutional cultures that shape the work of individual organizations and the broader environmental breast cancer movement. As part of their efforts, activists must negotiate these different—yet often intersecting—contexts, which encompass an array of social; cultural; political; ideological; economic; and organizational forces, values, and conditions.

Organizational Priorities and Limitations

Such kinship priorities reflect the organizational identity of the groups that constitute the environmental breast cancer movement. Given that many of these groups view breast cancer prevention as a primary objective, it makes sense that they emphasize children's health over the health of men and wildlife. After all, a growing body of scientific research demonstrates that exposure to toxic chemicals—especially endocrine disrupters—in utero, infancy, and early adolescence contributes to the development of the disease during adulthood. From this perspective, breast cancer prevention is a children's health issue, as risk reduction measures could be taken during the early phases of a female's life cycle.

Limited financial and staff resources further prevent such groups from straying too far from their primary focus on breast cancer. Zero Breast Cancer, for example, employs four full-time and one half-time staff. It relies on external grants for much of its funding. Even if the organization wanted to take on other issues, it would face significant time limitations, given that it has a small staff, and its members run the outreach programs, direct the educational programs, sit on advisory boards, network with scientists, and do the administrative work.[49] Similarly, the Huntington Breast Cancer Action Coalition's limited budget makes it difficult for it to pay its rent, phone bills, and other expenses. It depends on the financial support of local community and business leaders to help cover these expenses.[50] Lorraine Pace of Breast Cancer Help does not even draw a salary, to help the organization stay financially afloat.[51] Women's Community Cancer Center never had paid staff members, relying solely of the efforts of volunteers. In fact, it does not even have its own office space; volunteers do their work from home. The group no longer maintains a Web site or publishes a regular newsletter because of its limited human and financial resources.[52]

Framing Strategies

Another set of factors shaping the ways in which environmental breast cancer activists forge disease kinships relates to the politics of issue framing. To promote and implement their health agendas, activists need public support. To cultivate that support, they must frame the meaning and significance of their objectives in ways that align with the values, beliefs, and experiences of citizens, grant foundations, and policy makers, among others.[53] The focus on children's environmental health is significant from this perspective, especially given that breast cancer activists are not the only ones to emphasize such a focus. Many other organizations that work on environmental health issues, such as Physicians for Social Responsibility, World Resources Institute, Environmental Working Group, Public Interest Research Group, Clean Water Action, and Natural Resources Defense Council, often view their agendas through this lens. Groups such as the Children's Health Environmental Coalition and the Children's Environmental Health Network have been formed specifically to address children's health issues. Indeed, children's health is one of the most popular ways to frame environmental health issues. It is also a popular way in which to frame other contemporary health issues such as universal health care, as illustrated by the recent political debates surrounding the federal S-CHIP program.[54]

The focus on children's environmental health results from the belief that this strategy benefits not only children but humans in general. By protecting the lives of those most biologically vulnerable, the argument goes, everybody is protected. This is especially true with diseases such as breast cancer that researchers increasingly link to early toxic exposures. Moreover, activists connect the protection of children's health to the sustainability of the human race. According to 1 in 9's Geri Barish, "We need to take precaution, not for us but for the next generation. Otherwise, we won't have one."[55] Similarly, Nancy Evans explained that children's health is such a big focus because "children are our future."[56] The children's health frame also has the potential to bolster public and political support because issues of children's health "tug," as Breast Cancer Action's Brenda Salgado put it, at people's emotions in a way that those on the health of adults do not. Indeed, she notes that a number of health and religious organizations agreed to work with Breast Cancer Action on various children's health campaigns because they appealed to these types of sensibilities.[57] Some environmental health activists state that they use the children's health frame in their policy efforts because it increases the chances that their bills will pass; elected officials do not want to seem cold hearted by voting against measures to protect children. As MBCC's Deborah Shields explained, "Let's face it. No one wants to appear that they are against children's health."[58]

The public's concern about children's health is connected to the status of children in contemporary society. Childhood is a socially constructed category. In past centuries, children in Western cultures were viewed as "miniature adults." Only in recent generations have children been seen as biologically, emotionally, psychologically, and socially different from their elders. Two dominant conceptions of children exist in contemporary culture. The first, the Dionysian, views children as inherently naughty and lacking any internal moral or ethical compass. The second conception, the Apollonian, sees children as inherently good, virtuous, and innocent individuals who as they age become corrupted by adults and societal forces. Although these perspectives on childhood fundamentally contradict one another, they share an important assumption: because children cannot take care of themselves, adults must take responsibility for them and guide them into adulthood. From the Dionysian perspective, it is up to adults to socialize children to become "fully human"—that is, to become upstanding, responsible, and moral citizens. From the Apollonian viewpoint, adults and social institutions must take on the responsibility to protect children's inherent goodness by limiting their exposure to negative influences. Both discourses are present in the contemporary political arena, but the latter view is especially prevalent in the public health, advocacy, and policy debates surrounding the protection of children from harmful toxic exposures.[59]

Activists invoke the children's health frame in the context of many environmental issues. At the same time, the growing focus on endocrine disrupters—fueled by the growing body of knowledge that exposure to these chemicals is particularly harmful during early stages of development—strengthened the power of this frame. We might look at the congressional voting record for evidence of this. From 1972 to 1992, Congress introduced not one bill related to children's environmental health. Between 1993 and 2001, they introduced thirty-two.[60] Whereas some of the increased attention resulted from growing congressional concern with children's health in general, much of it resulted from worries in Congress about endocrine disrupters, particularly those found in pesticides. Not coincidentally, 1993 was the year that Theo

Colborn and other scientists, as well as environmental health activists, began testifying at congressional hearings about the need for increased federal funds to examine endocrine disrupters.[61] That same year, some of the first major studies linking endocrine disrupters to children's health disorders appeared. Significantly, some of the earliest legislation related to endocrine disrupters focused on children's health, including California Democratic representative Henry Waxman's 1994 bill to protect children from pesticides, the 1995 introduction of the Food Quality and Protection Act, and the development of the EPA's Endocrine Disrupter Screening and Testing Program.

The Biopolitics of Gender

Another factor that it is important to discuss is gender politics. Breast cancer is a highly gendered disease, as women constitute the vast majority of those afflicted with it. They have spearheaded and continue to lead the bulk of breast cancer organizations and the breast cancer movement more generally. Most breast cancer–related outreach efforts, educational campaigns, support services, biomedical services, policy reform, and corporate fund-raising efforts are geared toward women. Not surprisingly, the gender politics that shape our culture and social institutions also influence the biopolitical terrain of breast cancer, including the kinship strategies taken by the environmental breast cancer movement. Tellingly, such gender politics shape the activist focus on children's health. As women, many breast cancer activists are mothers or potential mothers who care about the health of their children. Moreover, mainstream culture blurs the line between womanhood and motherhood—an identity conflation that leads to the social, psychological, institutional, and political burden of children's health being placed on women and mothers. This burden is especially significant in the context of breast cancer, which links, via pregnancy and breastfeeding, the health of women to that of their children.

Gender politics inform the environmental breast cancer movement's relationship to men's health, particularly male reproductive health issues. To some extent, the fact that breast cancer activists focus relatively little on male reproductive health results from the fact that such issues have historically received little attention from environmental health and public health activists. Instead, most advocacy efforts to address the relationship between environmental exposures and reproductive health—including those put forth by many of the groups attending the AAAS workshop—generally focus on women or children. Indeed, it was because of this lack of attention to the impact of endocrine disrupters and other toxic substances on male reproductive health that Davis proposed her saves the male campaign.

One particularly powerful reason why environmental health activism focuses little on male reproductive health relates to the historical equation of reproductive health with women's health, especially when it comes to understanding the role of hormones in physiological development. Sociologist Nelly Oudshoorn notes that the "hormonal body" that emerged in the early to mid-twentieth century as an object of scientific study, biomedical treatment, and pharmaceutical intervention was assumed to be a woman's body. From the perspective of these research and biomedical fields, hormones influenced women's physiological and emotional development but not the development of men's.[62] This equation of reproductive health with women's health is especially apparent in the controversies surrounding the push to develop a male contraceptive pill—a "technology in the making" that, notes Oudshoorn, problematizes not only scientific and biomedical assumptions about men's reproductive health but also a culture that places the burden of family planning and parenthood on women.[63]

Another reason why environmental health groups pay little attention to male reproductive health issues is that men's health groups have not jumped on the environmental health bandwagon to the extent that breast cancer, women's health, and children's health groups have. To my knowledge, there is no male disease constituency leading the charge to address issues such as decreased sperm count or hypospadias. Even the men's health groups that exist tend to forgo environmental health issues. One notable example is the prostate cancer movement. Some researchers have argued that compelling links exist between the disease and hormone disrupters.[64] For the most part, however, the prostate cancer movement embraces a biomedical approach, working to raise public awareness about the disease; promote support; and encourage early detection, increased funding for basic research, and the development of better treatments and a cure. The movement's preventative efforts tend to focus on diet, smoking, exercise, and other behavioral factors.[65]

Yet another factor shaping how, and to what extent, breast cancer activists address men's health relates to the feminism that has been integral to the environmental breast cancer movement. On the one hand, some breast cancer activists believe that working on behalf of men—as well as other affected populations such as children and wildlife—promotes the health of women. Devra Davis argues that because much of the evidence linking endocrine disrupters to breast cancer is limited, situating breast cancer within a broader framework of wildlife and men's health builds a stronger case for why concern about xeno-estrogens and breast cancer is warranted. Similarly, Mary O'Brien believes that breast cancer will only be eradicated by working to eliminate the environmental health problems faced by all humans, animals, and the earth itself. For O'Brien, a total-ecology approach is a feminist approach. On the other hand, feminist values lead some activists to be critical of such connections. One activist worries that coalitions with men's health groups would lead their (presumably) male activists to rely on female breast cancer activists to do their work. Her concern is provoked by her work with prostate cancer activists who started to mobilize in the wake of the breast cancer movement's early success in the 1990s.[66] Referring to the specific context of endocrine disrupter theory, this activist also went on to say that forging links between breast cancer in women and male reproductive health disorders may make intellectual sense to scientists but would not make emotional sense to the public.[67]

The feminist roots of the environmental breast cancer movement may act as a catalyst for the movement's attention to the health issues of populations perceived as socially, politically, and economically vulnerable—such as women and children—as opposed to the health concerns of men, who, as a group, hold disproportionate levels of social, political, and economic power. The title of Nancy Evan's 1993 article, "The Persistence of Pesticides: Women and Children First," not only refers to the fact that women and children may have particular biological susceptibilities to pesticides and other endocrine-disrupting chemicals; it also suggests that their health deserves protection because of their marginalized position in society.[68] From this perspective, the empathy of activists with vulnerable and marginalized populations other than women explains why the efforts that they do take in the environmental health issues of men often involve addressing the environmental injustices facing low-income communities, especially those that are also communities of color.

Anthropocentrism

Another factor inhibiting wider efforts of activists is anthropocentrism. The lack of attention to conservation and wildlife health issues by environmental breast cancer activists results from the human-centered focus of environmental health activism in general. To some extent, this anthropocentrism reflects growing activist attention to the impact of environmental toxins on human health that occurred during the 1980s and 1990s. Before this time, environmental activism focused primarily on wildlife and conservation issues, whereas public health and consumer activism focused on human health issues. During this period, however, the separation between environmental issues and human health issues began to dissolve, especially in relation to increased understanding of endocrine disrupters and other environmental exposures. Not only did public health, community, and consumer groups begin to address environmental causes of human disorders; long-standing wildlife and conservation groups such as the Sierra Club and Greenpeace also began to take on human health issues. This increased activist attention to human environmental health issues results from political and scientific factors, including—but not limited to—the efforts by environmental justice activists to address environmental racism in low-income neighborhoods and communities of color; the attempts by cancer, women's cancer, and breast cancer activists to determine why the U.S. War on Cancer has failed to cure cancer and prevent it from occurring; and the efforts of Theo Colborn and others to raise public and political awareness about the implications of endocrine disrupter theory for human health.[69]

The anthropocentrism within environmental health activism reflects long-standing belief systems in Euro-American and industrial societies that place more value on the well-being and needs of humans than on those of nonhuman species. In addition to shaping activism and policies related to environmental health, these belief systems have shaped religious institutions, economic systems, political ideologies, technoscience, biomedical practices, and sociocultural values related to notions of progress and modernization. According to many environmental, spiritual, and feminist thinkers, this anthropocentric bias has led to the contamination and destruction of the earth's ecosystems and resources. Such anthropocentrism led Mary O'Brien to call on breast cancer activists and other audience members at her 1999 keynote speech to avoid forcing children "into a world that has no room for anything but humans."[70]

Interestingly, anthropocentrism also influences both wildlife and conservation activism. Although environmental breast cancer and other human-focused environmental health activists tend not to take on wildlife and conservation issues, many groups that focus on the health of nonhuman species actively work on human health campaigns. Besides joining coalitions working on behalf of human health, such organizations often highlight the relevance that their campaigns hold for human health. The World Wildlife Federation, for instance, runs a toxics program that seeks to eradicate the dangers posed by harmful chemicals in the environment for not only wildlife but also people: "Wherever scientists look—the tropics, marine systems, industrial regions, the Arctic—they find the effects of toxic chemicals. Wildlife, people and entire ecosystems are threatened by chemicals that can alter sexual and neurological development, impair reproduction, and undermine immune systems."[71] Among its efforts to reduce the burden of such chemicals, the group recently promoted alternatives to the use of pesticides in agricultural practices because of their impact on the health and biodiversity of wildlife that live in toxic-laden agricultural regions. As part of these efforts, the organization pointed to the health impacts of pesticides for human consumers, farmworkers, and other individuals who also live in these regions.[72]

In other cases, wildlife conservation groups strive to protect wildlife through initiatives aimed at improving human health. As part of its toxics program, the World Wildlife Foundation encourages consumers to eliminate endocrine disrupters and other toxic chemicals in their homes and communities through strategies such as buying organic produce and clothing, relying on nontoxic pest management, and using chemical-free cleaning products. Such measures benefit wildlife because human actions are embedded within broader ecosystems.[73] Similarly, the National Audubon Society argues that to protect the destruction of natural habitats and the animals that live in them, the "population momentum" among humans, particularly those in developing countries, must decrease. The organization supports international family planning efforts, as well as the social, cultural, political, and economic empowerment of women worldwide. The more power women have in their personal lives, families, and communities, the fewer children they tend to have.[74]

When it comes to addressing diseases other than breast cancer and affected populations besides women, it is certainly the case that environmental breast cancer organizations can only do so much. The assorted barriers and social contexts faced by such organizations make it difficult to take on a broad array of health issues that go beyond their primary focus on breast cancer and women's health. At the same time, it is also true that most, if not all, groups extend their focus beyond breast cancer, albeit to different degrees and in varying ways. Thus, it is important to assess the impact (intended or not) of activists' kinship choices on their everyday work, their professional relationships, and their political and public health goals.

In a broader sense, examining the kinship choices made by environmental breast cancer activists points to potential sites of cultural intervention. Bringing an increased focus to men's reproductive health and wildlife health, for example, may not only provide other frameworks through which to address the breast cancer problem but also help to broaden the gendered scope of reproductive health and allow the public to increasingly imagine a world that makes room for other beings besides humans, as Mary O'Brien might put it. To be sure, most environmental breast cancer groups are not necessarily willing or able make men's health and wildlife health priorities. That said, the social, political, scientific connections that activists already make between breast cancer and these other types of concerns have helped to put environmental health issues on the public, political, and scientific agenda.

Chapter 8

Still in the Making

In November 2006, my husband and I began in vitro fertilization (IVF) treatments after several years of unsuccessfully trying to start a family. As much as I tried to focus on the process for its own sake, I often found myself filtering it through the lens of breast cancer. Given that I was writing a book that dealt with synthetic estrogens—and that I had done my best to avoid them since beginning my research in the mid-1990s—it was difficult not to think about the treatments in these terms. I felt uneasy about the various synthetic hormones—birth control pills, estrogen replacement patches, progesterone oil, ovarian suppression drugs, and ovarian stimulation drugs—that I had to use during the IVF cycles. The absence of definitive evidence for a link between infertility treatments and breast cancer did not alleviate my worries, as I knew that absence of proof did not necessarily mean absence of harm.[1] At the same time, I worried about not getting pregnant, given that this would mean not experiencing pregnancy and not having the opportunity to breastfeed—both of which I wanted to experience on their own, as well as for the sake of reducing my breast cancer risk.

I also considered my fertility treatments in relation to my broader risk profile. It is true that I did not have many established risk factors for the disease. Up to 50 percent of all women with the disease, however, had no such factors. Moreover, I had concerns about various emerging—if not necessarily proven—risk factors. Specifically, I had had significant exposure to home pesticides during a two-year period that coincided with my puberty, as well as daily exposure to secondhand smoke during my childhood. On some days I felt excitement about the IVF; on others I was scared.

In many respects, my ruminations about IVF demonstrate how far environmental breast cancer activism has come since its inception. Over the past two decades, this movement in the making has changed how I—and many others—think about the problem of breast cancer. Since I began my research, I have added new toxins to my list of health risks to avoid or, at the very least, about which to be concerned. I have become more cognizant of past exposures to toxic chemicals, especially during my early childhood and adolescence, and it has empowered me to take actions to reduce my risk of developing the disease through healthy dietary choices and the avoidance of harmful personal care products, household cleaners, and other sources of exposure. Indeed, the movement has influenced the way I conceptualize risk by making the case for why it is important to take preventative actions when definitive proof of harm is lacking. It has helped me to recognize that breast cancer is only one facet of a broader set of environmental health problems facing men, women, children, animals, and the earth itself.

At the same time, my thoughts about IVF highlight that the environmental breast cancer movement is a work in progress. Activists and their allied scientists still have much to learn about the causes of breast cancer and the best methods for studying them. They still must work to implement more stringent environmental regulations locally, nationally, and globally. They must ensure that all women, not merely those who, like me, are socially and economically privileged, can take action to reduce their breast cancer risk and work for broader environmental health change. Just as the movement has evolved socially, culturally, politically, and scientifically over the past twenty years, so will it continue to evolve in the future. "Turning up the volume" on the movement's emerging directions of action provides important insights into where it is heading and what this may mean for women's health and societal health more generally, in the United States and beyond.[2]

Emerging Causes and Risk Factors

The environmental breast cancer movement has played—and continues to play—an important role in advancing the production of scientific knowledge regarding suspected environmental causes of the disease, especially endocrine disrupters. Indeed, its early efforts to identify such causes still resonate today. One example is research on cadmium, the xenoestrogen that Lorraine Pace and other activists identified as a possible cause of high breast cancer rates on Long Island. In June 2006, investigators from the University of Wisconsin Comprehensive Cancer Center conducted the first epidemiological study demonstrating that women with breast cancer had higher levels of cadmium in their urine than those of women without the disease.[3] Twenty years after Ana Soto and Carlos Sonneschein discovered that seemingly benign materials contained xenoestrogenic compounds, public health officials, policymakers, the media, and the public are finally taking notice and demanding regulatory action, most notably with regard to bisphenol A and phthalates.

One of the most compelling directions for future research, however, relates not so much to specific chemicals as to the timing of exposure. Bourgeoning research on early exposures is transforming the terrain of breast cancer science significantly. As it becomes increasingly evident that exposures during childhood and adolescence increase the risk for developing breast cancer later in life, it is also becoming clear that conventional epidemiological methods are inadequate for understanding breast cancer risk. Indeed, Zero Breast Cancer's Janice Barlow believes that "the model of studying the levels of chemicals in adult women's bodies is over."[4] This realization has led activists and scientists to devise better methods for assessing the nature and impact of early exposures through approaches such as the historical construction of risk. For example, they continue to refine geographic information system technology, analyses of past industrial and environmental records, and cognitive strategies for jogging women's memories of their past exposures. Still, reconstructing exposures that took place years if not decades ago is inherently fraught with difficulties and limitations. Moreover, it is often difficult to receive funding to develop such methods, given that this type of research tends to be policy driven rather than propelled by hypothesis. Thus, other types of methods are needed for assessing the effects of early exposures.

An alternative to historical reconstruction measurement is the study of exposures as they take place during the early stages of the life cycle. This innovative approach guides the epidemiological and experimental research taking place at the federally funded Breast Cancer and Environmental Research Centers run by Michigan State University, the University of California at San Francisco, the University of Cincinnati, and the Fox Chase Cancer Center in Philadelphia. It also partly drives the recent push for biomonitoring, which tracks the presence of levels of chemicals in the bodies of adults and children. As EPA cancer epidemiologist Ruth Allen explains, "We won't know how to prevent breast cancer if we don't know what is in people's bodies."[5] As shown by the passage of California Senate Bill 1379 in 2006, some biomonitoring efforts take place at the state level. More recently, activists have expanded their focus to the national level. The Breast Cancer Fund worked with Senator Hillary Clinton of New York and Speaker of the House Nancy Pelosi of California, both Democrats, to introduce the Coordinated Environmental Public

Health Network Act of 2007. This legislation (S. 2082 and H.R. 3643), if passed, would expand programs that conduct biomonitoring, provide for the compiling of public health data, and establish a service to assess and address disease clusters and regional environmental exposures. Ultimately, the development and coordination of such programs will allow public health officials to make connections between geographic exposures, disease clusters, and chemicals found in people's bodies.[6]

The growing attention to early exposures also shapes prevention efforts. Beyond focusing on adult women at risk for the disease, activists increasingly gear their prevention efforts toward girls, their parents, teachers, and pediatricians. This approach aims to reduce some of the early risk factors that girls face. Zero Breast Cancer's Breast Cancer and Environment Peer Toolkit educates teens in local schools about modifiable risk factors for the disease, presenting behavioral risk factors and risk reduction strategies, identifying environmental risk factors such as exposure to phthalates, and discussing ways to avoid them. Zero Breast Cancer's Web site links to the program's curriculum materials for use by other activists and educators.[7] Taking an even broader approach, the Babylon Breast Cancer Coalition (BBCC) runs Be Smart About Your Health, a program designed to teach children in grades one through six about the chemicals in their environment. The program focuses not on the specific disease outcomes associated with the chemicals but on the identification of such chemicals and the reasons for why, in a general sense, it is healthier to avoid them. BBCC provides the children with information packets to bring home to their parents explaining what they learned and how to take steps to minimize their children's exposure to toxic substances, and the group leaves information with the teachers for them to integrate into their curricula. BBCC's Time for Change program further targets children by reaching out to parents, women's groups, and PTA meetings.[8]

As environmental breast cancer research continues to evolve, so too does the relationship between activists and scientists. In the movement's early years, activists were the ones reaching out to scientists, asking them to take their research concerns seriously. Long Island activists, for example, demanded not only that scientists carry out a study of the region's breast cancer rates but also that the activists be allowed to play a role in the research process. Similarly, Zero Breast Cancer cold-called local scientists to ask them to serve as coinvestigators for the Adolescent Risk Factor Study. It took numerous tries before they found an epidemiologist who agreed to participate in the project. During this early phase of the movement, many activists saw themselves as scientific novices, not fully understanding how the research process worked. This naïveté, as numerous activists characterized it, led to mistakes and caused them to take aspects of the research process for granted. On Long Island activists assumed that biological samples collected by the scientists with whom they collaborated belonged to the community, as they came from the bodies of local residents. Only later did they realize that the scientists owned the samples. Zero Breast Cancer was "surprised to learn" that the community would not have control of certain types of data that was collected during the Adolescent Risk Factors study. After the organization took the matter up with the project's funder, however, the community became the data's repository.[9]

Since then, activists have become more scientifically savvy. Many have a strong grasp of environmental breast cancer and can assess the strengths and weaknesses of particular research methods and study designs. They know how to position themselves as legitimate participants in the research process. Before agreeing to collaborate with researchers, Zero Breast Cancer insists on their signing a contract stating that the community owns whatever samples they collect. For its part, the scientific community takes activists more seriously. Increasingly, scientists take the initiative and ask activists to participate in their research projects. Given that Zero Breast Cancer now receives so many requests of this sort, the organization screens scientists to make sure that their perspectives and goals align with its own. In fact, it turned down one offer because the researcher did not believe that environmental factors played a role in breast cancer.[10] Similarly, the National Cancer Institute and the National Institute of Environmental Health Sciences regularly ask activists to participate in their studies and sit on their advisory boards. In short, many scientists recognize that taking activists seriously, especially during a project's design phase, will help the progress of their research. As Karen Miller explains, "We [activists] keep our ear to the ground. We are well aware of the health concerns and questions that are paramount to our communities. Scientists should address these concerns. With increased opportunities for open dialogue, there will be increased trust and transparency between community and researchers, as well as the sharing of information among various disciplines that equates to needed change and continuance of environmental research."[11]

Fifteen years after activists proposed their first environmental breast cancer research projects, they continue to develop new ones. The Massachusetts Breast Cancer Coalition, the Silent Spring Institute, and the University of Massachusetts at Lowell are working to establish a state-funded environmental breast cancer research program. If the state legislature approves the $1 million annual budget to run the program, scientists from Massachusetts could apply for funds to conduct environmental health research in communities across the state. Ideally, the findings from this research would spur future studies by other investigators in the state and across the nation. In the meantime, Silent Spring and the University of Massachusetts at Lowell are conducting the Breast Cancer Prevention Project, which maps breast cancer incidence across the state over time. The findings from this project will be a foundation for future research efforts on possible environmental factors implicated in the state's high breast cancer rates.[12]

The California Breast Cancer Research Program, founded in 1992 as a collaborative research venture between activists, scientists, survivors, clinicians, and researchers across the state, is a model for the type of program that the Massachusetts groups seek to establish. Since 1992, the California program has spent more than $200 million on breast cancer research, including research on environmental exposures, which has had national and international impact. Yet just as the Massachusetts Breast Cancer Coalition, Silent Spring, and the university hope to start their program, California activists are scrambling to save theirs. In 2008, the University of California Office of the President (UCOP) proposed that it gut the California Breast Cancer Research Program by eliminating its planning, evaluation, and information dissemination functions. This cut would weaken the most innovative aspect of the program's research decision-making process—the collaborative effort by "survivors, advocates and activists, scientists, clinicians, and researchers"—by putting funding decisions into the hands of what Breast Cancer Action calls "UCOP bureaucrats."[13] Time will tell whether efforts to save the innovative and collaborative aspects of program are successful.

Broadening the Movement's Social and Geographic Focus

Although the most powerful and extensive networks of environmental breast cancer activism are in the San Francisco Bay Area, in Greater Boston, and on Long Island, it is important not to overlook the efforts by other environmental breast cancer groups around the country. For example, Ithaca, New York, is home to the Cancer Resource Center of the Finger Lakes. Founded in 1994 as the Ithaca Breast Cancer Alliance, the organization changed its name in 2007 to reflect its focus on "everybody affected by cancer." Since its inception, the organization has worked on various breast cancer issues, including prevention. In 1996, the organization was asked to serve on the advisory board of the New York State Program on Breast Cancer and Environmental Risk Factors. Many of the group's annual meetings have featured prominent speakers—among them Sandra Steingraber (2000) and Devra Davis (2003)—who study and write about breast cancer and other environmental health issues.[14] Also located in Ithaca is the Program on Breast Cancer and Environmental Risk Factors at Cornell University, funded by the New York State Departments of Health and Environmental

Conservation and the U.S. Department of Agriculture that conducts research on risk perception and risk communication strategies. Established in 1995, it translates research conducted on environmental factors associated with breast cancer into forms of knowledge that can be used by health professionals, policymakers, educators, activists, other scientists, and the general public. In addition to housing such information on its extensive Web site in the form of fact sheets, resource pages, geographic maps, bibliographies, and a research database, the program publishes several newsletters a year, holds public meetings, and sends representatives to activist and scientific conferences.[15]

It is also important to recognize that new regions of activism continue to form. Washington State is a compelling example. A 2005 federal study found that the state has the highest breast cancer incidence rates in the country (147.8 cases per one hundred thousand women compared with 124.9 cases nationally). King, Ferry, Island, San Juan, and Garfield counties—all in the Seattle metro area—have the state's highest rates. Disproportionate levels of childlessness, wide spread use of hormone replacement therapy, heavy alcohol consumption, deficiencies of Vitamin D and sunlight, exposure to household toxics, and circadian disruption are factors named as possible causes of Seattle's high rates. Significant air pollution in King County, where Seattle is located, puts residents at 100 times greater risk for cancer than the goal established by the U.S. Clean Air Act, and the lower Duwamish River is considered one of the most contaminated sites in the county, containing PCBs, mercury, and other persistent toxic chemicals. The state as a whole also contains several hundred toxic sites contaminated with dioxin, PAHs, PCBs, and other chemicals.[16]

To address the environmental dimensions of Washington's growing breast cancer problem, the Breast Cancer Fund teamed with state activists, scientists, and health professionals as part of the Washington Toxic-Free Legacy Coalition. To conduct this work, the organization hired a Washington state coordinator.[17] Along with the Washington State Departments of Ecology and Health, the Washington State Nurses Association, the Washington State Medical Association, and other groups, the Breast Cancer Fund helped to spearhead the passage of legislation prohibiting the use of toxic flame retardants known as PBDEs. This bill, the first of its kind in the nation, bans the use of such chemicals by 2008 or 2011, depending on the type. The EPA classifies one type of PBDE, deca, as a possible carcinogen, and in vitro studies have found that PBDEs function as xenoestrogens, making them a possible risk factor for breast cancer.[18] In October 2007, the Breast Cancer Fund organized talks in Seattle and Olympia at which Sandra Steingraber discussed her new publication (co-written with the group), "The Falling Age of Puberty in U.S. Girls: What We Know, What We Need to

Know." The organization encourages its members and other citizens to participate in its Washington-based efforts.[19]

Environmental breast cancer organizations work to mobilize citizens and activists in other regions around the country, as well. The Breast Cancer Fund (BCF), for example, provides a "legislative tool kit" that citizens can apply to their own local and state-based campaigns, in working toward policy reform related to biomonitoring, chemical regulations, safe cosmetics, and toxic toys. BCF also provides a list of "tips on becoming an advocate for prevention," including strategies for "[using] your voice" to raise public awareness about environmental breast cancer issues; meeting with political representatives; and joining the Strong Voice Leadership Development Program, a "nationwide network of women and men who share their personal stories while inspiring the public to take action to end the breast cancer epidemic."[20] Similarly, Breast Cancer Action disseminates guides for individuals and organizations seeking to pass Stop Cancer Where It Starts resolutions in their own cities as a way to promote and implement the precautionary principle nationwide.[21]

While the environmental breast cancer movement expands geographically, it also continues to grow socially and culturally. Activists are developing new strategies for incorporating the needs ands perspectives of women of color and low-income women in the movement via advisory boards, leadership positions, town halls, forums, and other venues. Of particular note is the work to identify the environmental factors that may contribute to high levels of breast cancer incidence and mortality in communities of color, especially among younger African American women. As part of the state-funded environmental breast cancer research program that it hopes to establish, the Silent Spring Institute plans to extend its household assessment research to low-income communities and communities of color across the state.[22] The California Breast Cancer Research Program has created initiatives to examine "environmental exposures and breast cancer among large and diverse groups of women at several points through their life" and to find the reasons "why people from different racial and ethnic groups have different survival outcomes, despite being diagnosed with breast cancer at the same stage."[23] When it comes to protecting the health of women of color and low-income women, activists have already broadened their approaches to prevention through strategies such as focusing on workers, in addition to consumers, and devising inexpensive strategies for reducing one's personal risks. The findings from these emerging lines of research could have significant implications for the direction of future prevention efforts.

The increasing environmental efforts by so-called mainstream organizations reflect another change in the environmental breast cancer movement's social terrain. Groups such as Susan G. Komen for the Cure and the American Cancer Society have taken bigger steps to support environmental health and prevention issues through measures such as lobbying for the for federal funds for environmental breast cancer research, funding the scientific and political work of other environmental breast cancer groups, and developing their own environmental health materials. Even Avon—the company that activists criticize for its refusal to remove chemicals linked to breast cancer from its products, its perpetuation of mainstream breast cancer culture through its awareness and fund-raising efforts, and its lack of financial oversight with regard to its annual 2-Day Walk—has gotten involved. In July 2008, the Avon Foundation contributed five hundred thousand dollars to the California Breast Cancer Research Program, a grant that will fund, among other things, research on environmental links to breast cancer.[24]

The growing interest in environmental health issues by these sorts of institutions is, in many respects, a positive development. Such institutions not only reach a vast array of women across the country but also possess substantial financial resources and political clout and therefore have the potential to effect change. Plus, the more organizations that work on environmental breast cancer issues, the better. Indeed, the efforts by these groups may reflect that environmental health concerns have already begun to seep into mainstream culture. Yet the fact that the dominant breast cancer paradigm has historically guided and continues to guide the bulk of their work raises legitimate concerns about their overall commitment to environmental issues. It begs the question of whether these recent initiatives reflect a bona fide change of focus on the part of the institutions, the hard-won efforts of a few board members or staff, a need for the organizations to respond strategically to a growing body of criticism of their inattention to environmental factors and prevention, or some of each. There is also the potential for the groups to co-opt the environmental breast cancer issue, watering down its more radical elements—particularly its critiques of corporate, political, and other structural forms of power—and constructing it primarily through the lens of individual behavior and choice. Perhaps cautious optimism about these efforts is warranted, especially given that paradigm shifts within institutions tend to take place incrementally over time.

Going Global

Working to pass more stringent environmental regulations at the local and state levels is an important political strategy, as it is often easier to get environmental health legislation passed there than at the federal level. It is also true that local and state legislation not only helps to protect the people who live in particular areas, but also puts pressure on other cities, counties, states, and even the federal government to follow suit. The success of this strategy is illustrated by the San Francisco Bay Area's Stop Cancer Where It Starts ordinances; California's Safe Cosmetics and Safe Toys Acts; the Safe and Sustainable Purchasing Bill, passed by Long Island's Suffolk County in March 2007; and the Green Procurement Policy, passed by Nassau County in April 2008. These last two bills require that the counties review their use of harmful products and purchase safer alternatives. Seattle, San Francisco, and New York City had passed similar legislation earlier.[25] Another piece of proposed legislation that the Alliance for a Healthy Tomorrow helped to develop has made significant progress toward becoming law in Massachusetts. In June 2007, the Joint Committee on Environment, Natural Resources, and Agriculture held a key hearing on the "Safer Alternatives Bill." Seven months later, the legislation passed the Massachusetts Senate. As of July 2008, the bill was under consideration by the House Committee on Ways and Means.[26]

Yet activists also recognize the need to develop a global perspective when it comes to environmental policy reform and breast cancer prevention. Taking a global approach to the environmental breast cancer problem is important for various reasons. Breast cancer is the most commonly diagnosed cancer among women worldwide, with an estimated 1.3 million new cases of invasive breast cancer occurring in 2007. That year, there were 465,000 deaths from the disease. The United States has the highest incidence rates, but other countries are catching up. In Western countries, incidence rates have increased around 30 percent over the past twenty-five years. In England, there were 56 cases per 100,000 women in 1975; in 2004, there were 88. Incidence rates are also rising in developing countries, where they have historically been relatively low. Indeed, cases in developing countries will constitute 70 percent of all breast cancer cases by 2020.[27] In part what is behind the growing global breast cancer problem is the spread of Western culture. Western cuisine is replacing traditional, often healthier, diets. Increased industrialization and reliance on technology lead to decreased levels of physical activity and greater body weight. Changing gender roles mean that more women delay childbirth or have fewer children to pursue educational and professional opportunities. Biological factors may intermingle with these behavioral risks. Asian women, for example, tend to have particularly dense breasts, a greater risk for carrying BRCA1 and BRCA2, and a higher chance of developing the so-called triple negative form of the disease.[28] Toxic exposures may also play a role in the global rise of breast cancer rates, especially in countries with lax environmental regulations and expanding industrialization.

One important strategy that U.S. activists use to understand and address environmental breast cancer issues facing other countries is networking with their international counterparts. Some U.S. groups have already formed international coalitions, such as Prevention First, to tackle health and policy issues of relevance to multiple countries. U.S. activists also network via conferences. Of particular note is the World Conference on Breast Cancer organized by the Canadian-based World Conference on Breast Cancer Foundation. This conference, which the foundation has hosted four times since 1997, seeks "to build and strengthen international networks involved with breast cancer" and "to move forward and advance global and local action related to breast cancer issues."[29] All past conferences featured activists and scientists who spoke about, among other topics, environmental breast cancer issues around the world. In October 2007, Deborah Shields and Erin Boles of the Massachusetts Breast Cancer Coalition flew to Béthune, France, to participate in a conference focused solely on breast cancer and the environment. This area is known for its heavy industrialization and high breast cancer incidence rates. Although France has more stringent environmental health protection than does the United States, health activists and public health officials have not addressed the link between breast cancer and toxic substances to the degree that their U.S. counterparts have. The Massachusetts Breast Cancer Coalition spoke at the conference not only to learn about the environmental breast cancer problem in this region but also to provide local activists with ideas, information, and strategies for mobilizing around the issue.[30]

A global perspective is especially important given the ubiquitous nature of toxic exposures. Although policy reform at the local, state, and federal levels are beneficial, they do not stop the transnational flow of chemicals and other harmful substances, which I call "toxicscapes." Toxicscapes are similar to the five types of global cultural flows—ethnoscapes, technoscapes, mediascapes, ideoscapes, and financescapes—identified by anthropologist Arjun Appadurai.[31] Chemicals can cross national borders by air, waterways, precipitation, and wind, as well as through food products, toys, household products, and other commercial goods imported and exported as part of the expanding networks of global economies and trade. From this perspective, it is important to promote not only stronger environmental regulations in certain countries but also international treaties to eliminate the worldwide production and use of toxic chemicals. One such treaty addresses persistent organic pollutants (POPs): the Stockholm Convention on Persistent Organic Pollutants, which seeks to end the production of "intentionally produced" POPs (such as DDT, PCBs, and other industrial chemicals and pesticides) as well as the release of "unintentionally produced" POPs (such as dioxin and furans). The convention also calls for the management and disposal of existing POPs in a "safe, effective, and environmentally sound manner."[32] The United Nations treaty was adopted at the May 2001 Conference of Plenipotentiaries in Stockholm. One hundred eighty-four countries participated, and 152 of the participants ratified the treaty. The United States signed on to the convention in May 2001 but Congress has yet to ratify it.[33]

A global perspective further encourages activists to look at other countries as role models for how chemical regulation in the Unites States should work. In April 2008, Canada became the first country to define bisphenol A as a toxic substance, and it banned the "sale, import, and advertising" of baby bottles containing the chemical.[34] Many U.S. environmental breast cancer groups point to Canada's decision when putting pressure on the federal government to take a similar stand. On a broader scale, they look to the European Union as a model for U.S. environmental health policy more generally. In 2001, the European Union developed a new chemical regulatory system named REACH (Registration, Evaluation, and Authorisation of Chemicals). This system seeks to manage the "production, import, and use of chemicals in Europe." REACH requires companies to register chemicals that they produce or import in excess of one ton, and companies must provide scientific information regarding the health hazards associated with such chemicals. Based on the information, the European Union determines to what extent, if at all, companies can use the registered chemicals in their products. It also determines which consumer uses, if any, of these chemicals are acceptable. In regard to chemicals of high concern, authorization for specific purposes is time limited. Thus, they must go through another review after their authorization expires. Companies must also classify and label all chemicals on their products. Ultimately, REACH places the burden of responsibility on chemical manufacturers when it comes to guaranteeing the public's safety.[35]Although REACH did not go into effect until 2007, in January 2003 the European Union amended the Cosmetic Directive to ban the use of chemicals—including phthalates—in cosmetics that caused or were "strongly suspected" of causing cancer, birth defects, or mutations. The ban, which went into effect in January 2004, applies to cosmetics produced in Europe, as well as to imports from other countries.[36]

Reforming Industry

Not surprisingly, the administration of President George W. Bush and the U.S. chemical industry dislike the REACH program, including the specific ban on harmful compounds in cosmetics. Both fought against its passage by arguing that the program would "interfere with trade, increase, costs, discourage innovation, and hamper commerce," as well as discourage sales of products that contain hazardous toxins, because the public would not want to buy them. They also challenged the chemical testing and evaluation process, as it could increase costs for U.S. companies that market their products in Europe; they would be forced to follow REACH's requirements in order to continue exporting to Europe. The implementation of REACH puts pressure on the U.S. government to pass similar regulatory reform—a move that the chemical industry and the Bush administration resist.[37]

The economic worries of the Bush administration and the chemical industry are not necessarily well founded, however. After the European Union passed the cosmetics ban, companies simply reformulated their products, which sold as usual.[38] Moreover, public awareness of and concern about the presence of toxic chemicals in daily life is growing. U.S. media coverage of phthalates, bisphenol A, and other harmful substances found in home, personal care, and children's products has dramatically increased in the past few years.[39] The *Milwaukee Journal Sentinel*, for example, ran fourteen, mostly front-page articles between November 2007 and April 2008 on bisphenol A and other endocrine disrupters. Taken together, these articles not only discussed the ubiquitous presence of such chemicals in our everyday products, homes, and bodies, but also criticized industry and the federal government for downplaying the risk associated with them. The series examined the efforts of health groups, consumer organizations, and stakeholders to pressure policymakers and industry to regulate more stringently the production and use of endocrine disrupters and other chemicals.[40]

Opinion polls demonstrate that consumers are increasingly concerned about the presence of toxic substances in products they use every day and are interested in purchasing safer alternatives. In a 2003 Princeton Survey Research Associates poll, 50 percent of respondents said that advertising grooming products as natural or organic would make them more interested in buying them.[41] In March 2004, the Prevention Magazine/Food Marketing Institute found that 34 percent of those polled would like their grocery stores to offer more organic food options.[42] Similarly, 32 percent of participants in a Harris Poll conducted in October 2007 stated that their purchase of organic food products had increased a great deal or increased somewhat over the preceding year.[43] It also appears that consumers increasingly desire other types of safe products. After the *Milwaukee Journal Sentinel* published its series on the dangers of bisphenol A, residents of southeastern Wisconsin began to demand that local businesses sell baby bottles, especially made of glass, that did not contain the chemical. Numerous businesses, among them Whole Foods, Babies R Us, and Happy Bambino, expanded their supply of safe bottles in response to consumer demands. At the national level, many companies have noted that sales for both glass and bisphenol A–free plastic bottles rose in recent months. NuturePure, a company that sells glass bottles online, reported that sales of their product increased by more than 500 percent from May to November 2007.[44]

Proponents of chemical policy reform work directly with industry to help companies understand that, contrary to widely held beliefs, protecting the health of people and the environment can exist together with making a profit. One strategy consists of helping companies develop and use safer technologies, manufacturing processes, and materials. The Lowell Center for Sustainable Production focuses much of its efforts on this approach. As part of its Sustainable Production and Consumption program, the center "assist[s] producers to redesign goods and services to improve their environmental and social impacts."[45] Its Clean Production and Research Training program develops "technical innovations in materials (biodegradability, for example), products (such as designing for reuse and disassembly), and facility design (zero discharge facilities)." The center runs specific projects that focus on the development of safe and sustainable toys, hospital products, and other materials in Massachusetts.[46]

A second strategy for pushing companies to embrace healthier practices is to endorse those that manufacture safe products and encourage consumers to buy these goods. The Campaign for Safer Cosmetics encourages companies to sign its Compact for Safe Cosmetics. The six hundred companies that have endorsed the contract "pledge not to use chemicals that are known or strongly suspected of causing cancer, mutation, or birth defects in their products and to implement substitution plans that replace hazardous materials with safer alternatives in every market they serve." Consumers can search the list of signees on the campaign's Web site and link to the companies' Web sites to learn more about their products. The campaign identifies some of the major companies—OPI, Avon, Estée Lauder, L'Oreal, Revlon, Proctor and Gamble, and Unilever—that have not signed the contract, to exert pressure on them to sign on.[47]

A third strategy entails making change from within. Over the past few years, company shareholders have increasingly demanded healthier products. Shareholder groups have developed more than two dozen resolutions calling on corporations to change their chemical uses and practices. In 2002, Breast Cancer Action bought one share of stock in Avon. Since then, it has worked with other breast cancer groups, health organizations, and socially responsible investment firms to develop shareholder resolutions requesting that Avon remove parabens (2003 and 2004), phthalates (2003 and 2004), and nanoparticles (2008) from its products, as well as "reformulate cosmetics products sold in the United States and other world markets to meet tougher European standards (2006)."[48] Although corporate responses to such shareholder resolutions have been modest, the strategy is gaining momentum. In 2004, Avon agreed to remove dibutyl phthalates from some of its products. Whole Foods and Walmart recently agreed to remove baby bottles, canned food, and other products containing bisphenol A from its stores, and Sears, Kmart, and Walmart have agreed to stop selling products containing PVC. On the production end, Nalgene agreed to stop using bisphenol A in its widely used water bottles, while companies such as Hasbro; CVS; and Bed, Bath, and Beyond agreed to meet with their shareholders to discuss demands that they remove phthalates, PVC, and other chemicals from their products. Many of these companies' shareholder groups have altruistic goals; they believe in industry being socially responsible. At the same time, they recognize that there is growing public demand for safe products and consequently, a new avenue for financial profit.[49]

Beyond Breast Cancer

A common theme that I came across over the course of my research was that the environmental breast cancer movement needs to go "beyond breast cancer," as several activists put it. In some cases, this means focusing on the broader category of cancer. Zero Breast Cancer's Janice Barlow emphasizes the need to "think outside of the organ." Breast cancer research, she maintains, is limited by its strict focus on the diseased organ itself, and research would benefit from further attention to the more general process of carcinogenesis and the relationship between breast cancer and other organ systems. Barlow notes that estrogen receptors are found in not only the breast but also other organs, such as the thyroid and the brain.[50] Similarly, 1 in 9's Geri Barish believes that we need to better understand the relationship between breast cancer and other cancers, including prostate cancer, because their development may have genetic— and generational—connections.[51] The category of cancer continues to shape environmental breast cancer science, politics, and prevention at the institutional level. In 2004, Devra Davis became the inaugural director of the world's first Center for Environmental Oncology at the University of Pittsburgh Cancer Center. The center conducts and assesses research on the environmental causes of cancer, educates the public about its findings, and proposes policies to reduce cancer's environmental risks.[52]

Still, most efforts to go beyond breast cancer situate the disease within the broader context of environmental health. Some efforts emphasize particular chemicals or groups of chemicals linked to breast cancer and other diseases. Davis's earlier calls for a Save the Males campaign, the 2000 American Association for the Advancement of Science Environment and Fertility meeting, and other efforts centered on endocrine disrupters reflect this strategy. Other activist work takes an even wider view of environmental health. The Prevention Is the Cure campaign forges connections between diseases—breast cancer, Alzheimer's, autism, and Parkinson's, among others—that are not necessarily linked to the same types of chemicals. The group's founder, Karen Miller, takes this strategy because she likes her work to be "inclusive." Yet she also seeks to highlight the extent to which links between toxic substances and health problems exist because doing so has the potential to increase public attention to environmental health issues, to lead to a growing number of allies and constituents to push for change, and to bring about a more comprehensive implementation of preventative efforts in daily life.[53]

Another organization that takes a broad approach is the Collaborative on Health and the Environment. This group, which is administrated by Commonweal in Bolinas, California, was created as a result of discussions that took place in May 2002 at a meeting of the San Francisco Medical Society. The collaborative brings together scientists, health professionals, activists, and other concerned citizens to addresses the preventable causes of chronic disease, especially in regard to environmental toxicants.[54] Guided by the precautionary principle, it seeks to share "scientific research information about the links between environmental contaminants and human disease; [foster] interdisciplinary and inclusive collaboration among diverse constituencies interested in those links; and [facilitate] appropriate actions to reduce exposure to contaminants and to improve care of those affected."[55] The organization runs thirteen working groups that focus on such issues as asthma, fertility/early pregnancy, learning and developmental disabilities, electromagnetic fields, Parkinson's disease, integrative health, and breast cancer.[56]

The environmental breast cancer movement serves as a compelling lens through which to examine the broader terrain of environmental health activism, science, and prevention. This terrain provides breast cancer activists with scientific and political frameworks for legitimating their concerns about xenoestrogens and other toxic substances. It provides them with key allies with whom to form coalitions and joint campaigns around issues of common concern. It offers innovative frameworks for taking precautionary action. At the same time, environmental breast cancer activism contributes to the broader field of environmental health. The early research on xenoestrogens, for example, brought about important insights into the nature of endocrine disrupters.

Scientists have used the research methods developed to assess the relationship between xenoestrogens and breast cancer to study the relationship between the chemicals and other diseases. Furthermore, environmental breast cancer activism brings public attention to the dangers of toxic exposures via a disease that holds a prominent place within the contemporary cultural and political landscape. At the Breast Cancer Fund's press conference on Capitol Hill in October 1999, Speaker Nancy Pelosi predicted that environmental health would become one of the most important issues of the twenty-first century. There is no doubt that breast cancer activists have played a central role in making this prediction a reality.

In the years to come, the environmental breast cancer and environmental health movements will continue to evolve socially, politically, and scientifically, both separately and in tandem. The disease kinships that will inevitably deepen—if not newly develop—as a result of this ongoing relationship will surely benefit the health of women by contributing to better understandings of environmental causes of breast cancer; providing breast cancer activists with new allies; and continuing to cultivate a societal infrastructure that takes toxic exposures, precaution, and disease prevention seriously. Just as important, the environmental breast cancer movement is well positioned to use its breast cancer work as a way to contribute not only to the eradication of the disease itself but also to the environmental health of all humans and other living beings.

Notes

Chapter 1 — A Movement in the Making

1. For the updated version of the postcard, see http://www.womensart.com/artists/liroff/pages/postcard.htm (accessed February 22, 2008).

2. Joan H. Fujimura, "Future Imaginaries: Genome Scientists as Sociocultural Entrepreneurs," in *Genetic Nature/Culture: Anthropology and Science Beyond the Two-Culture Divide*, ed. Alan H. Goodman, Deborah Heath, and M. Susan Lindee (Berkeley and Los Angeles: University of California Press, 2003). Fujimura states that "imagination is a social practice deployed in the production of science and technology. Creating future imaginaries is a major part of scientists' work" (176). I extend this notion to activists' work.

3. National Heart, Lung, and Blood Institute, "Women's Fear of Heart Disease Has Almost Doubled in Three Years," http://www.nhlbi.nih.gov/health/hearttruth/press/fear_doubled.htm (accessed June 22, 2008).

4. American Cancer Society, *Breast Cancer Facts and Figures, 2007–2008* (Atlanta: American Cancer Society, 2007), 1, http://www.cancer.org/downloads/STT/BCFF-Final.pdf (accessed February 20, 2008).

5. *Inflammatory Breast Cancer: Are You at Risk?* (Summit, N.J.: Susan G. Komen for the Cure North Jersey, 2007).

6. James S. Olson, *Bathsheba's Breast: Women, Cancer, and History* (Baltimore: Johns Hopkins University Press, 2002), 1–26.

7. Nancy Evans, ed., *State of the Evidence: What Is the Connection between the Environment and Breast Cancer?* 4th ed. (San Francisco: Breast Cancer Fund and Breast Cancer Action, 2006), 13, http://www.breastcancerfund.org/atf/cf/{DE68F7B2-5F6A-4B57-9794-AFE5D27A3CFF}/State%20of%20the%20Evidence%202006.pdf (accessed December 6, 2008).

8. One percent of all breast cancers occur in men. In 2007, 2,030 men were expected to be diagnosed and 450 were expected to die from the disease. *Breast Cancer Facts and Figures*, 2–6.

9. From 2000 to 2004, white women suffered the highest overall incidence rates, at 132.5 per 100,000 women, followed by African Americans, at 118.3; Asian Americans/Pacific Islanders, at 89.0; Latinas, at 89.3; and American Indians/Alaska Natives, at 69.8. *Breast Cancer Facts and Figures*, 1–5.

10. African Americans suffered the highest overall mortality rates, between 2000 and 2004, at 33.8 per 100,000, followed by white women, at 25.0; Latinas, at 16.1; Native Americans, at 13.9; and Asian Americans, at 12.6. See *Breast Cancer Facts and Figures*, 4–9.

11. Olson, *Bathsheba's Breast*, 22; *Breast Cancer Facts and Figures*, 10.

12. Patricia A. Newman, "Perspective: Cancer Research in the 1980s," *Journal of the National Cancer Institute* 82, no. 3 (1990): 178; John C. Bailar III, "The Case for Cancer Prevention," *Journal of the National Cancer Institute* 62, no. 4 (1979): 727–731; Richard Doll and Richard Peto, "The Causes of Cancer: Quantitative Estimates of Avoidable Risks of Cancer in the United States Today," *Journal of the National Cancer Institute* 66, no. 6 (1981): 1191–1308.

205

13. Newman, "Perspective," 176–177; Joan H. Fujimura, *Crafting Science: A Sociohistory of the Quest for the Genetics of Cancer* (Cambridge, Mass.: Harvard University Press, 1996).

14. *Breast Cancer Facts and Figures*, 9–10; Shobita Parthasarathy, *Building Genetic Medicine: Breast Cancer, Technology, and the Comparative Politics of Health Care* (Cambridge, Mass.: MIT Press, 2007).

15. *Breast Cancer Facts and Figures*, 8–12.

16. In the broadest sense, *environmental factors* refers to behavioral choices and exposure to toxic substances. Here and throughout the book, I use the term more narrowly to refer to the latter, which is how those working on such issues tend to use the phrase.

17. Program on Breast Cancer and Environmental Risk Factors, "Ionizing Radiation and Breast Cancer Risk," http://envirocancer.cornell.edu/factsheet/physical/fs52. radiation.cfm (accessed July 18, 2008).

18. Phil Brown and Stephen Zavestoski, "Social Movements in Health: An Introduction," in *Social Movements in Health*, ed. Phil Brown and Stephen Zavestoski (Oxford, U.K.: Blackwell, 2005), 1–9; David J. Hess, "Medical Modernisation, Scientific Research Fields and the Epistemic Politics of Health Social Movements," in *Social Movements in Health*, 17–30.

19. Phil Brown et al., "Embodied Health Movements: New Approaches to Social Movements in Health," *Sociology of Health and Illness* 26, no. 1 (2004): 64. Other embodied health movements of note focus on conditions such as asthma (Phil Brown et al., "Policy Issues in Environmental Health Disputes," *Annals of the American Academy of Political and Social Science* 584, no. 1 [2002]: 175–202); Down syndrome (Rayna Rapp, Deborah Heath, and Karen-Sue Taussig, "Genealogical Dis-ease: Where Heredity, Abnormality, Biomedical Explanation, and Family Responsibility Meet," in *Relative Values: Reconfiguring Kinship Studies*, ed. Sarah Franklin and Susan McKinnon [Durham: Duke University Press, 2001], 384–409); dwarfism (Karen-Sue Taussig, Rayna Rapp, and Deborah Heath, "Flexible Eugenics: Technologies of the Self in the Age of Genetics," in *Genetic Nature/Culture: Anthropology and Science Beyond the Two-Culture Divide*, ed. Alan H. Goodman, Deborah Heath, and M. Susan Lindee [Berkeley and Los Angeles: University of California Press, 2003], 58–76); epidermolysis bullosa (Deborah Heath et al., "Nodes and Queries: Linking Locations in Networked Fields of Inquiry," *American Behavioral Scientist* 43, no. 3 [1999]: 450–463); Gulf War syndrome (Brown et al., "Policy Issues"; Stephen Zavestoski et al., "Patient Activism and the Struggle for Diagnosis: Gulf War Illness and Other Medically Unexplained Symptoms in the U.S.," *Social Science and Medicine* 58, no. 1 [2004]: 161–175); HIV/AIDS (Steven Epstein, *Impure Science: AIDS, Activism, and the Politics of Scientific Knowledge* [Berkeley and Los Angeles: University of California Press, 1996]); Marfan's syndrome (Deborah Heath, "Bodies, Antibodies, and Modest Interventions," in *Cyborgs and Citadels: Anthropological Interventions in Emerging Sciences and Technologies*, ed. Gary Lee Downey and Joseph Dumit [Santa Fe, N.M.: School of American Research Press, 1997], 67–82); multiple chemical sensitivity (Steve Kroll-Smith and H. Hugh Floyd, *Bodies in Protest: Environmental Illness and the Struggle over Medical Knowledge* [New York: New York University Press, 1997]).

20. Maren Klawiter, "Racing for the Cure, Walking Women, and Toxic Touring: Mapping Cultures of Action within the Bay Area Terrain of Breast Cancer," *Social Problems* 46, no. 1 (1999): 104–126.

21. Evans, *State of the Evidence*, 5.

22. Michael Jerrett and Murray Finkelstein, "Geographies of Risk in Studies Linking Chronic Air Pollution Exposure to Health Outcomes," *Journal of Toxicology and Environmental Health, Part A* 68, no. 13–14 (2005): 1214.

23. Epstein, *Impure Science.*

24. Ibid., 3.

25. Simon S. Shackley and Brian E. Wynne, "Global Climate Change: The Mutual Construction of an Emergent Science-Policy Domain," *Science and Public Policy* 22, no. 4 (1995): 221–228.

26. Phil Brown et al., "'A Lab of Our Own': Environmental Causation of Breast Cancer and Challenges to the Dominant Epidemiological Paradigm," *Science, Technology, and Human Values* 31, no. 5 (2006): 524–528.

27. Brown et al., "Embodied Health Movements," 63–64.

28. Geoffrey C. Bowker and Susan Leigh Star, *Sorting Things Out: Classification and Its Consequences* (Cambridge, Mass.: MIT Press, 2000), 1–32.

29. See, for example, Bowker and Star, *Sorting Things Out*; Alberto Cambrosio and Peter Keating, "Matter of FACS: Constituting Novel Entities in Immunology," *Medical Anthropology Quarterly* 6, no. 4 (1992): 362–384; Adele E. Clarke and Monica J. Casper, "From Simple Technology to Complex Arena: Classification of Pap Smears, 1917–1990," *Medical Anthropology Quarterly* 10, no. 4 (1996): 601–623; Kroll-Smith and Floyd, *Bodies in Protest.*

30. Donna J. Haraway, *Modest_Witness@Second_Millenium.FemaleMan_Meets_OncoMouse™: Feminism and Technoscience* (New York: Routledge, 1997), 52–53.

31. Paul Rabinow, "Artificiality and Enlightenment: From Sociobiology to Biosociality," in *Essays on the Anthropology of Reason* (Princeton: Princeton University Press, 1996), 99.

32. Maren Klawiter, "Breast Cancer in Two Regimes: The Impact of Social Movements on Illness Experience," in *Social Movements in Health* (see note 18, above), 166.

33. Maren Klawiter, "Chemicals, Cancer, and Prevention: The Synergy of Synthetic Social Movements," in *Synthetic Planet: Chemical Politics and the Hazards of Modern Life*, ed. Monica J. Casper (New York: Routledge, 2003), 174.

34. Within Euro-American and other industrial societies, the concept of kinship has historically been based on shared biological substances, such as blood or genes (David M. Schneider, *American Kinship: A Cultural Account* [Chicago: University of Chicago Press, 1980]). In recent decades, however, scholars have approached the study of Euro-American kinship from new theoretical directions, highlighting how biomedical and technoscientific developments complicate notions of biogenetic relatedness and the relationship between biology and culture; rethinking what kinds of bonds count as kinship; and describing how such bonds shape and are shaped by systems of sociocultural, political, and economic power. See Sarah Franklin and Susan McKinnon, eds. *Relative Values: Reconfiguring Kinship Studies* (Durham: Duke University Press, 2001); Haraway, *Modest_Witness*; Rayna Rapp, *Testing Women, Testing the Fetus: The Social Impact of Amniocentesis in America* (New York: Routledge, 2000). My notion of disease kinship builds on this lineage by emphasizing the common biosocial characteristics that link health conditions together within a particular classification.

35. Paul Rabinow, *French DNA: Trouble in Purgatory* (Chicago: University of Chicago Press, 2001). "From time to time, and always in time," Rabinow writes, "new forms emerge that catalyze previously existing actors, things, temporalities, or spatialities into a new mode of existence, a new assemblage, one that makes things work in a different manner and produces and instantiates new capacities" (180).

36. George E. Marcus, "Ethnography in/of the World System: The Emergence of Multi-sited Ethnography," *Annual Review of Anthropology* 24 (1995): 95–117.

37. Akhil Gupta and James Ferguson, "Discipline and Practice: 'The Field' as Site, Method, and Location in Anthropology," in *Anthropological Locations: Boundaries and Grounds of a Field Science*, ed. Akhil Gupta and James Ferguson (Berkeley and Los Angeles: University of California Press, 1997), 39.

38. Heath, "Bodies, Antibodies, and Modest Interventions." Heath defines "modest interventions" as "translocal engagements that reveal, perturb, and perhaps transform the constructed boundaries between local, situated knowledges" (68).

39. Rapp, *Testing Women*, 20.

40. Gary Lee Downy and Joseph Dumit, "Locating and Intervening: An Introduction," in *Cyborgs and Citadels* (see note 19, above), 27.

Chapter 2 — "End the Silence": Uncertainty Work and the Politics of the Cancer Industry

1. Chela Zabin, "Support for Women with Cancer," *Register-Pajaronian*, April 26, 1993; Deb Abbott, oral history, cond. Regan Brashear, ed. Irene Reti, in Out in the Redwoods: Gay, Lesbian, Bisexual, Transgender History Oral History series, Regional History Project of the University Library, University of California, Santa Cruz, 2004, http://library.ucsc.edu/reg-hist/oir.exhibit/deb_abbott.html (accessed May 30, 2008).

2. Wendy Traber, "My Body, the Planet," *WomenCARE Newsletter*, no. 1 (Fall 1994): 1.

3. Sandra Morgen, *Into Our Own Hands: The Women's Health Movement in the United States, 1969–1990* (New Brunswick: Rutgers University Press, 2002).

4. Roberta Altman, *Waking Up, Fighting Back: The Politics of Breast Cancer* (Boston: Little, Brown, 1996), 291–312.

5. Theresa Montini and Sheryl Ruzek, "Overturning Orthodoxy: The Emergence of Breast Cancer Treatment Policy," *Research in the Sociology of Health Care* 8 (1989): 3–32. For additional information about the history of breast cancer surgery, see Ellen Leopold, *A Darker Ribbon: Breast Cancer, Women, and Their Doctors in the Twentieth Century* (Boston: Beacon Press, 1999).

6. Altman, *Waking Up*, 296; Leopold, *A Darker Ribbon*, 234–237.

7. Mary Anglin, "Working from the Inside Out: Implications of Breast Cancer Activism for Biomedical Politics and Practices," *Social Science and Medicine* 44 (1997): 1403–1415; Sharon Batt, *Patient No More: The Politics of Breast Cancer* (Charlottetown, Canada: gynergy books 1994); Leopold, *A Darker Ribbon*, 72–138; R. Ruth Linden, "Re-inventing Treatment Activism," *Breast Cancer Action Newsletter*, no. 33 (December 1995): 3–4.

8. Altman, *Waking Up*, 107–158; Batt, *Patient No More*, 31–54; John W. Gofman, *Preventing Breast Cancer: The Story of a Major, Proven, Preventable Cause of This Disease*, 2nd ed. (San Francisco: Committee for Nuclear Responsibility, 1996).

9. In 2003, the organization broadened its mission beyond cancer to address a range of health needs experienced by lesbian, bisexual, and transgendered women. See Mautner Project, "The Mautner Project—Who We Are," http://www.mautnerproject.org/about_us/Mission___History/index.html (accessed September 21, 2007).

10. Midge Stocker, ed., *Cancer as a Women's Issue: Scratching the Surface* (Chicago: Third Side Press, 1991); Midge Stocker, ed., *Confronting Cancer, Constructing Change: New Perspectives on Women and Cancer* (Chicago: Third Side Press, 1993). See especially Jackie Winnow, "Lesbians Evolving Health Care: Cancer and AIDS,"

in *1 in 3: Women with Cancer Confront an Epidemic*, ed. Judy Brady (San Francisco: Cleis Press, 1991), 233–244.

11. Suzanne Haynes has stated that lesbians have a one in three chance of developing breast cancer at some point in their lifetime. In 2002, however, Suzanne Dibble found that lesbians had only a slightly higher risk (11.1 percent) of developing breast cancer than heterosexual women (10.6 percent). See Sacramento Area Lesbian Health Resource Guide, "Lesbians and Breast Cancer," http://www. saclesbianhealth.com/healthinfo/lesbiansbreastcancer2.htm (accessed January 28, 2008).

12. Maureen Hogan Casamayou, *The Politics of Breast Cancer* (Washington, D.C.: Georgetown University Press, 2001), 1–7.

13. Altman, *Waking Up*, 10; Casamayou, *The Politics of Breast Cancer*, 57–59.

14. Audre Lorde, *The Cancer Journals* (San Francisco: aunt lute books, 1980), 16.

15. Rachel Carson is the author of *Silent Spring* (New York: Houghton Mifflin, 1962), one of the first books to raise public awareness about the health dangers from DDT and other pesticides.

16. Judy Brady, in discussion with the author, April 17, 2008.

17. Women's Cancer Resource Center, "Who We Are," http://wcrc.org/who.htm (accessed September 21, 2007); Women's Cancer Resource Center, "Key Facts," http://www. wcrc.org/downloads/bod/WCRCKeyFacts.doc (accessed September 21, 2007); Margo Rivera-Weiss, in discussion with the author, February 19, 2008.

18. Rita Arditti, in discussion with the author, May 9, 2008; Women's Review of Books, "Biology Is Not Destiny: An Interview with the Women's Community Cancer Project," *Women's Review of Books* 11, no. 10–11 (1994): 7; Susan Shapiro, "Cancer as a Feminist Issue," *Sojourner: The Women's Forum* (September 1989): 18.

19. Giovanna DiChiro, "Nature as Community: The Convergence of Environmental and Social Justice," in *Uncommon Ground: Rethinking the Human Place in Nature*, ed. William Cronon (New York: W. W. Norton, 1995), 298–320; Rosi Braidotti et al., *Women, the Environment, and Sustainable Development: Towards a Theoretical Synthesis* (London: Zed Books, 1994); Chris J. Cuomo, *Feminism and Ecological Communities: An Ethic of Flourishing* (New York: Routledge, 1998); Joni Seager, "Rachel Carson Died of Breast Cancer: The Coming of Age of Feminist Environmentalism," *Signs: The Journal of Women in Culture and Society* 28, no. 1 (2003): 445–472.

20. This is a loose definition; medical and scientific experts differ on the characteristics shared by all cancers.

21. In fiscal year 2007, the NCI received a total of $4.79 billion dollars. The NIH institute that received the second-highest allocation was the National Institute of Allergy and Infectious Diseases at $4.41 billion, followed by the National Heart, Lung, and Blood Institute at $2.92 billion. By contrast, the National Institute of Nursing Research received $137.34 million. See U.S. Department of Health and Human Services (USD-HHS), *National Institutes of Health: FY 2008 Performance Budget Overview* (Washington, D.C., 2007), 19, http://officeofbudget.od.nih.gov/FY07/Overview.pdf (accessed January 30, 2008).

22. The NCI's cumulative budget, from its establishment in 1938 to the present, totals $76,838,833,200. See USDHHS, *NCI 2007 Fact Book* (Washington, D.C., 2007), H-1, http://obf.cancer.gov/financial/attachments/07Factbk.pdf (accessed July 20, 2008).

23. James T. Patterson, *The Dread Disease: Cancer and Modern American Culture* (Cambridge, Mass.: Harvard University Press, 1987); American Cancer Society,

Cancer Facts and Figures, 2008 (Atlanta: American Cancer Society, 2008), 1, http://www.cancer.org/downloads/STT/2008CAFFfinalsecured.pdf (accessed December 5, 2007)

24. For conventional versus alternative cancer treatments, see David J. Hess, *Can Bacteria Cause Cancer? Alternative Medicine Confronts Big Science* (New York: New York University Press, 1997); Ralph Moss, *Cancer Therapy: The Independent Consumer's Guide to Non-toxic Treatment and Prevention* (New York: Equinox Press, 1992); Ralph Moss, *Questioning Chemotherapy* (New York: Equinox Press, 1995). For the health benefits of chemotherapy, see Moss, *Cancer Therapy* and *Questioning Chemotherapy*. For diet and cancer, see Steven Hiltgartner, *Science in Public Discourse: The Diet and Cancer Debate* (Ithaca, N.Y.: Cornell University Press, 1988); Evelleen Richards, *Vitamin C and Cancer: Medicine or Politics?* (New York: St. Martin's Press, 1991).

25. Samuel Epstein reissued *The Politics of Cancer* (San Francisco: Sierra Club Books, 1978) as *The Politics of Cancer, Revisited* (Fremont Center, N.Y.: East Ridge Press, 1998). Ralph Moss's *The Cancer Syndrome* (New York: Grove Press, 1980) was reissued as *The Cancer Industry: The Classic Exposé on the Cancer Establishment* (New York: Paragon House, 1989).

26. Judy Brady, in discussion with the author, April 17, 2008; Judy Brady, e-mail message to the author, April 29, 2008.

27. Women's Review of Books, "Biology Is Not Destiny," 7.

28. In 2003, overall deaths from cancer declined for the first time since the tracking of such deaths in 1930. See National Cancer Institute, "Welcome to the National Cancer Institute," http://www.cancer.gov/directorscorner/welcome (accessed June 24, 2008). For a statistical breakdown of current U.S. cancer incidence and mortality rates, see American Cancer Society, *Cancer Facts and Figures, 2008*, 2–3.

29. Sylvia Noble Tesh, *Hidden Arguments: Political Ideology and Disease Prevention Policy* (New Brunswick: Rutgers University Press, 1988).

30. Moss, *The Cancer Industry*, 417.

31. Daniel Faber, foreword to *The Struggle for Ecological Democracy: Environmental Justice Movements in the United States*, ed. Daniel Faber (New York: Guilford Press, 1998), ix–xi.

32. Daniel Faber, introduction to *The Struggle for Ecological Democracy* (see note 31, above), 7; Christopher H. Foreman Jr., *The Promise and Peril of Environmental Justice* (Washington, D.C.: Brookings Institution, 1998), 15–17.

33. Faber, foreword, ix.

34. Luke W. Cole and Sheila R. Foster, *From the Ground Up: Environmental Racism and the Rise of the Environmental Justice Movement* (New York: New York University Press, 2001), 31–32.

35. U.S. Environmental Protection Agency, "Basic Information," http://www.epa.gov/compliance/basics/ejbackground.html (accessed September 27, 2007).

36. Ibid., "National Environmental Justice Advisory Council," http://www.epa.gov/compliance/environmentaljustice/nejac/index.html (accessed September 27, 2007).

37. Ibid., "Basic Information."

38. American Cancer Society, "ACS Mission Statements," http://www.cancer.org/docroot/AA/content/AA_1_1_ACS_Mission_Statements.asp (accessed September 25, 2007).

39. Ibid., "ACS Fact Sheet," http://www.cancer.org/docroot/AA/content/AA_1_2_ACS_Fact_Sheet.asp?sitearea=&level (accessed September 25, 2007).

40. Ibid., "International Program," http://www.cancer.org/docroot/AA/content/AA_2_5_International_Program.asp?sitearea=AA (accessed September 25, 2007).

41. American Cancer Society, *Breast Cancer Facts and Figures, 2007–2008* (Atlanta: American Cancer Society, 2007), 23, http://www.cancer.org/downloads/STT/BCFF-Final.pdf (accessed December 14, 2007).

42. Gerald D. Dodd, "American Cancer Society Guidelines from the Past to the Present," *Cancer*, suppl. 72, no. 4 (1993): 1429.

43. American Cancer Society, "Breast Cancer Resources," http://www.cancer.org/docroot/PAR/Content/PAR_2_3_Breast_Cancer_Resources.asp (accessed September 25, 2007).

44. Ibid., "Making Strides Against Breast Cancer," http://www.cancer.org/docroot/PAR/PAR_2_Making_Strides_Against_Breast_Cancer.asp (accessed June 24, 2008); ibid., "About Making Strides Against Breast Cancer," http://www.cancer.org/docroot/PAR/Content/PAR_2_1_About_Making_Strides.asp (accessed June 24, 2008).

45. For example, see Batt, *Patient No More*, 213–238.

46. Amber Coverdale Sumrall, in discussion with the author, March 31, 2008.

47. American Cancer Society, "What Causes Breast Cancer?" http://www.cancer.org/docroot/CRI/content/CRI_2_2_2X_What_causes_breast_cancer_5.asp?sitearea=(accessed September 25, 2007).

48. American Cancer Society, *Breast Cancer Facts and Figures*, 9.

49. American Cancer Society, "Known and Probable Carcinogens," http://www.cancer.org/docroot/PED/content/PED_1_3x_Known_and_Probable_Carcinogens.asp?sitearea=PED (accessed September 25, 2007). The International Agency for Research on Cancer, based in France, is a division of the World Health Organization. The National Toxicology Program is jointly run by several government agencies, including the NIH, CDC, and FDA.

50. Ibid., "Environmental Carcinogens," http://www.cancer.org/docroot/PED/ped_1_1.asp (accessed September 25, 2007).

51. Samuel S. Epstein, David Steinman, and Suzanne LeVert, *The Breast Cancer Prevention Program* (New York: Macmillan, 1997), 306–309.

52. *Special Touch: Patient's Guide* (Sacramento, Calif.: California Division of the American Cancer Society, 1996).

53. Moss, *The Cancer Industry*, 402–403; Robert N. Proctor, *Cancer Wars: How Politics Shapes What We Know and Don't Know about Cancer* (New York: Basic Books, 1995), 266.

54. Cancer Prevention Coalition, "The American Cancer Society: the World's Wealthiest 'Nonprofit' Institution," http://preventcancer.com/losing/acs/wealthiest_links.htm (accessed July 22, 2008).

55. Judy Brady, "The Goose and the Golden Egg," in *1 in 3* (see note 10, above), 17; Breast Cancer Fund, "Chemical Fact Sheet: 1, 3-Butadiene," http://www.breastcancerfund.org/site/pp.asp?c=kwKXLdPaE&b=3956619 (accessed May 31, 2008).

56. Proctor, *Cancer Wars*, 255–257.

57. Brian Campbell, "Uncertainty as Symbolic Action in Disputes among Experts," *Social Studies of Science* 15, no. 3 (1985): 429–453.

58. I discuss these strategies in subsequent chapters. See also Proctor, *Cancer Wars*, 54–74.

59. For credibility in expert disputes, see Campbell, "Uncertainty as Symbolic Action"; Michael Lynch, "The Discursive Production of Uncertainty: The OJ Simpson 'Dream Team' and the Sociology of Knowledge Machine," *Social Studies of Science* 28, no. 5/6 (1998): 829–868. For managing professional relationships, see Simon Shackley and Brian Wynne, "Representing Uncertainty in Global Climate Change Science and Policy: Boundary Ordering Devices and Authority," *Science, Technology, and*

Human Values 21, no. 3 (1996): 275–303. For negotiating disciplinary boundaries, see Sheila S. Jasanoff, "Contested Boundaries in Policy-Relevant Science," *Social Studies of Science* 17, no. 2 (1987):195–230.

60. Judy Brady, ed., *1 in 3: Women with Cancer Confront an Epidemic* (San Francisco: Cleis Press, 1991); Stocker, *Cancer as a Women's Issue*; Stocker, *Confronting Cancer*; Terri Tempest Williams, *Refuge: An Unnatural History of Family and Place* (New York: Vintage Books, 1991).

61. Batt, *Patient No More*; Virginia M. Soffa, *The Journey beyond Breast Cancer: From the Personal to the Political* (Rochester, Vt.: Healing Arts Press, 1994); Altman, *Waking Up*; Leopold, *A Darker Ribbon*.

62. Liane Clorfene-Casten, *Breast Cancer: Poisons, Profits, and Prevention* (Monroe, Maine.: Common Courage Press, 1996); Epstein, Steinman, and LeVert, *The Breast Cancer Prevention Program*; Cathy Read, *Preventing Breast Cancer: The Politics of an Epidemic* (San Francisco: Pandora Press, 1995); Janette D. Sherman, *Life's Delicate Balance: Causes and Prevention of Breast Cancer* (New York: Taylor and Francis, 2000).

63. Cynthia Robins, "Acting on Anger about Breast Cancer," *San Francisco Examiner*, March 11, 1993.

64. *Breast Cancer Action Newsletter*, no. 2 (October 1990), http://bcaction.org/index.php?page=1990-newsletters (accessed March 31, 2008).

65. Women's Community Cancer Project, "Cancer Activists Demonstrate at American Cancer Society's National Breast Cancer Conference," *Women's Community Cancer Project Newsletter* (Fall 1993): 1.

66. Massachusetts Breast Cancer Coalition, "MBCC History and Accomplishments," http://mbcc.org/content.php?id=17 (accessed September 28, 2007); Rita Arditti, in discussion with the author, May 9, 2008.

67. Beverly Baccelli, past president of the Massachusetts Breast Cancer Coalition, in discussion with the author, May 20, 2008.

68. National Breast Cancer Awareness Month, "NBCAM Facts," http://www.nbcam.org/newsroom_nbcam_facts.cfm (accessed September 25, 2007).

69. Greenpeace, *October: National Cancer Industry Awareness Month* (San Francisco: Greenpeace, 1995), 1–2.

70. National Breast Cancer Awareness Month, "Board of Sponsors," http://nbcam.org/about_board_of_sponsors.cfm (accessed September 25, 2007).

71. Ibid., "NBCAM Facts."

72. Michael W. DeGregorio and Valerie J. Wiebe, *Tamoxifen and Breast Cancer: What Everyone Should Know about the Treatment of Breast Cancer* (New Haven: Yale University Press, 1995).

73. Greenpeace, *October*, 1.

74. Ibid., 2; Jean Powers, "National Cancer Industry Awareness: WCCP, MBCC, and Greenpeace Protest Breast Cancer Awareness Month," *Women's Community Cancer Project Newsletter*, Winter 1995/1996, 5.

75. Rita Arditti, "Fight Back! Stop It Before It Starts!" *Women's Community Cancer Project Newsletter*, Winter 1995/1996, 1.

76. Greenpeace, *October*, 2.

77. Toxic Links Coalition, "Home Page," http://toxiclinks.net (accessed September 25, 2007). The coalition is considering regrouping for October 2008 events. Bradley Angel, executive director of Green Action for Health and Environmental Justice, in discussion with the author, April 2, 2008.

78. Toxic Links Coalition, "Home Page."

79. Bradley Angel, in discussion with the author, April 2, 2008.
80. Robins, "Acting on Anger."
81. Breast Cancer Fund, "The Mission and History of the Breast Cancer Fund," http://www.breastcancerfund.org/site/pp.asp?c=kwKXLdPaE&b=46951 (accessed September 26, 2007).

Chapter 3 — From Touring the Streets to Taking On Science

1. Maren Klawiter, "Racing for the Cure, Walking Women, and Toxic Touring: Mapping the Cultures of Action within the Bay Area Terrain of Breast Cancer," *Social Problems* 46, no. 1 (1999): 104–126.
2. Klawiter, "Racing for the Cure," 121; Judy Brady, in discussion with the author, April 17, 2008.
3. Sharon Batt, *Patient No More: The Politics of Breast Cancer* (Charlottetown, Canada: gynergy books, 1994), 203.
4. Theo Colborn, Dianne Dumanoski, and John Peterson Myers, *Our Stolen Future: Are We Threatening Our Fertility, Intelligence, and Survival? A Scientific Detective Story* (New York: Plume Books, 1997), 122–130, 140; Ana Soto et al., "*P*-Nonyl-phenol: An Estrogenic Xenobiotic Released from 'Modified' Polystyrene," *Environmental Health Perspectives* 92 (1991): 167–173; Carlos Sonnenschein and Ana Soto, "Control of Estrogen-Target Cell Proliferation, Environmental Estrogens, and Breast Tumorigenesis," *Comments on Toxicology* 5, no. 4–5 (1996): 425–433.
5. Devra Davis, *When Smoke Ran Like Water: Tales of Environmental Deception and the Battle against Pollution* (New York: Basic Books, 2002), 176–179.
6. Devra L. Davis et al., "Medical Hypothesis: Xeno-Estrogens as Preventable Causes of Breast Cancer," *Environmental Health Perspectives* 101, no. 5 (1993): 372–377.
7. Samuel S. Epstein, David Steinman, and Suzanne LeVert, *The Breast Cancer Prevention Program* (New York: Macmillan, 1997), 25–27.
8. Devra L. Davis et al., "Environmental Influence on Breast Cancer Risk," *Science and Medicine* 4, no. 3 (1997): 56–63; Devra Lee Davis et al., "Rethinking Breast Cancer Risk and the Environment: The Case for the Precautionary Principle, *Environmental Health Perspectives* 106, no. 9 (1998): 523–529.
9. Mary S. Wolff et al., "Blood Levels of Organochlorine Residues and Risk of Breast Cancer," *Journal of the National Cancer Institute* 85, no. 8 (1993): 648–652.
10. Nancy Krieger et al., "Breast Cancer and Serum Organochlorines: A Prospective Study among White, Black, and Asian Women," *Journal of the National Cancer Institute* 86, no. 8 (1994): 589–599; Kathy A. Fackelman, "Breast Cancer Risk and DDT: No Verdict Yet," *Science News* (April 23, 1997), http://findarticles.com/p/articles/mi_m1200/is_n17_v145/ai_15209847 (accessed July 28, 2008).
11. Jennifer L. Kelsey and Leslie Bernstein, "Epidemiology and Prevention of Breast Cancer," *Annual Review of Public Health* 17 (1996): 47–67.
12. At the same time, some research indicates that certain forms of phytoestrogens, especially genistein—may contribute to mammary tumor development. Nancy Evans, ed., *State of the Evidence: What Is the Connection between the Environment and Breast Cancer?* 4th ed. (San Francisco: Breast Cancer Fund and Breast Cancer Action, 2006), 29, http://www.breastcancerfund.org/atf/cf/{DE68F7B2-5F6A-4B57-9794-AFE5D27A3CFF}/State%20of%20the%20Evidence%202006.pdf (accessed December 6, 2008).
13. American Cancer Society, "What Causes Breast Cancer?" http://www.cancer.org/docroot/CRI/content/CRI_2_2_2X_What_causes_breast_cancer_5.asp?sitearea=(accessed January 4, 2008); Susan G. Komen for the Cure, "Current or Recent Use of

Birth Control Pills," http://cms.komen.org/komen/AboutBreastCancer/RiskFactors Prevention/AbcBirthControlPillUse?ssSourceNodeId=290&ssSourceSiteId=Komen (accessed January 4, 2008).

14. American Cancer Society, "What Causes Breast Cancer?"

15. Writing Group for the Women's Health Initiative Investigators, "Risks and Benefits of Estrogen Plus Progestin in Healthy Postmenopausal Women: Principal Results from the Women's Health Initiative Randomized Controlled Trial," *Journal of the American Medical Association* 288, no. 3 (2002): 321–333.

16. Karla Kerlikowske et al., "Declines in Invasive Breast Cancer and Use of Postmenopausal Hormone Therapy in a Screening Mammography Population," *Journal of the National Cancer Institute* 99, no. 17 (2007): 1335–1339.

17. Ted Schettler et al., *Generations at Risk: Reproductive Health and the Environment* (Cambridge, Mass.: MIT Press, 1999), 151–156.

18. Sheldon Krimsky, *Hormonal Chaos: The Scientific and Social Origins of the Environmental Endocrine Hypothesis* (Baltimore: Johns Hopkins University Press, 2000). Krimsky defines a public hypothesis as "that stage in the development of a scientific hypothesis during which segments of the public feel they have a stake in the outcome of the scientific debates and therefore make increasing demands in order to establish a clearer understanding of the conflicting views" (56–57).

19. Joan H. Fujimura, *Crafting Science: A Sociohistory of the Quest for the Genetics of Cancer* (Cambridge, Mass.: Harvard University Press, 1996), 2–3.

20. Sabrina McCormick, Phil Brown, and Stephen Zavestoski, "The Personal Is Scientific, the Scientific Is Political: The Public Paradigm of the Environmental Breast Cancer Movement," *Sociological Forum* 18, no. 4 (2003): 547–548.

21. Mary K. Anglin, "Working from the Inside Out: Implications of Breast Cancer Activism for Biomedical Policies and Practices," *Social Science and Medicine* 44, no. 9 (1997): 1403–1415.

22. Steven Epstein, *Impure Science: AIDS, Activism, and the Politics of Scientific Knowledge* (Berkeley and Los Angeles: University of California Press, 1996), 208–234; Ulrike Boehmer, *The Personal and the Political: Women's Activism in Response to the Breast Cancer and AIDS Epidemics* (Albany: State University of New York Press, 2000).

23. Maureen Hogan Casamayou, *The Politics of Breast Cancer* (Washington, D.C.: Georgetown University Press, 2001), 103–152; National Breast Cancer Coalition, "History Goals and Accomplishments," http://www.stopbreastcancer.org/index. php?option=com_content&task=view&id=45&Itemid=62 (accessed January 4, 2008).

24. Alan Irwin, *Citizen Science: A Study of People, Expertise, and Sustainable Development* (London: Routledge, 1995).

25. Luke W. Cole and Sheila R. Foster, *From the Ground Up: Environmental Racism and the Rise of the Environmental Justice Movement* (New York: New York University Press, 2000), 28–29.

26. See, for example, Steven J. Milloy, "Our Stolen Future: How They Are Insulting Our Intelligence," Junk Science, http://www.junkscience.com/news/stolen.html (accessed July 8, 2008).

27. Colborn, Dumanoski, and Myers, *Our Stolen Future*, xvii.

28. Krimsky, *Hormonal Chaos*, 202–203.

29. Ibid., 82–84.

30. Ibid., 203–207.

31. Sabrina McCormick et al., "Public Involvement in Breast Cancer Research: An Analysis and Model for Future Research, *International Journal of Health Services* 34, no. 4 (2004): 628. Phil Brown originally coined the term "popular epidemiology," which he outlined in "Popular Epidemiology: Community Response to Toxic Waste–Induced Disease in Woburn, Massachusetts," *Science, Technology and Human Values* 12, no. 3–4 (1987): 76–85.

32. Liam R. O'Fallon and Allen Dearry, "Community-Based Participatory Research as a Tool to Advance Environmental Health Sciences," *Environmental Health Perspectives* 110, suppl. 2 (2002): 155–159.

33. As the state's overall breast cancer rates increased during the late 1980s and early 1990s, so too did Long Island's rates. Whereas 121.8 per 100,000 women across the state developed breast cancer annually between 1988 and 1992, Nassau County had 137.8 cases and Suffolk County had 133 cases. See Deborah M. Winn, "The Long Island Breast Cancer Study Project," *Nature Reviews Cancer* 5, no. 12 (2005): 986, http://epi.grants.cancer.gov/documents/LIBCSP/nrc1755.pdf (accessed June 3, 2008).

34. Geri Barish, in discussion with the author, April 21, 2008.

35. Ibid.; 1 in 9: The Long Island Breast Cancer Action Coalition, "Mile by Mile," http://1in9.0rg/milebymile.htm (accessed March 31, 2008).

36. 1 in 9, "Mile by Mile."

37. Lorraine Pace, in discussion with the author, October 18, 2007. Also see West Islip Breast Cancer Coalition for Long Island, "Mission/Brief History," http://wibcc.org/mission.htm (accessed October 4, 2007).

38. Lorraine Pace, in discussion with the author, October 18, 2007; West Islip Breast Cancer Coalition, "Mission/Brief History."

39. Lorraine Pace, in discussion with the author, October 18, 2007.

40. Breast Cancer Help, "Initiatives," http://breastcancerhelpinc.org/initiatives. php (accessed June 3, 2008); ibid., "About Breast Cancer Help, Inc.," http://breastcancerhelpinc.org/about.php (accessed June 3, 2008).

41. Geri Barish, in discussion with the author, April 21, 2008.

42. 1 in 9, "Mile by Mile."

43. Geri Barish, in discussion with the author, April 21, 2008.

44. U.S. Department of Health and Human Services (USDHHS) et al., *Report to the U.S. Congress: The Long Island Breast Cancer Study Project* (Washington, D.C., November 2004), iii. http://epi.grants.cancer.gov/documents/LIBCSP/RepttoCong_1104.pdf (accessed July 8, 2008).

45. Ibid., 10–23.

46. Karen Joy Miller, in discussion with the author, November 13 and 14, 2007.

47. Ibid.; Karen Joy Miller, e-mail message to the author, June 26, 2008.

48. Department of Health and Human Services et al., "Report," 29–30.

49. Karen Joy Miller, e-mail message to the author, August 1, 2008.

50. Ibid., in discussion with the author, November 13 and 14, 2007; Deborah Basile, in discussion with the author, April 15, 2008; USDHHS et al., *Report*, 29–30.

51. USDHHS et al., *Report*, 29.

52. Jan Beyea and Maureen Hatch, "Geographic Exposure Modeling: A Valuable Extension of Geographic Information Systems for Use in Environmental Epidemiology," *Environmental Health Perspectives* 107, suppl. 1 (1999): 181–190.

53. Silent Spring Institute, *Findings of the Cape Cod Breast Cancer and Environment Study* (Newton, Mass.: Silent Spring Institute, 2006), 4; Winn, "The Long Island

Breast Cancer Study Project," 990, http://library.silentspring.org/publications/pdfs/report_web_v2.pdf (accessed January 29, 2008)

54. Cheryl Osimo, in discussion with the author, May 19, 2008.

55. Beverly Baccelli, in discussion with the author, May 20, 2008; Julia Green Brody, Joel Tickner, and Ruthann Rudel, "Community-Initiated Breast Cancer and Environmental Studies and the Precautionary Principle," *Environmental Health Perspectives* 113, no. 8 (2005): 921.

56. Phil Brown et al., "'A Lab of Our Own': Environmental Causation of Breast Cancer and Challenges to the Dominant Epidemiological Paradigm," *Science, Technology, and Human Values* 31, no. 5 (2006): 527–530.

57. Silent Spring Institute, "About Us: Staff," http://silentspring.org/neweb.about/staff.html (accessed July 22, 2008); ibid., "About Us: Board of Directors," http://silentspring.org/about/board/html (accessed July 22, 2008).

58. Ruthann Rudel, in discussion with the author, November 30, 2008.

59. Silent Spring Institute, "Silent Spring Institute Funding Sources," http://www.silentspring.org/newweb/about/funders.html (accessed September 14, 2007).

60. Julia Brody, in discussion with the author, February 20, 2008.

61. Wikipedia, "Hanford Site," http://en.wikipedia.org/wiki/Hanford_Site (accessed April 8, 2008).

62. *Findings of the Cape Cod Breast Cancer and Environment Study*, 5; Ruthann Rudel, e-mail message to the author, July 28, 2008.

63. *Findings of the Cape Cod Breast Cancer and Environment Study*, 10.

64. Silent Spring Institute, "Household Exposure Study," http://www.silentspring.org/newweb/research/household.html (accessed September 16, 2007); *Findings of the Cape Cod Breast Cancer and Environment Study*, 12.

65. Silent Spring Institute, "Ground Water and Drinking Water Initiatives," http://www.silentspring.org/newweb/research/water.html (access September 16, 2007).

66. Ibid., "The Newton Breast Cancer Study," http://www.silentspring.org/newweb/research/newton/html (accessed September 16, 2007).

67. Ibid., "Breast Cancer and Environmental Justice," http://www.silentspring.org/newweb/research/ej.html (accessed March 5, 2008).

68. Ibid., "Silent Spring Institute Board of Directors," http://www.silentspring.org/newweb/about/board.html (accessed September 14, 2007).

69. Cheryl Osimo, in email message to the author, July 31, 2008.

70. *Grassroots Breast Cancer Advocacy and the Environment: A Report on Interviews with Grassroots Leaders* (Newtown, Mass.: Silent Spring Institute, 2004), 1, http://www.silentspring.org/newweb/activists/SSI_grassroots_advocacy_report.pdf (accessed June 30, 2007).

71. Also see Ruthann Rudel, "Predicting Health Effects of Exposure to Compounds with Estrogenic Activity: Methodological Issues," *Environmental Health Perspectives* 105, suppl. 3 (1997): 655–663.

72. Janice Barlow, in discussion with the author, November 12, 2007. Whereas the average national incidence rate between 1995 and 1999 was 144 cases per 100,000 white, non-Hispanic women and the San Francisco Bay Area averaged 155 cases, the rate in Marin County was 199 cases. By 2000, rates in Marin County were 7 percent higher than those in the rest of the Bay Area and 18 percent higher than in the United States as a whole. See Margaret Wrensch et al., "Risk Factors for Breast Cancer in a Population with High Incidence Rates," *Breast Cancer Research* 5, no. 4 (2003): R88–R102.

73. Nancy Evans, in discussion with the author, December 11, 2007.
74. Janice Barlow, in discussion with the author, November 12, 2007.
75. Ibid. See also Zero Breast Cancer, "Research," http://www.zerobreastcancer.org/research.html#2 (accessed September 14, 2007).
76. Zero Breast Cancer, "The Adolescent Risk Factors Study," http://zerobreastcancer.org/research/r_arfs.html (accessed September 14, 2007).
77. Janice Barlow, in discussion with the author, November 12, 2007; Zero Breast Cancer, "Educating the Community," http://zerobreastcancer.org/education/ed_comm.html (accessed January 4, 2008); Janice Barlow, e-mail message to the author, July 7, 2008.
78. Janice Barlow, in discussion with the author, November 12, 2007. See also Zero Breast Cancer, "Breast Cancer and Personal Environmental Risk Factors in Marin County—Pilot Study (PERFS)," http://zerobreastcancer.org/research/r_perfs.html (accessed January 4, 2008); ibid., "Marin Environmental Data Study (MEDS)," http://zerobreastcancer.org/research/r_meds.html (accessed January 4, 2008).
79. Zero Breast Cancer, "The Adolescent Risk Factor Study"; ibid., "Marin Environmental Data Study."
80. Janice Barlow, in discussion with the author, November 12, 2007.
81. Ibid., e-mail message to the author, July 7, 2008.
82. Zero Breast Cancer, "Research," http://zerobreastcancer.org/research.html#3 (accessed July 30, 2008).
83. USDHHS et al., *Report*, v; Marilie Gammon et al., "Environmental Toxins and Breast Cancer on Long Island. I. Polycyclic Aromatic Hydrocarbon DNA Adducts," *Cancer Epidemiology, Biomarkers, and Prevention* 12, no. 1 (2003), 677–685.
84. USDHHS et al., *Report*, 18–19; Erin S. O'Leary et al., "Pesticide Exposure and Risk of Breast Cancer: A Nested Case-Control Study of Residentially Stable Women Living on Long Island," *Environmental Research* 94, no. 2 (2004): 134–144.
85. USDHHS et al., *Report*, 15–17; Steven D. Stellman et al., "Breast Cancer Risk in Relation to Adipose Concentrations of Organochlorine Pesticides and Polychlorinated Biphenyls in Long Island, New York," *Cancer Epidemiology, Biomarkers, and Prevention* 9, no. 11 (2000): 1241–1249; Joshua E. Muscat et al., "Adipose Concentrations of Organochlorine Compounds and Breast Cancer Recurrence in Long Island, New York," *Cancer Epidemiology, Biomarkers, and Prevention* 12, no. 12 (2003): 1474–1478.
86. USDHHS et al., *Report*, v.
87. Ibid., 18–19.
88. Silent Spring Institute, "The Newton Breast Cancer Study."
89. For particular toxins, researchers found twenty-three pesticides in the air and twenty-seven in dust. The most common compounds were from plastics, detergents, disinfectants, and personal care products, with most homes exceeding the EPA health-based guidelines for PAHs and DEHP, a phthalate used to make plastics. Investigators also found traces of substances that had been banned several decades ago—including PCBs, DDT, chlordane, dieldrin, heptachlor, and lindane—demonstrating that persistent chemicals break down slowly indoors. *Findings of the Cape Cod Breast Cancer and Environment Study*, 12.
90. Ibid., 17–21.
91. Zero Breast Cancer, "The Adolescent Risk Factors Study"; Wrensch et al., "Risk Factors."
92. Zero Breast Cancer, "Other Bay Area Breast Cancer Projects," http://zerobreastcancer.org/research/r_marinresearch.html (accessed January 4, 2008).

93. Trevor J. Pinch and Wiebe E. Bijker, "The Social Construction of Facts and Artifacts: Or How the Sociology of Science and the Sociology of Technology Might Benefit Each Other," in *The Social Construction of Technological Systems*, ed. Wiebe E. Bijker, T. P. Hughes, and Trevor J. Pinch (Cambridge, Mass.: MIT Press, 1987), 27. Pinch and Bijker define interpretive flexibility as when scientific facts "are open to more than one interpretation."

94. American Cancer Society, "Breast Cancer on Long Island: Experts Find Some Answers, Seek More," October 9, 2002, http://www.cancer.org/docroot/NWS/content/NWS_1_1x_Breast_Cancer_On_Long_Island_Researchers_Find_Some_Answers_Seek_More.asp (accessed June 27, 2007).

95. Winn, "The Long Island," 988–989, 992.

96. Huntington Breast Cancer Action Coalition, "Reported Residential Pesticide Use and Breast Cancer Risk on Long Island, New York," *Huntington Breast Cancer Action Newsletter*, Winter/Spring 2007, http://hbcac.org/newsletter/winterspring2007/reportedpesticide.html (accessed June 26, 2007).

97. Evans, *State of the Evidence*, 5.

98. Ibid., 33.

99. Silent Spring Institute, "Environment and Breast Cancer: Science Review," http://sciencereview.silentspring.org/index.cfm (accessed January 4, 2008).

100. Saunders-Matthey Cancer Coalition Prevention, "Critique," http://www.stopcancer.org/default2.asp?active_page_id=83 (accessed September 18, 2007). See also Janette D. Sherman, *Life's Delicate Balance: Causes and Prevention of Breast Cancer* (New York: Taylor and Francis, 2000), 178.

101. Evans, *State of the Evidence*, 32.

102. Julia Green Brody et al., "Environmental Pollutants and Breast Cancer: Epidemiologic Studies," *Cancer* suppl. 109, no. 12 (2007): 2668, http://www3.interscience.wiley.com/cgi-bin/fulltext/114261513/PDFSTART (accessed January 4, 2008).

103. Brody et al., "Environmental Pollutants," 2668; *State of the Evidence*, 15, 43.

104. Theo Colborn, "From Silent Spring (1962) to Wingspread (1991)," *Comments on Toxicology* 5, no. 4–5 (1996): 320–321.

105. Nancy Evans, *State of the Evidence: What Is the Connection between the Environment and Breast Cancer?* 2nd ed. (San Francisco: Breast Cancer Fund and Breast Cancer Action, 2002), 6.

106. American Cancer Society, *Breast Cancer Facts and Figures, 2007–2008* (Atlanta: American Cancer Society, 2007), 9, http://www.cancer.org/downloads/STT/BCFF-Final.pdf (accessed December 6, 2008).

107. Ruthann A. Rudel et al., *Summary of "Animal Mammary Gland Carcinogens": Chemicals Causing Mammary Gland Tumors in Animals Signals New Directions for Epidemiology, Chemical Testing, and Risk Assessment for Breast Cancer Prevention* (Newton, Mass.: Silent Spring Institute, 2006), 1, http://sciencereview.silentspring.org/PDFs/lay_Mammary%20Carinogens%20FINAL.pdf (accessed July 10, 2008).

Chapter 4 — "We Should Not Have to Be the Bodies of Evidence": The Precautionary Principle in Policy, Science, and Daily Life

1. Nancy Evans, ed. *State of the Evidence: What Is the Connection between the Environment and Breast Cancer?* 4th ed. (San Francisco: Breast Cancer Fund and Breast Cancer Action, 2006), 49, http://www.breastcancerfund.org/atf/cf/{DE68F7B2-5F6A-4B57-9794-AFE5D27A3CFF}/State%20of%20the%20Evidence%202006.pdf (accessed December 6, 2008).

2. Carolyn Raffensperger and Joel Tickner, "Appendix A: Lessons from Wingspread," in *Protecting Public Health and the Environment: Implementing the Precautionary Principle*, ed. Carolyn Raffensperger and Joel Tickner (Washington, D.C.: Island Press, 1999), 353.

3. Joel Tickner, in discussion with the author, October 23, 2007.

4. Wikipedia, "Lowell, Massachusetts," http://en.wikipedia.org/wiki/Lowell%2C_Massachusetts (accessed September 20, 2007); Wikipedia, "History of Lowell, Massachusetts," http://en.wikipedia.org/wiki/History_of_Lowell%2C_Massachusetts (accessed September 20, 2007).

5. Lowell Center for Sustainable Production, "About the Center," http://sustainableproduction.org/abou.brie.shtml (accessed September 20, 2007).

6. Joel Tickner, in discussion with the author, October 23, 2007.

7. Science and Environmental Health Network, "About SEHN," http://sehn.org/about.html (accessed September 20, 2007).

8. Precautionary language has been invoked—albeit often weakly and without actual implementation—in an array of federal environmental policymaking procedures since the 1970s. For examples, see Raffensperger and Tickner, *Protecting Public Health* (see note 2, above), 177–180. For a history of the precautionary principle in Europe, see Poul Harremoës et al., *Late Lessons from Early Warnings: The Precautionary Principle, 1896–2000* (Copenhagen: European Environment Agency, 2001), http://www.genok.org/filarkiv/File/late_response.pdf (accessed June 25, 2008).

9. See, for example, Nicholas A. Ashford, "A Conceptual Framework for the Use of the Precautionary Principle in Law," in *Protecting Public Health* (see note 2, above), 198–206; Peter L. deFur, "The Precautionary Principle: Application to Policies Regarding Endocrine Disrupting Chemicals," in *Protecting Public Health* (see note 2, above), 337–348; Sandra Steingraber, "Why the Precautionary Principle? A Meditation on Polyvinyl Chloride (PVC) and the Breasts of Mothers," in *Protecting Public Health* (see note 2, above), 362–365.

10. Devra L. Davis et al., "Rethinking Breast Cancer Risk and the Environment: The Case for the Precautionary Principle," *Environmental Health Perspectives* 106, no. 9 (1998): 523–529; Ted Schettler, "Where's the Evidence?" (paper presented at the annual meeting for the American Public Health Association, Washington, D.C., November 15–19, 1998).

11. Theo Colborn, Dianne Dumanoski, and John Peterson Myers, *Our Stolen Future: Are We Threatening Our Fertility, Intelligence, and Survival? A Scientific Detective Story* (New York: Plume Books, 1997), xviii–xx.

12. Ibid., 258.

13. See many of the articles in *Comments on Toxicology* 54, no. 4–5 (1996).

14. Julian Morris, "Defining the Precautionary Principle," in *Rethinking Risk and the Precautionary Principle*, ed. Julian Morris (Oxford, U.K.: Butterworth Heinemann Press, 2000), 1–21. See also Cass R. Sunstein, *Laws of Fear: Beyond the Precautionary Principle* (Cambridge, U.K.: Cambridge University Press, 2005).

15. Susan Leigh Star and James R. Griesemer, "Institutional Ecology, 'Translations,' and Boundary Objects: Amateurs and Professionals in Berkeley's Museum of Vertebrate Zoology, 1907–39," *Social Studies of Science* 19, no. 3 (1989): 393.

16. For further discussion of AHT, see Phil Brown, *Toxic Exposures: Contested Illnesses and the Environmental Breast Cancer Movement* (New York: Columbia University Press, 2007), 202–227.

17. Alliance for a Healthy Tomorrow, "About the Alliance for a Healthy Tomorrow," http://healthytomorrow.org/about.html (accessed October 8, 2007).
18. Ibid.
19. Joel Tickner, e-mail message to the author, July 16, 2008.
20. Alliance for a Healthy Tomorrow, "Our Coalition," http://healthytomorrow.org/members.htm (accessed October 8, 2007).
21. Ibid., "Home Page," http://healthytomorrow.org/campaign.html (accessed May 15, 2003).
22. Ibid., "Actions to Protect Our Health: A Memorandum for the Patrick-Murray Administration," http://www.healthytomorrow.org/PDF/Final_PatrickMemo.pdf (accessed October 8, 2007).
23. The formal title of the Mercury Products Bill is An Act Relative to Mercury Management (H-4319 and S-2464). Alliance for a Healthy Tomorrow, "Mercury Bill Updates," http://healthytomorrow.org/LegUpd_mercury.htm (accessed October 8, 2007).
24. Ibid., "The Safer Alternatives Bill: An Act for a Healthy Massachusetts," 1, http://www.healthytomorrow.org/PDF/factsheet-10-SAbi11200705final.pdf (accessed June 25, 2008). The bill's formal title is An Act for a Healthy Massachusetts: Safer Alternatives to Toxic Chemicals (H-783 and S-558). Representative Jay Kaufman and Senator Steve Colman first filed the bill in 2002. Eighty-two representatives (of 160) and 30 (of 40) senators had co-sponsored it. After a series of vetoes, legislators revised and reintroduced the bill in January 2007. See ibid., "Current Legislative Priorities, 2007–08," http://healthytomorrow.org/currentleg.html (accessed April 2, 2008).
25. The formal titles of the Safer Cleaning Products Bill are An Act to Require Environmentally Safe Alternatives to Harmful Cleaning Products (H-2246) and An Act to Reduce Asthma Rates and their Associated Costs (S-2201). See ibid.
26. Breast Cancer Action, "Stop Cancer Where It Starts," http://www.bcaction.org/index.php?page=stop-cancer (accessed April 2, 2008).
27. Berkeley City Council, "Berkeley 'Stop Cancer Where It Starts' Resolution," http://www.bcaction.org/index.php?page=Berkeley-resolution (accessed April 2, 2008).
28. Breast Cancer Action, "Stop Cancer Where It Starts."
29. The eight founding groups were Boston Women's Health Book Collective, Breast Cancer Action (San Francisco), Center for Medical Consumers (New York), DES Action (Oakland, Calif.), Massachusetts Breast Cancer Coalition, National Women's Health Network (Washington, D.C.), Women's Community Cancer Project, and Women and Health Protection/Breast Cancer Action Montreal. See Prevention First, "Founding Members," http://www.preventionfirstcoalition.org/AboutUs/FoundingMembers.html (accessed October 8, 2007).
30. Prevention First, "About Us," http://www.preventionfirstcoalition.org/Endorsing Orgs/EndorsingOrgs.html (accessed October 8, 2007).
31. Ivan Illich, "The Medicalization of Life," in *Medical Nemesis: The Expropriation of Health* (New York: Pantheon, 1982).
32. Prevention First, "Prevention First," http://preventionfristcoalition.org (accessed October 8, 2007).
33. Prevention First, "Prevention First."
34. They are called SERMs because they also act like estrogens in other tissues. This explains why they may be useful for conditions such as osteoporosis and why they are being investigated as menopausal drugs. See National Cancer Institute,

"Estrogen Receptors/SERMS," http://www.cancer.gov/cancertopics/understanding-cancer/estrogenreceptors (accessed October 8, 2007).

35. Also, the category of "high-risk women" is socially constructed. See Maren Klawiter, "Risk, Prevention, and the Breast Cancer Continuum: The NCI, the FDA, Health Activism, and the Pharmaceutical Industry," *History and Technology* 18, no. 4 (2002): 309–353; Jennifer Fosket, "Constructing 'High Risk Women': The Development and Standardization of a Breast Cancer Risk Assessment Tool," *Science, Technology, and Human Values* 29, no. 3 (2004): 291–313.

36. National Cancer Institute, "The Study of Tamoxifen and Raloxifene (STAR): Questions and Answers," http://www.cancer.gov/Templates/doc.aspx?viewid=0123E12E-CCD6–47BC-9964-D5DD6CB0399E (accessed October 11, 2007); National Women's Health Network, "Chemoprevention: A 21st Century Shell Game," http://www.nwhn.org/newsletter/article.cfm?content_id=102 (accessed June 25, 2008).

37. National Cancer Institute, "STAR"; United States Food and Drug Administration, "FDA Approves New Uses for Evista (raloxifene hydrochloride)," http://www.fda.gov/cder/Offices/OODP/whatsnew/raloxifene.htm (accessed October 11, 2007).

38. Prevention First, "Drug Ads Have Nasty Side Effects," http://preventionfirstcoalition.org/PDF/Brochure.pdf (accessed October 11, 2007).

39. National Women's Health Network, "Chemoprevention."

40. U.S. General Accounting Office, *Prescription Drugs: FDA Oversight of Direct-to-Consumer Advertising Has Limitations*, Report no. GAO-03-177 (Washington, D.C.: GAO, 2002), 6–8.

41. Prevention First, "Drug Ads"; Prevention First, "Will Breast Cancer Prevention Come in a Pill?" http://www.preventionfirstcoalition.org/PDF/PPFAd.pdf (accessed October 8, 2007).

42. International Summit on Science and the Precautionary Principle, "Statement from the International Summit on Science and the Precautionary Principle," http://sustainableproduction.org/precaution/stat.summ.html (accessed April 3, 2007). Also see Katherine Barrett and Carolyn Raffensperger, "Precautionary Science," in *Protecting Public Health* (see note 2, above), 106–122; Joel Tickner, ed., *Precaution, Environmental Science, and Preventative Public Policy* (Washington, D.C.: Island Press, 2003).

43. International Summit on Science and the Precautionary Principle, "Summit Participants and Collaborator Signatories," http://sustainableproduction.org/precaution/supp.html (accessed October 11, 2007); "Additional Signatories," http://sustainableproduction.org/precaution/supp.html (accessed June 25, 2008).

44. For DDT's disruption of breast cell communication, see Kyung-Sun Kang et al., "Inhibition of Gap Junctional Intercellular Communication in Normal Human Breast Epithelial Cells after Treatment with Pesticides, PCBs, and PBBs, Alone or in Mixtures," *Environmental Health Perspectives* 104, no. 2 (1996): 192–200. For DDT's stimulation of breast cancer cell growth, see Craig Dees et al., "DDT Mimics Estradiol Stimulation of Breast Cancer Cells to Enter the Cell Cycle, *Molecular Carcinogenesis* 18, no. 2 (1997), 107–114.

45. For cancer risk in Scandinavian women, see Lars Rylander and Lars Hagmar, "Mortality and Cancer Incidence among Women with a High Consumption of Fatty Fish Contaminated with Persistent Organochlorine Compounds," *Scandinavian Journal of Work, Environment, and Health* 21, no. 6 (1995): 419–426. For the correlations between increased risk of breast cancer and DDT exposure, see Mary S. Wolff et al., "Blood Levels of Organochlorine Residues and Risk of Breast Cancer," *Journal*

of the National Cancer Institute 85, no. 8 (1993): 648–652; Eric Dewailly et al., "High Organochlorine Body Burden in Women with Estrogen Receptor-Positive Breast Cancer," *Journal of the National Cancer Institute* 86, no. 3 (1994): 232–234; Nancy Krieger et al., "Breast Cancer and Serum Organochlorines: A Prospective Study among White, Black, and Asian Women," *Journal of the National Cancer Institute* 86, no. 8 (1994): 589–599.

46. Erin S. O'Leary et al., "Pesticide Exposure and Risk of Breast Cancer: A Nested Case-Control Study of Residentially Stable Women Living on Long Island," *Environmental Research* 94, no. 2 (2004): 134–144.

47. Devra L. Davis, Michelle B. Gottlieb, and Julie R. Stampnitzky, "Reduced Ratio of Male to Female Births in Several Industrialized Countries: A Sentinel Health Indicator?" *Journal of the American Medical Association* 279, no. 13 (1998): 1018–1023; Bruce B. Allan et al., "Declining Sex Ratios in Canada," *Canadian Medical Association Journal* 156, no. 1 (1997): 37–41; Paolo Mocarelli et al., "Change in Sex Ratio with Exposure to Dioxin," *Lancet* 348, no. 9024 (1996): 409; Paolo Mocarelli et al., "Paternal Concentrations of Dioxin and Sex Ratio of Offspring," *Lancet* 355, no. 9218 (2000): 1858–1863.

48. Niels E. Skakkebaek, Ewa Rajpert-De Meyts, and Katharina M. Main, "Testicular Dysgenesis Syndrome: An Increasingly Common Developmental Disorder with Environmental Aspects," *Human Reproduction* 16, no. 5 (2001): 972–978; Niels E. Skakkebaek and Gitte Meyer, "Health of Male Reproduction and Environmental Estrogens," *Comments on Toxicology* 5, no. 4–5 (1996): 415–424; Stuart Hosie et al., "Is There a Correlation between Organochlorine Compounds and Undescended Testes?" *European Journal of Pediatric Surgery* 10, no. 5 (2000): 304–309.

49. Devra Lee Davis, "Environmental Health and the Precautionary Principle" (keynote address, Massachusetts Precautionary Principle kick-off meeting, Framingham, Mass., May 15, 1999), http://www.sustainableproduction.org/precaution/back.brie.envi.html (accessed June 25, 2008).

50. For limb malformations and abnormal sex concentrations in frogs, see Stacia A. Sower, Karen L. Reed, and Kimberly J. Babbitt, "Limb Malformations and Abnormal Sex Hormone Concentrations in Frogs," *Environmental Health Perspectives* 108, no. 11 (2000):1085–1090. For deformed frogs and declining frog populations, see United States Geological Services, "Amphibian Research and Monitoring Initiative—Amphibian Decline," http://www.umesc.usgs.gov/terrestrial/amphibians/armi/stressors.html (accessed July 22, 2008).

51. Edward F. Orlando and Louis J. Guillette Jr., "Developmental and Reproductive Abnormalities Associated with Endocrine Disrupters in Wildlife," in *The Handbook of Environmental Chemistry, Volume 3, Part M: Endocrine Disrupters, Part II*, ed. Manfred Metzler (Berlin: Springer Berlin-Heidelberg, 2002), 249–270; Louis J. Guillette Jr. and D. Andrew Crain, "Endocrine- Disrupting Contaminants and Reproductive Abnormalities in Reptiles," *Comments on Toxicology* 5, no. 4–5 (1996): 381–399; Louis J. Guillette Jr., Endocrine Disrupting Contaminants and Alligator Embryos: A Lesson from Wildlife?" in *Hormonally Active Agents in Food: A Deutsche Forschungsgemeinschaft Symposium*, ed. G. Eisenbrand et al. (Weinheim, Germany: Wiley-VCH, 1998), 72–88.

52. Guillette and Crain, "Endocrine Disrupting Contaminants."

53. Also see Samuel S. Epstein, David Steinman, and Suzanne LeVert, *The Breast Cancer Prevention Program* (New York: Macmillan, 1997), 188–199; Sheldon Krimsky, *Hormonal Chaos*, 205–206; John Wargo, *Our Children's Toxic Legacy: How*

Science and Law Fail to Protect Us from Pesticides (New Haven, Conn.: Yale University Press, 1996), 162–168.

54. *Rachel's Daughters: Searching for the Causes of Breast Cancer*, VHS, directed by Irving Saraf and Allie Light (San Francisco: Light-Saraf-Evans Productions, 1997); Lorraine Pace, in discussion with the author, October 18, 2007.

55. Ruthann Rudel, in discussion with the author, November 30, 2007; ibid., e-mail message to the author, July 28, 2008.

56. Joan H. Fujimura, *Crafting Science: A Sociohistory of the Quest for the Genetics of Cancer* (Cambridge, Mass.: Harvard University Press, 1996), 10–11. Fujimura describes "doable" research problems as "sociotechnical achievements." That is, scientific research trajectories become doable as the social, economic, institutional, and technical infrastructures inside and outside the lab emerge to support them.

57. Ruthann Rudel, in discussion with the author, October 26, 1999, and November 30, 2007.

58. For the history of simple living in the Unites States, see Mary Grigsby, *Buying Time and Getting By: The Voluntary Simplicity Movement* (Albany: State University of New York Press, 2004).

59. See also Mary O'Brien, *Making Better Environmental Decisions: An Alternative to Risk Assessment* (Cambridge, Mass.: MIT Press, 2000), 139–214.

60. Linda L. Layne, "The Cultural Fix: An Anthropological Contribution to Science and Technology Studies," *Science, Technology and Human Values* 25, no. 4 (2000), 492–519. As Layne describes, "The notion of the cultural fix focuses attention on changed meanings as a vehicle for identifying problems and solving them, which shifts the significance of cultural meanings for people and social action from broader underlying assumptions to specific configurations of meanings that challenge individuals in specific contexts" (509).

61. Sharon Koshar, in discussion with the author, October 23, 1999, and December 3, 2008.

62. Ayurveda is an approach to health that was founded in India several thousand years ago. It combines dietary changes, lifestyle regimes, cleansing techniques, and spiritual practices to ensure physical, emotional, and spiritual well-being. Health practitioners such as Deepak Chopra have brought Ayurveda to contemporary Western audiences.

63. Prevention Is the Cure, "Toxic Triggers," http://www.preventionisthecure.org/ToxicTriggers1.pdf (accessed October 11, 2007).

64. Ibid., "2008 Prevention Is the Cure Week," http://www.preventionisthecure.org/preventionisthecureweek.html (accessed June 25, 2008).

65. Ibid., "Home," http://www.preventionisthecure.org (accessed October 8, 2007).

66. National Institute of Environmental Health Sciences Public Meetings for Comments on the Working Group Report, San Francisco, October 1, 1998, http://www.niehs.nih.gov/emfrapid/html/EMF_MTGS/SanFrancisco.html (accessed March 13, 2005).

Chapter 5 — The Cultural Politics of Sisterhood

1. Breast Cancer Fund to President Bill Clinton, letter, October 27, 1999.

2. Ibid.

3. Representative Pelosi (the current Speaker of the House) and Senator Snowe have long supported women's health issues during their congressional tenures. See http://www.house.gov/pelosi and http://snowe.senate.gov. Both were scheduled to speak at the press conference, but Senator Snowe canceled because of an unexpected meeting, and Andrea Martin read a prepared statement by the senator.

4. For further discussion about the cultural politics of DES, see Susan Bell, "From Local to Global: Resolving Uncertainty about the Safety of DES in Menopause," *Research in the Sociology of Health Care* 11 (1994), 41–56; Susan Bell, "Narratives and Lives: Women's Health Politics and the Diagnosis of Cancer for DES Daughters," *Narrative Inquiry* 9, no. 2 (1999): 347–389.

5. American Cancer Society, *Breast Cancer Facts and Figures, 2007–2008* (Atlanta: American Cancer Society, 2007), 3, http://www.cancer.org/downloads/STT/BCFF-Final.pdf (accessed May 30, 2008).

6. Patricia Ireland, "NOW Press Release," October 27, 1999, http://now.org/10–99/1–27–99.html (accessed February 1, 2003).

7. Phil Brown et al., "Embodied Health Movements: New Approaches to Social Movements in Health," *Sociology of Health and Illness* 26, no. 1 (2004): 67–71; Stephen Zavestoski, Sabrina McCormick, and Phil Brown, "Gender, Embodiment, and Disease: Environmental Breast Cancer Activists' Challenges to Science, the Biomedical Model, and Policy," *Science as Culture* 13, no. 4 (2004): 563–586.

8. Barbara Ehrenreich, "Welcome to Cancerland: A Mammogram Leads to a Cult of Pink Kitsch," *Harper's Magazine*, November 2001, 47.

9. Ibid., 46.

10. Ibid., 48.

11. Ibid., 49.

12. Ibid., 53.

13. Gayatri Spivak states, "It is not possible, within discourse, to escape essentializing somewhere, . . . you have to be aware that you are going to essentialize anyway. So then strategically you can look at essentialisms, not as descriptions of the way things are, but as something one must adapt to produce a critique of anything." Gayatri Chakravorty Spivak and Walter Adamson, "The Problem of Self Representation," in *The Post-colonial Critic: Interviews, Strategies, and Dialogues*, ed. Sarah Harasym (New York: Routledge, 1990), 51.

14. Ehrenreich, "Welcome to Cancerland," 45–46.

15. Ibid., 51.

16. In 2007, Follow the Money members included After Breast Cancer Surgery (New Jersey), Babylon Breast Cancer Coalition (New York), Breast Cancer Action (San Francisco), Breast Cancer Resource Center of Santa Barbara (California), Huntington Breast Cancer Action Coalition (New York), The Mautner Project for Lesbians with Cancer (Washington, D.C.), New York State Breast Cancer Network, Rachel's Friends Breast Cancer Coalition (Oregon), and Women's Cancer Resource Center (Minneapolis). See Massachusetts Breast Cancer Coalition, "Follow the Money," http://mbcc.org/content.php?id=10 (accessed September 19, 2007).

17. Breast Cancer Action, "Critical Questions to Ask," http://www.thinkbeforeyoupink.org/Pages/CriticalQuestions.html (accessed September 19, 2007).

18. Appliance Design, "Eureka Announces New Partnership and New Product Line," http://www.appliancedesign.com/CDA/Archives/7a2275132f938010VgnVCM100000f932a8c0 (accessed September 19, 2007).

19. Massachusetts Breast Cancer Coalition, "Against the Tide," http://mbcc.org/swim (accessed September 19, 2007).

20. Breast Cancer Fund, "Climb Against the Odds," http://www.breastcancerfund.org/site/pp.asp?c=kwKXLdPaE&b=85494&msource=EVNT0905&tr=y&auid=1128718 (accessed September 19, 2007).

21. Ibid., "Subscribe to *Utne Magazine* and Support TBCF!" e-mail action alert to Breast Cancer Fund mailing list, October 15, 2002.

22. LunaBar, "You + Community," http://www.lunabar.com/pages/hchw (accessed April 2, 2008).

23. Breast Cancer Fund, "Breast Cancer Fund Store," http://www.breastcancerfund.org/site/pp.asp?c=kwKXLdPaE&b=378913 (accessed September 19, 2007); *Art.Rage.Us: Art and Writing by Women with Breast Cancer* (San Francisco: Chronicle Books, 1998).

24. Sandy M. Fernandez, "Pretty in Pink: The Life and Times of the Ribbon That Tied Breast Cancer to Corporate Giving," *MAMM* (June/July 1998), 54.

25. Ehrenreich, "Welcome to Cancerland," 46.

26. Zillah Eisenstein, *Manmade Breast Cancers* (Ithaca: Cornell University Press, 2001), 127.

27. Breast Cancer Action, "Frequently Asked Questions about Think Before You Pink," http://www.thinkbeforeyoupink.org/Pages/FAQ.html (accessed July 28, 2008). For a discussion about corporate greenwashing, see Joshua Karliner, *The Corporate Planet: Ecology and Politics in the Age of Globalization* (San Francisco: Sierra Club Books, 1997).

28. Appliance Design, "Eureka Announces."

29. BMW North America, "Pink Ribbon Collection," http://www.bmw-online.com/BMWRA_products.asp?mm=Gift+Ideas&c=Pink+Ribbon+Collection&sc=&m=Automotive&i1=ON&p1=50&p2=50&r1=&ref=cat (accessed March 1 2007).

30. Ehrenreich, "Welcome to Cancerland," 48.

31. Barbara Ehrenreich, keynote address, "Beyond the Pink Ribbon: Challenging the Culture of Breast Cancer," Breast Cancer Action town hall meeting, April 20, 2002, http://www.bcaction.org/Pages/LearnAboutUs/TownMeetingsArchive.html (accessed September 18, 2007).

32. Barbara Brenner, "Let Them Lick Stamps," *Breast Cancer Action Newsletter*, no. 37 (August/September 1996), http://www.bcaction.org/Pages/SearchablePages/1996Newsletters/Newsletter037B.html (accessed September 19, 2007).

33. Ibid. The original stamp was replaced in 1998 by a semipostal depicting Whitney Sherman's illustration of a mythical "goddess of the hunt." The ethnically ambiguous woman on the stamp wears a toga, outlining her breasts. When the United States Postal Service first released the stamp, it cost forty cents. In 2008, it cost fifty-five cents. Since 1998, the postal service has raised more than $54 million for research, with 70 percent going to the National Institutes of Health and 30 percent going to the Department of Defense's Medical Research program. See United States Postal Service, "Fundraising Stamps (Semipostal Stamp Program)," http://usps.com/communications/community/semipostals.htm (accessed June 28, 2008).

34. Janice Barlow, in discussion with the author, November 12, 2007.

35. Erin Boles and Deborah Shields, in discussion with the author, April 24, 2008; Beverly Baccelli, in discussion with the author, May 20, 2008.

36. Eisenstein, *Manmade Breast Cancers*, 109–130.

37. Deborah Basile, in discussion with the author, April 15, 2008.

38. Babylon Breast Cancer Coalition, "Lend A Helping Hand," http://www.babylonbreastcancer.org/lahh.html (accessed June 26, 2008).

39. Ibid., "SOS—Sense of Security Program," http://www.babylonbreastcancer.org/sos.html (accessed June 26, 2008).

40. Massachusetts Breast Cancer Coalition, *Stop The Epidemic! The Newsletter of the Massachusetts Breast Cancer Coalition*, no. 23 (Summer 2001).

41. Fernandez, "Pretty in Pink," 64.

42. Ehrenreich, "Welcome to Cancerland," 53.

43. Sandra Steingraber, "Lifestyles Don't Kill: Carcinogens in Air, Food, and Water Do; Imagining Political Responses to Cancer," in *Cancer as a Women's Issue: Scratching the Surface*, ed. Midge Stocker (Chicago: Third Side Press, 1991), 96–97.

44. Barbara Brenner, "Hope, Politics, and Living with Breast Cancer," *Breast Cancer Action Newsletter*, no. 71 (May/June 2002): 2, http://bcaction.org/uploads/PDF/71.pdf (accessed June 26, 2008).

45. Sandra Steingraber, "Lifestyles Don't Kill," 97.

46. Judy Brady, "The Goose and the Golden Egg," in *1 in 3: Women with Cancer Confront an Epidemic*, ed. Judy Brady (San Francisco: Cleis Press, 1991), 27.

47. Ehrenreich, keynote address.

48. Brenda Salgado, in discussion with the author, November 19, 2007.

49. Brenner, "Hope, Politics, and Living with Breast Cancer," 2.

50. Nancy Brinker, "Susan G. Komen's Story," http://cms.komen.org/komen/AboutUs/SusanGKomensStory/index.htm (accessed September 19, 2007).

51. Susan G. Komen for the Cure, "Our Work." http://cms.komen.org/komen/AboutUs/OurWork/index.htm (accessed September 19, 2007).

52. Ibid., "Grants Program," http://cms.komen.org/komen/grantsprogram/index.htm (accessed June 28, 2008).

53. Ibid., "Public Policy," http://cms.komen.org/komen/PublicPolicy/index.htm (accessed September 19, 2007).

54. Ibid., "Komen Race for the Cure," http://cms.komen.org/komen/NewsEvents/RacefortheCure/index.htm (accessed September 19, 2007).

55. Ibid., "Passionately Pink for the Cure," http://cms.komen.org/komen/NewsEvents/PassionatelyPinkfortheCure/index.htm (accessed September 19, 2007).

56. Ibid., "Promise Shop," http://apps.komen.org/PromiseShop/ (accessed April 2, 2008).

57. Ibid., "Charlie Sheen Urges America to Don Denim for a Cause," http://cms.komen.org/Komen/NewsEvents/KomenNews/LNDD_2004 (accessed September 19, 2007).

58. Ibid., "'Desperate' Men Ask Fans for $10 Million," http://cms.komen.org/Komen/NewsEvents/KomenNews/LNDD_05 (accessed September 19, 2007).

59. Susan G. Komen for the Cure, *Many Faces One Voice: 2005–2006 Annual Report* (Dallas, Tex.: Susan G. Komen for the Cure, 2006), 5, http://cms.komen.org/komen/AboutUs/FinancialInformation/index.htm (accessed June 3, 2008).

60. Susan G. Komen for the Cure, "Corporate Partners," http://cms.komen.org/komen/Partners/CorporatePartners/index.htm (accessed September 19, 2007 and June 27, 2008).

61. Ibid., "Million Dollar Council," http://cms.komen.org/komen/Partners/MillionDollarCouncil/index.htm (accessed June 27, 2008).

62. Susan G. Komen for the Cure, "Breast Cancer Research," http://cms.komen.org/komen/PublicPolicy/BreastCancerResearch/index.htm (accessed September 19, 2007).

63. Rodriquez died two years later from the disease at age thirty-one. Barbara Waters, in discussion with the author, October 22, 2007.

64. *Reduce Your Risk* (Summit, N.J.: North Jersey Affiliate of Susan G. Komen for the Cure, 2007).

65. James Clifford, "Traveling Cultures," in *Cultural Studies*, ed. Lawrence Grossberg, Cary Nelson, and Paula Treichler (New York: Routledge, 1992), 100.

66. Susan G. Komen for the Cure, "Global Initiatives," http://cms.komen.org/komen/AboutUs/OurGlobalReach/GlobalInitiatives/index.htm (accessed September 19, 2007).

67. This approach resonates with David Hess's notion of "heterogeneous constructivism," which posits that "the content of science and technology is constructed along with the social relations and structures in the wider society. In other words, content and context co-constitute or mutually shape each other in a pattern that is sometimes called a seamless web." See David J. Hess, *Science Studies: An Advanced Introduction* (New York: New York University Press, 1997), 83.

68. Barbara Waters, in discussion with the author, October 22, 2007.

69. Nancy Evans, "From the President: One Baby Step Forward," *Breast Cancer Action Newsletter*, no. 27 (December 1994): 1.

70. Silent Spring Institute, "Breast Cancer and Environment: State of the Science Assessment," http://www.silentspring.org/newweb/research/ssa.html (accessed August 1, 2008).

71. Francesca Lyman, "You Can Run for the Cure but You Can't Run from the Cause," http://stopcancer.org (accessed July 18, 2003).

72. Massachusetts Breast Cancer Coalition, "Beyond the Headlines," May 2001, 2.

73. Susan G. Komen for the Cure, "Can Breast Cancer Be Prevented?" http://cms. komen.org/Komen/NewsEvents/KomenNews/SABCS-6_BCPrevention (accessed September 20, 2007); ibid., "Options for Women at Higher Risk of Breast Cancer," http://cms.komen.org/komen/AboutBreastCancer/RiskFactorsPrevention/ AbcHighRiskOptions?ssSourceNodeId=290&ssSourceSiteId=Komen (accessed September 19, 2007).

74. Eisenstein, *Manmade Breast Cancers*, 127.

75. Jennifer Keck, "Cult, Kitsch, or Political Movement: Breast Cancer Activism in the 21st Century," *Network News* 7, no. 1 (2002): 11, http://www.cbcn.ca/documents/ pdf/netnews-spring02.pdf (accessed September 19, 2007).

76. Hugh Gusterson provides a compelling example of the complexity of personal worldviews with regard to nuclear weapons scientists in *Nuclear Rites: A Weapons Laboratory at the End of the Cold War* (Berkeley and Los Angeles: University of California Press, 1996), 38–67.

Chapter 6 — Toxic Tours Move Indoors: Race, Class, and Breast Cancer Prevention

1. U.S. Environmental Protection Agency, "Hunters Point Naval Shipyard: California EPA ID# CA1170090087," http://yosemite.epa.gov/r9/sfund/r9sfdocw.nsf/vwsoalphabetic/Hunters+Point+Naval+Shipyard? (accessed June 20, 2008); Naval Facilities Engineering Command, "Hunters Point Shipyard," https://portal.navfac. navy.mil/portal/page?_pageid=181,3878667&_dad=portal&_schema=portal (accessed June 20, 2008); Masta Mind, "Masta Mind News Updates," http://www. mastamind.com/HP.htm (accessed June 20, 2008).

2. Allyce Bess and David Kaplowitz, "City, Navy Failed to Monitor Hunters Point Fire, Alert Residents to Risks," http://ecologycenter.org/terrain/article.php?id=13082 (accessed December 4, 2007).

3. Eva Glaser, Martha Davis, and Tomás Aragón, *Cancer Incidence among Residents of the Bayview–Hunters Point Neighborhood, San Francisco, California, 1993–1995* (San Francisco: San Francisco Department of Public Health, 1998), 2–4, http://www. sfdph.org/dph/files/reports/studiesdata/diseaseinjury/bvhuntca.pdf (accessed August 1, 2008).

4. A quick LexisNexis search on media coverage from 1995 to 2008 found that national media published 519 stories on Marin County, 109 stories on Hunters Point, and 88

on Bayview Hunters Point; state media published 351 stories on Marin County, 97 on Hunters Point, and 69 on Bayview Hunters Point; and San Francisco Bay Area media published 347 stories on Marin County, 91 on Hunters Point, and 77 on Bayview Hunters Point.

5. Susan Love, with Karen Lindsey, Dr. Susan Love's Breast Book (Reading, Mass.: Addison-Wesley, 1995), 184–185.

6. American Cancer Society, Breast Cancer Facts and Figures, 2007–2008 (Atlanta: American Cancer Society, 2008), 4–5.

7. Ibid., 8.

8. Triple Negative Breast Cancer Foundation, "Understanding Triple Negative Breast Cancer," http://www.tnbcfoundation.org/understandingtnbc.htm (accessed July 21, 2008).

9. Mary K. Anglin, "Working from the Inside Out: Implications of Breast Cancer Activism for Biomedical Policies and Practices," Social Science and Medicine 44, no. 9 (1997): 1403–1415.

10. Anglin, "Working from the Inside Out."

11. Lorraine Pace, in discussion with the author, October 18, 2007.

12. Activist, in discussion with the author, May 8, 2008.

13. Stephen Klaidman, "Roles and Responsibilities of Journalists," in Mass Communication and Public Health: Complexities and Conflicts, ed. Charles Atkin and Lawrence Wallack (New York: Sage, 1990), 60–70; David Pritchard and Karen D. Hughes, "Patterns of Deviance in Crime News," Journal of Communication 47, no. 3 (1997): 49–67.

14. Chaia Heller and Arturo Escobar, "From Pure Genes to GMOs: Transnationalized Gene Landscapes in the Biodiversity and Transgenic Food Networks," in Genetic Nature/Culture: Anthropology and Science Beyond the Two-Culture Divide, ed. Alan H. Goodman, Deborah Heath, and M. Susan Lindee (Berkeley and Los Angeles: University of California Press, 2003), 155–175; Sharon Stephens, "Physical and Cultural Reproduction in a Post-Chernobyl Norwegian Sami Community," in Conceiving the New World Order: The Global Politics of Reproduction, ed. Faye D. Ginsburg and Rayna Rapp (Berkeley and Los Angeles: University of California Press, 1995), 270–287; Brian Wynne, "Misunderstood Misunderstandings: Social Identities and Public Uptake of Science," in Misunderstanding Science? The Public Reconstruction of Science and Technology, ed. Alan Irwin and Brian Wynne (Cambridge, U.K.: Cambridge University Press, 2004), 19–46.

15. Sisters of Greater Long Island, "Welcome," http://sogli.org/ (accessed May 12, 2008).

16. Brenda Salgado, in discussion with the author, November 19, 2007; Nancy Evans, in discussion with the author, December 11, 2007; Barbara Waters, in discussion with the author, October 22, 2007.

17. Mitchell H. Katz, Health Programs in Bayview Hunters Point and Recommendations for Improving the Health of Bayview Hunters Point Residents (San Francisco: San Francisco Department of Public Health, 2006), 6–10, http://www.sfdph.org/dph/files/reports/StudiesData/BayviewHlthRpt09192006.pdf (accessed on July 14, 2008).

18. Ibid, 6–10.

19. Katz, Health Programs in Bayview Hunters Point, 7.

20. Barbara Waters, in discussion with the author, October 22, 2007. Brenda Salgado (in discussion with the author, November 19, 2007), Nancy Evans (in discussion with the author, December 11, 2007), and Deborah Shields (in discussion with the author, July 16, 2008) reinforced this point.

21. Karen Joy Miller, in discussion with the author, June 27, 2008.

22. Donna J. Haraway, *Simians, Cyborgs, and Women: The Reinvention of Nature* (New York: Routledge, 1991); Sandra Harding, *Whose Science? Whose Knowledge? Thinking from Women's Lives* (Ithaca, N.Y.: Cornell University Press, 1991); Sandra Harding, ed., *The "Racial" Economy of Science: Toward a Democratic Future* (Bloomington: Indiana University Press, 1993); Maralee Mayberry, Banu Subramaniam, and Lisa H. Weasel, eds., *Feminist Science Studies: A New Generation* (New York: Routledge, 2001).

23. *For Our Daughters: Breast Cancer Prevalence and Geographic Information Survey* (Huntington, N.Y.: Huntington Breast Cancer Action Coalition, 2005), 2.

24. Andrea R. Martin and Joan Reinhardt Reiss, "Update on Our Sign-On Letter" (San Francisco: Breast Cancer Fund, 2000), 2.

25. Breast Cancer and Environment Research Centers, "Background Information," http://bcerc.org/general.htm (accessed June 12, 2008).

26. Ibid., "Working Group Members," http://bcerc.org/wgmembers.htm (accessed June 12, 2008).

27. Ibid., "University of California, San Francisco (BABCERC)," http://bcerc.org/ucsf.htm (accessed June 12, 2008).

28. Ibid., "Community Outreach and Translation," http://bcerc.org/cotc.htm (accessed June 12, 2008).

29. Ibid., "Research Projects," http://bcerc.org/research.htm (accessed January 28, 2008).

30. Sandra Steingraber, *The Falling Age of Puberty in U.S. Girls: What We Know, What We Need to Know* (San Francisco: Breast Cancer Fund, 2007), 26–29.

31. Ibid., 10–11.

32. Ibid., 41–57.

33. Center for Environmental Oncology, *Environmental Risks of Breast Cancer in African American Women* (Pittsburgh: University of Pittsburgh Cancer Institute, 2007), 2, http://www.environmentaloncology.org/files/file/Publications/AA%20Brochure/websiteafamerbroch.pdf (accessed December 6, 2008).

34. Steingraber, *The Falling Age*, 23–25.

35. Ruthann Rudel, in discussion with the author, November 30, 2007.

36. Communities for a Better Environment, "Homepage," http://cbecal.org (accessed December 3, 2007).

37. Ruthann Rudel, in discussion with the author, November 30, 2007.

38. Silent Spring Institute, "Breast Cancer and Environmental Justice—Household Exposure Study," http://www.silentspring.org/newweb/research/ej.html (accessed January 28, 2008).

39. Ruthann Rudel, in discussion with the author, November 30, 2007

40. Rachel Morello-Frosh and Edmond D. Shenassa, "The Environmental 'Riskscape' and Social Inequity: Implications for Explaining Maternal and Child Health Disparities," *Environmental Health Perspectives* 114, no. 8 (2006): 1150–1153; Michael Jerrett and Murray Finklestein, "Geographies of Risk in Studies Linking Chronic Air Pollution Exposure to Health Outcomes," *Journal of Toxicology and Environmental Health Part A*, 68, no. 13–14 (2005): 1207–1242.

41. Donna Jurasits, in discussion with the author, April 15, 2008.

42. Nancy Evans and Andrea Ravinett Martin, *Pathways for Prevention: Eight Practical Steps—from the Personal to the Political—towards Reducing the Risk of Breast Cancer* (San Francisco: Breast Cancer Fund, 2000).

43. Sharon Koshar, in discussion with the author, December 3, 2007.

44. Chris Kenning and Jessie Halladay, "Cities Study Dearth of Healthy Food," *USA Today*, January 25, 2008; Amy Worden, "Wanted: Inner City Supermarkets," *Philadelphia Inquirer*, November 21, 2003.

45. Evans and Martin, *Pathways for Prevention*, 38.

46. Breast Cancer Action, "Comida saludable, cuerpo sano," *Saber es Poder*, edicion 19 (2007), http://bcaction.org/uploads/PDF/SEP19.pdf (accessed January 11, 2008).

47. Margo Rivera-Weiss, in discussion with the author, February 19, 2008.

48. Donna Jurasits, in discussion with the author, April 15, 2008.

49. Geri Barish, in discussion with the author, April 21, 2008.

50. Center for Environmental Oncology, "Environmental Risks," 2.

51. *Workplace and Cancer* (Houston: Intercultural Cancer Council, 2004), 2.

52. Breast Cancer Fund, "2005 California Legislative Summary," http://www.breastcancerfund.org/site/pp.asp?c=kwKXLdPaE&b=1486231 (accessed January 11, 2005).

53. Campaign for Safe Cosmetics, "Cosmetics Companies Lobby Against Safe Cosmetics Legislation," http://www.breastcancerfund.org/atf/cf/{DE68F7B2–5F6A-4B57–9794—AFE5D27A3CFF}/CaLegFactsheet.pdf (accessed January 11, 2008).

54. Alliance for a Healthy Tomorrow, "The Safe Alternatives Bill: An Act for a Healthy Massachusetts," 1, http://www.healthytomorrow.org/PDF/factsheet-10—SAbi 11200705final.pdf (accessed June 25, 2008).

55. Brenda Salgado, in discussion with the author, November 19, 2007; Nancy Evans, in discussion with the author, December 11, 2007; the California Healthy Nail Salon Collaborative, "Membership and Participation Guidelines, January 2008," http://ahschc.org/nailsalon.pdf (accessed May 15, 2008).

56. WAGES: Women's Action to Gain Economic Security, "Home Page," http://wagesco-operatives.org (accessed January 11, 2008).

57. Natural Home Cleaning Professionals, "Home Page," http://www.naturalhomeclean-ing.com/ (accessed January 11, 2008).

58. Breast Cancer Action, "Trabajo saludable, cuerpo sano," *Saber es Poder*, edición 19 (2007): 3, http://bcaction.org/index.php?page=saber-es-poder-no-19 (accessed July 15, 2008).

59. *Frameworks for Environmental Health, Rights, and Justice* (San Francisco: Breast Cancer Action, 2007). Breast Cancer Action's framework is based on Asian Communities for Reproductive Justice, *The New Vision for Advancing Our Movement for Reproductive Health, Reproductive Rights and Reproductive Justice* (Oakland, Calif.: Asian Communities for Reproductive Justice, 2005).

60. Melissa Checker, "'It's in the Air': Redefining the Environment as a New Metaphor for Old Social Justice Struggles," *Human Organization* 61, no. 1 (2002): 94–95.

61. Giovanna DiChiro, "Nature as Community: The Convergence of Environmental and Social Justice," in *Uncommon Ground: Rethinking the Human Place in Nature*, ed. William Cronon (New York: W. W. Norton, 1995), 298–320.

62. Massachusetts Breast Cancer Coalition, "Campaign for Safe Cosmetics," http://mbcc.org/content.php?id=8 (accessed November 9, 2007).

63. For an account of the politics of breast cancer and community-based studies in Bayview Hunters Point, see Jennifer Fishman, "Assessing Breast Cancer: Science and Environmental Activism in an 'At-Risk' Community," in *Ideologies of Breast Cancer: Feminist Perspectives*, ed. Laura K. Potts (London: Macmillan, 2000), 181–205.

64. Melissa Checker, "'But I Know It's True': Environmental Risk Assessment, Justice, and Anthropology," *Human Organization* 66, no. 2 (2007): 117–120; Reina Diaz, "The Harvest of Poison" in *1 in 3: Women with Cancer Confront an Epidemic*, ed. Judy Brady (San Francisco: Cleis Press, 1991), 77. Fishman, "Assessing Breast Cancer," 194–200.

65. Sara Shostak, "Environmental Justice and Genomics: Acting on the Futures of Environmental Health," *Science as Culture* 13, no. 4 (2004): 549–551.

66. Melissa Checker, "Environmental Justice through Citizen Science" (paper presented at the annual meeting of the American Anthropological Association, San Jose, California, November 2006); Checker, "But I Know It's True," 118.

67. Fishman, "Assessing Breast Cancer," 192.

68. Ruthann Rudel, in discussion with the author, November 30, 2007.

69. Ibid.

70. Activist, in discussion with the author, May 8, 2008. Also see Boston Public Health Commission, "Pink and Black Campaign," http://www.bphc.org/pinkblack/index2.asp (accessed July 28, 2008).

71. Fishman, "Assessing Breast Cancer," 190.

Chapter 7 — Beyond Breast Cancer, Beyond Women's Health

1. Sheryl Burt Ruzek, Virginia L. Olesen, and Adele E. Clarke, "Social, Biomedical, and Feminist Models of Women's Health," in *Women's Health: Complexities and Differences*, ed. Sheryl Burt Ruzek, Virginia L. Olesen, and Adele E. Clarke (Columbus: Ohio State University Press, 1997), 22.

2. Nancy Evans and Andrea Ravinett Martin, *Pathways to Prevention: Eight Practical Steps—from the Personal to the Political—toward Reducing the Risk of Breast Cancer* (San Francisco: Breast Cancer Fund, 2000).

3. *Rachel's Daughters: Searching for Causes of Breast Cancer*, VHS, directed by Irving Saraf and Allie Light (San Francisco: Light-Saraf-Evans Productions, 1997).

4. See Ted Schettler et al., *Generations at Risk: Reproductive Health and the Environment* (Cambridge, Mass.: MIT Press, 1999); Sandra Steingraber, *Having Faith: An Ecologist's Journey to Motherhood* (Cambridge, Mass.: Perseus, 2001).

5. Nancy Evans, "The Persistence of Pesticides: Women and Children First," *Breast Cancer Action Newsletter*, no. 20 (October 1993): 1.

6. Evans, "The Persistence of Pesticides," 2.

7. Breast Cancer Action, "August 2001 Email Alert," http://bcaction.org/pages/get-informed/emailalerts/aug2001alert.html (accessed January 2, 2003).

8. Toxic Links Coalition, "Victories in 2000 and 2001 for the Toxic Links Coalition and Our Participant Organizations," http://toxiclinks.net/victories%20in%202000%20 and%202001.html (accessed March 5, 2003).

9. Breast Cancer Action, "January 2002 Email Alert," http://bcaction.org/pages/getinformed/emailalerts/jan2002alert.html (accessed January 2, 2003).

10. Physicians for Social Responsibility, *Arsenic Fact Sheet* (Washington, D.C.: Physicians for Social Responsibility, 2001).

11. Breast Cancer Action, "November 2001 Email Alert," http://bcaction.org/pages/get-informed/emailalerts/nov2001alert.html (accessed January 2, 2003).

12. Breast Cancer Fund, "January 2002 E-Alert," http://breastcancerfund.org/jan2002_alert.html (accessed January 2, 2003).

13. Felix Aguilar, "The Importance of Using a Community-Based Approach to Conducting Biomonitoring: Using Breast Milk as a Marker to Measure Community

Health" (public testimony at the Joint Information Hearing on Breast Cancer and the Environment to the California Senate Health and Human Services Committee and Assembly Health Committee, October 23, 2002), http://breastcancerfund.org/environment_hearing_aguilar.htm (accessed January 2, 2003).

14. Jeanne Rizzo, "Summary of Policy Recommendations from the Field," ibid. I borrow the concept of nonhuman "actant" from Bruno Latour, *Science in Action: How to Follow Scientists and Engineers Through Society* (Cambridge, Mass.: Harvard University Press, 1987). Latour states, "Both people who talk and things unable to talk have spokesmen. I propose to call whoever and whatever is represented [an] actant," 83–84.

15. Steingraber, *Having Faith*, 251.

16. Understanding the movement of chemicals across generations and bodies resonates with Monica Casper's notion of "following the molecule" in "Introduction: Chemical Matters," in *Synthetic Planet: Chemical Politics and the Hazards of Modern Life*, ed. Monica J. Casper (New York: Routledge, 2003), xxii–xvii.

17. Breast Cancer Fund, "SB600-Measuring and Understanding the 'Pollution in People,'" http://www.breastcancerfund.org/site/pp.asp?c=kwKXLdPaE&b=1104425 (accessed November 9, 2007).

18. Ibid., "2006 Legislative Summary," http://www.breastcancerfund.org/site/pp.asp?c=kwKXLdPaE&b=2776125 (accessed November 9, 2007).

19. Prevention Is the Cure, "2008 Prevention Is the Cure Week," http://www.preventionisthecure.org/preventionisthecureweek.html (accessed June 30, 2008).

20. Ibid., "Power Plants' Mercury Pollution: Jeopardizing the Health and Future," http://www.preventionisthecure.org/pdf/powerplants.pdf (accessed November 7, 2007).

21. Devra L. Davis, "Environmental Health and the Precautionary Principle" (keynote address, Massachusetts Precautionary Principle kick-off meeting, Framingham, Mass., May 15, 1999), http://www.sustainableproduction.org/precaution/back.brie.envi.html (accessed June 30, 2008).

22. Andrea R. Martin and Joan Reinhardt Reiss, "Update on Our Sign-on Letter" (San Francisco: Breast Cancer Fund, May 12, 2000), 3.

23. John W. Brock et al., "Phthalate Monoester Levels in the Urine of Young Children," *Bulletin of Environmental Contamination and Toxicology* 68, no. 3 (2002): 309–314.

24. Susan M. Duty et al., "The Relationship between Environmental Exposures to Phthalates and DNA Damage in Human Sperm Using the Neutral Comet Assay," *Environmental Health Perspectives* 111, no. 9 (2003): 1164–1169.

25. Lennart Hardell et al., "Increased Concentrations of Polychlorinated Biphenyls, Hexachlorobenzene, and Chlordanes in Mothers to Men with Testicular Cancer," *Environmental Health Perspectives* 111, no. 7 (2003): 930–934.

26. Jane Houlihan, Charlotte Brody, and Bryony Schwan, *Not Too Pretty: Phthalates, Beauty Products, and the FDA* (Washington, D.C.: Environmental Working Group, Coming Clean, and Health Care Without Harm, 2002), http://www.safecosmetics.org/docUploads/NotTooPretty_r51.pdf (accessed November 9, 2007).

27. Women's Environmental Network, Swedish Society of Nature Conservation, and Health Care Without Harm, *Pretty Nasty: Phthalates in European Cosmetics* (n.p., Sweden: Health Care Without Harm, 2002), http://www.safecosmetics.org/docUploads/Prettynasty.pdf 1 (accessed November 9, 2007).

28. Not Too Pretty's Web site (http://nottoopretty.org) was terminated after the organization became the Campaign for Safe Cosmetics.

29. Women's Voices for the Earth, http://www.wildrockies.org/WVE (accessed January 22, 2003). The organization's new URL is http://www.womenandenvironment.org.

30. Campaign for Safe Cosmetics, "About the Campaign for Safe Cosmetics," http://www.safecosmetics.org/about (accessed November 9, 2007).

31. Ibid., "Policies and Legislation," http://www.safecosmetics.org/about/policies.cfm (accessed November 9, 2007).

32. Ibid., "The Compact for Safe Cosmetics," http://www.safecosmetics.org/companies/compact_with_america.cfm (accessed November 9, 2007).

33. The Skin Deep: Safe Cosmetics Database is located at http://www.cosmetic database.com/index.php?nothanks=1 (accessed November 9, 2007).

34. Campaign for Safe Cosmetics, "Get the Lead Out," http://safecosmetics.org (accessed June 15, 2007).

35. Breast Cancer Action, "August 2002 Email Alert," http://bcaction.org/pages/getin formed/emailalerts/aug2002alert.htm (accessed January 2, 2003).

36. Ibid., "December 2002 Email Alert," http://bcaction.org/pages/getinginformed/emailalerts/dec2002alert.html (accessed February 27, 2003); Breast Cancer Fund, "December 2002 E-Alert," http://breastcancerfund.org/dec2002_alert.html (accessed February 27, 2003).

37. Breast Cancer Fund, "Cosmetics and Breast Carcinogens," http://www.breastcancer-fund.org/site/pp.asp?c=kwKXLdPaE&b=3005277 (accessed November 9, 2007).

38. Massachusetts Breast Cancer Coalition, "Campaign for Safe Cosmetics," http://mbcc.org/content.php?id=8 (accessed November 9, 2007).

39. Prevention Is the Cure, "Mount Sinai Ads Campaign," http://preventionisthecure.org/ad4a.html (accessed November 7, 2007).

40. Mary O'Brien, "Racing towards the Starting Line: The Radical Nature of Precaution" (keynote address, "At the Heart of Primary Prevention: Breast Cancer and the Precautionary Principle," Boston, October 23, 1999), http://www.sehn.org/ppintan-drevessays.html (accessed June 15, 2008).

41. Huntington Breast Cancer Action Coalition, "I Am Fed Naturally," http://hbcac.org/fednaturally.html (accessed June 3, 2008).

42. Breast Cancer Fund, "December 2002 E-Alert," http://breastcancerfund.org/dec2002_alert.html (accessed January 2, 2003); ibid., "November 2002 E-Alert," http://breastcancerfund.org/nov2002_alert.html (accessed January 2, 2003); ibid., "October 2002 E-Alert," http://breastcancerfund.org/oct2002_alert.html (accessed January 2, 2003); ibid., "September 2002 E-Alert," http://breastcancerfund.org/sep2002_alert.html (accessed January 2, 2003).

43. Ibid., "October 2002 E-Alert."

44. Ibid., "November 2002 E-Alert," http://breastcancerfund.org/nov2002_alert.html (accessed January 2, 2003).

45. National Audubon Society, "Clean Water," http://www.audubon.org/campaign/cleanWater2.html (accessed November 9, 2007).

46. Clean Water Network, "Home," http://www.cleanwaternetwork.org (accessed November 9, 2007).

47. National Audubon Society, "Help Combat Global Warming," http://www.audubon.org/globalWarming (accessed November 9, 2007).

48. Ibid., "Protect the Artic Refuge," http://www.protectthearctic.com; ibid., *Toxic Tundra: Oil Drilling in an Alaskan Wildlife Refuge Leaves a Toxic Legacy of Oil Spills and Pollution* (Washington, D.C.: National Audubon Society, 2002), CIThttp://www.audubon.org/campaign/arctic_report/Arctic_Refuge_final_2–13.pdf.

49. Janice Barlow, in discussion with the author, November 12, 2007.

50. Karen Joy Miller, in discussion with the author, November 13 and 14, 2007.

51. Lorraine Pace, in discussion with the author, October 18, 2007.

52. Rita Arditti, in discussion with the author, May 9, 2008.

53. David A. Snow et al., "Frame Alignment Processes, Micromobilization, and Movement Participation," *American Sociological Review* 51, no. 4 (1986): 464.

54. Brenda Salgado, in discussion with the author, November 19, 2007.

55. Geri Barish, in discussion with the author, April 21, 2008.

56. Nancy Evans, in discussion with the author, December 11, 2007.

57. Brenda Salgado, in discussion with the author, November 19, 2007.

58. Deborah Shields, in discussion with the author, April 24, 2008.

59. Sarah L. Holloway and Gill Valentine, *Cyberkids: Children in the Information Age* (London: Routledge/Falmer, 2003), 3–5.

60. In January 2003, I conducted an online search of the Thomas congressional database to track the number children's environmental health bills that congressional members introduced to the House and Senate over the past thirty years. I searched the database with the terms *children's health, children's health and the environment, children's environmental health,* and *children's health and pesticides.* In 1972–1973, there were 32 bills related to children's health introduced in Congress. In 1991–1992, the number increased to 78. In 1993–1994, it jumped to 115; and in 2001–2002, it grew to 263.

61. Sheldon Krimsky, *Hormonal Chaos: The Scientific and Social Origins of the Environmental Endocrine Hypothesis* (Baltimore: Johns Hopkins University Press, 2000), 61–63.

62. Nelly Oudshoorn, *Beyond the Natural Body: An Archeology of Sex Hormones* (London: Routledge, 1994).

63. Ibid., *The Male Pill: A Biography of a Technology in the Making* (Durham: Duke University Press, 2003).

64. Maricel V. Maffini et al., "Endocrine Disruptors and Reproductive Health: The Case of Bisphenol-A," *Molecular and Cellular Endocrinology* 254–255 (2006): 179–186; Shuk-Mei Ho et al., "Developmental Exposure to Estradiol and Bisphenol A Increases Susceptibility to Prostate Carcinogenesis and Epigenetically Regulates Phosphodiesterase Type 4 Variant 4," *Cancer Research* 66, no. 11 (2006): 5624–5632.

65. This approach is exemplified by the National Prostate Cancer Coalition. See http://fightprostatecancer.org (accessed November 15, 2007).

66. See also Susan H. Dimock, "Demanding Disease Dollars: How Activism and Institutions Shape Medical Research Funding for Breast Cancer and Prostate Cancer" (PhD diss., University of California at San Diego, 2003).

67. Activist, in discussion with the author, May 16, 1999.

68. Evans, "The Persistence of Pesticides."

69. For low-income neighborhoods and communities of color, see Giovanna DiChiro, "Nature as Community: The Convergence of Environmental and Social Justice," in *Uncommon Ground: Rethinking the Human Place in Nature,* ed. William Cronon (New York: W. W. Norton, 1995), 298–320. For the War on Cancer, see Samuel Epstein, *The Politics of Cancer* (San Francisco: Sierra Club Books, 1978); Ralph W. Moss, *The Cancer Industry: The Classic Exposé of the Cancer Establishment* (New York: Equinox Press, 1996); Judy Brady, "The Goose and the Golden Egg," in *1 in 3: Women with Cancer Confront an Epidemic,* ed. Judy Brady (San Francisco: Cleis Press, 1991), 13–35.

70. O'Brien, "Racing Towards the Starting Line."
71. World Wildlife Foundation, "Toxic Chemicals," http://wordlwildlife.org/toxics (accessed November 12, 2007).
72. Ibid., "Agricultural Pesticides," http://worldwildlife.org/toxics/proareas/ap/index.htm (accessed March 4, 2007).
73. Ibid., "Reducing Toxic Chemicals," http://worldwildlife.org/consumer/rtc.cfm (accessed November 12, 2007).
74. National Audubon Society, "Population and Habitat: Making the Connection," http://www.audubon.org/campaign/population_habitat/ (accessed July 1, 2008); ibid., "Tell Your Representatives That Family Planning Benefits Women and the Environment," http://audubonaction.org/campaign/hr1225 (accessed November 12, 2007).

Chapter 8 — Still in the Making

1. Itzhak Pappo et al., "The Possible Association between IVF and Breast Cancer Incidence," *Annals of Surgical Oncology* 15, no. 4 (2008): 1048–1055; M. Salhab, W. Al Sarakbi, and Kefah Mokbel, "In Vitro Fertilization and Breast Cancer Risk: A Review," *International Journal of Fertility and Women's Medicine* 50, no. 6 (2005): 259–266.
2. Adele Clarke and Theresa Montini, "The Many Faces of RU-486: Tales of Situated Knowledges and Technological Contestations," *Science, Technology, and Human Values* 18, no. 1 (1993): 42–78.
3. Jane A. McElroy et al., "Cadmium Exposure and Breast Cancer Risk," *Journal of the National Cancer Institute* 98, no. 12 (2006): 869–873.
4. Janice Barlow, in discussion with the author, November 12, 2007.
5. Ruth Allen, in discussion with the author, November 20, 2007.
6. Breast Cancer Fund, "Urge Congress to Connect Diseases with Causes and Solutions," http://www.breastcancerfund.org/siteapps/advocacy/ActionItem.aspx?c=kwKXLdPaE&b=3558771 (accessed November 29, 2007).
7. Zero Breast Cancer, "The Breast Cancer and Environment—Peer Education Tool Kit," http://zerobreastcancer.org/education/zbc_ap_coverpage.html (accessed January 26, 2008).
8. Deborah Basile, in discussion with the author, April 15, 2008; Donna Jurasits, in discussion with the author, April 15, 2008.
9. Janice Barlow, in discussion with the author, November 12, 2007; Karen J. Miller, in discussion with the author, November 13 and 14, 2007.
10. Janice Barlow, in discussion with the author, November 12, 2007.
11. Karen Joy Miller, in discussion with the author, November 13 and 14, 2007.
12. Erin Boles and Deborah Shields, in discussion with the author, April 24, 2008; Beverly Baccelli, in discussion with the author, May 20, 2008; University of Massachusetts at Lowell, "Breast Cancer Prevention Project," http://gis.uml.edu/mediawiki/index.php/Breast_Cancer_Prevention_Project (accessed July 26, 2008).
13. Breast Cancer Action, "Action Alert! Help Save the California Breast Cancer Research Program," http://app.e2ma.net/campaign/126913cf28aebda4eec485b5ca9b56fb (accessed July 15, 2008).
14. Cancer Resource Center of the Finger Lakes, "History and Timeline," http://www.ibca.net/about_us/history&timeline.php (accessed November 27, 2007).
15. Program on Breast Cancer and Environmental Risk Factors, "Home," http://envirocancer.cornell.edu/ (accessed November 27, 2007). See also ibid., "About

BCERF," http://envirocancer.cornell.edu/program/aboutUS.cfm (accessed November 27, 2007).

16. Breast Cancer Fund, "Washington State Advocacy," http://www.breastcancerfund. org/site/pp.asp?c=kwKXLdPaE&b=71146 (accessed November 26, 2007).

17. Ibid., "Washington State Advocacy."

18. Ibid., "Washington State Legislative Effort," http://www.breastcancerfund.org/site/ pp.asp?c=kwKXLdPaE&b=2560087 (accessed November 27, 2007); Washington Toxics Coalition, "Toxic Flame Retardants," http://www.watoxics.org/issues/pbde (accessed July 11, 2008).

19. Breast Cancer Fund, "RSVP for the Falling Age of Puberty," http://www. breastcancerfund.org/site/apps/ka/ct/contactus.asp?c=kwKXLdPaE&b=3293845& en=ghLHLSOCJiKMKRMDJlJNJRPBJlKTLYPILmKRI300JrK5H (accessed November 27, 2007).

20. Ibid., "Tips on Becoming an Advocate for Prevention," http://www.breastcancer-fund.org/site/pp.asp?c=kwKXLdPaE&b=2061055 (accessed November 27, 2007).

21. Breast Cancer Action, "Starting a Stop Cancer Where It Starts Where You Live: You Can Do It Too!" http://bcaction.org/uploads/PDF/SCWISGuide.pdf (accessed January 28, 2008).

22. Deborah Shields, in discussion with the author, July 16, 2008; Ruthann Rudel, e-mail message to author, July 30, 2008.

23. California Breast Cancer Research Program, "California Breast Cancer Research Program Receives $500,000 from Avon Foundation," http://www.cbcrp.org/media/ pr/071408.php (accessed July 26, 2008).

24. Ibid., "California Breast Cancer."

25. Prevention Is the Cure, "Nassau County Unanimously Passes a Green Procurement Policy," http://preventionisthecure.org/green_procurement.htm (accessed July 8, 2008); Legislator Steven H. Stern, "Legislator Stern Applauds Passage of Safe and Sustainable Procurement Policy," http://www.co.suffolk.ny.us/legis/ press/d016/2007/d016PR%20031307%20procurement%20dh.htm (accessed July 8, 2008).

26. Alliance for a Healthy Tomorrow, "Current Legislative Priorities, 2007–08," http:// healthytomorrow.org/currentleg.html (accessed April 2, 2008); ibid., "Legislative Updates," http://www.healthytomorrow.org/Leg_Updates.html (accessed June 25, 2008).

27. Kathleen Kingsbury, "The Changing Face of Breast Cancer," *Time*, October 2007, http://www.time.com/time/specials/2007/article/0,28804,1666089_1666563_16684 77,00.ht (accessed July 11, 2008).

28. Kingsbury, "The Changing Face"; American Cancer Society, *Global Cancer Facts and Figures, 2007* (Atlanta: American Cancer Society, 2007), 10, http://www.can-cer.org/downloads/STT/Global_Cancer_Facts_and_Figures_2007_rev.pdf (accessed July 11, 2008).

29. World Conference on Breast Cancer Foundation, "Profile," http://www.wcbcf.ca/ foundation/profile (accessed January 28, 2008).

30. Deborah Shields and Erin Boles, in discussion with the author, April 24, 2008; Tout en Ronduer, "Prévention cancer du sein, une asso qui se bouge dans le Pas de Calais!!!" http://toutenrounduer.over-blog.com/article-12482210.html (accessed July 12, 2008).

31. Arjun Appadurai, "Disjuncture and Difference in the Global Cultural Economy," in *Modernity at Large: The Cultural Dimensions of Globalization* (Minneapolis: University of Minnesota Press, 1997).

32. *The Hazardous Chemicals and Wastes Conventions* (Geneva: United Nations Environmental Programme, 2003), 1, http://www.pops.int/documents/background/hcwc.pdf, 1 (accessed April 9, 2008).

33. Stockholm Convention on Persistent Organic Pollutants (POPs), "Status of Ratification," http://chm.pops.int/Countries/StatusofRatification/tabid/252/language/en-US/Default.aspx (accessed July 15, 2008); Collaborative on Health and the Environment, "Consensus Statement on Breast Cancer and the Environment 2006," http://www.breastcancerfund.org/site/pp.asp?c=kwKXLdPaE&b=2065995 (accessed January 28, 2008).

34. Meg Kissinger and Susanne Rust, "Canada Says Plastic in Water Bottles Is Unsafe," *Milwaukee Journal Sentinel*, April 18, 2008.

35. Lowell Center for Sustainable Development, "REACH—the New EU Chemicals Strategy: A New Approach to Chemicals Management," http://chemicalspolicy.org/reach.shtml (accessed January 28, 2008); Campaign for Safe Cosmetics, "Are Your Products Safe?" http://www.safecosmetics.org/your_health/index.cfm (accessed January 28, 2008); Committee on Government Reform—Minority Office, "A Special Interest Case Study: The Chemical Industry, the Bush Administration, and European Efforts to Regulate Chemicals." (Washington, D.C.: U.S. House of Representatives, April 1, 2004), 1–2, http://www.safecosmetics.org/docUploads/waxman%2Epdf (accessed January 28, 2008).

36. Campaign for Safe Cosmetics, "Are Your Products Safe?"

37. Committee on Government Reform—Minority Office, "A Special Interest Case Study," 2.

38. Nancy Evans, in discussion with the author, December 11, 2007.

39. On December 13, 2007, I conducted a LexisNexis search. Specifically, I searched U.S. newspapers and newswire services for their coverage on phthalates and bisphenol A. Between December 13, 2001, and December 13, 2004, I found 171 newspaper articles and 106 newswire reports on phthalates and 29 newspaper articles and 29 newswire releases on bisphenol A. After December 13, 2004, these numbers jumped. I found 622 articles and 211 releases on phthalates, and 290 articles and 171 releases on bisphenol A.

40. Susanne Rust, "Chemical's Use Extensive," *Milwaukee Journal Sentinel*, November 9, 2007; Susanne Rust, Meg Kissinger, and Cary Spivak, "Chemical Fallout Part 1: Are Your Products Safe? You Can't Tell," *Milwaukee Journal Sentinel*, November 25, 2007; ibid., "Chemical Fallout Part Two: Bisphenol A Is in You," *Milwaukee Journal Sentinel*, December 2, 2007; Meg Kissinger, "Formula Concerns Arise," *Milwaukee Journal Sentinel*, December 6, 2007; Cary Spivak, "Investors Take Aim at Plastic Products," *Milwaukee Journal Sentinel*, December 10, 2007; Cary Spivak, "Sears, Kmart to Remove Products with Polyvinyl Chloride," *Milwaukee Journal Sentinel*, December 13, 2007; Susanne Rusk and Cary Spivak, "Area Parents Switching to Glass for Baby's Bottles," *Milwaukee Journal Sentinel*, December 26, 2007; Meg Kissinger, Cary Spivak, and Susanne Rust, "Plastics Report Reviewed," *Milwaukee Journal Sentinel*, January 10, 2008; Susanne Rust and Cary Spivak, "Baby Products under Scrutiny," *Milwaukee Journal Sentinel*, January 18, 2008; Susanne Rust, "Chemical Ingested, Study Finds," *Milwaukee Journal Sentinel*, January 23, 2008; ibid., "Chemicals in Lotion May Enter Babies' Skin," *Milwaukee Journal Sentinel*, February 4, 2008; Cary Spivak and Susanne Rust, "Panel to Question Plastics Consultant," *Milwaukee Journal Sentinel*, February 7, 2008; Susanne Rust, "FDA Relied on Industry Studies to Judge Safety," *Milwaukee Journal Sentinel*, March 22, 2008; Kissinger and Rust, "Canada Says Plastic in Water Bottles Is Unsafe."

41. Princeton Survey Research Associates, http://poll.orspub.com/document.php?id=quest04.0ut_18720&type=hitlist&num=0 (accessed December 11, 2007).

42. Prevention Magazine/Food Marketing Institute, http://poll.orspub.com/document.php?id=quest04.0ut_16674&type=hitlist&num=14 (accessed December 11, 2007).

43. Harris Poll, http://poll.orspub.com/document.php?id=quest07.0ut_17907&type=hitlist&num=287 (accessed July 11, 2008).

44. Rust and Spivak, "Area Parents Switching to Glass."

45. Lowell Center for Sustainable Production, "Sustainable Production and Consumption Program," http://www.sustainableproduction.org/proj.spro.abou.shtml (accessed January 28, 2008).

46. Ibid., "Clean Production Research and Training," http://www.sustainableproduction.org/proj.clea.abou.shtml (accessed January 28, 2008).

47. Campaign for Safe Cosmetics, "Signers of the Compact for Safe Cosmetics," http://www.safecosmetics.org/companies/signers.cfm (accessed December 11, 2007).

48. Brenda Salgado, "Beauty and the Beast: Activists Work for Safer Cosmetics," *Satya Magazine*, January 2005, http://stayamag.com/jan05/salgado.html (accessed July 28, 2008); Campaign for Safe Cosmetics, "Press Release—May 21, 2005," http://safecosmetics.org/newsroom/press.cfm?pressReleaseID=9 (accessed July 26, 2008); Richard A. Liroff, *Protecting Public Health, Increasing Profits, and Promoting Innovation by Benchmarking Corporate Governance of Chemicals in Products* (Washington, D.C.: World Wildlife Fund, 2005), 28; Investors Environmental Health Network, "Shareholder Resolutions," http://www.iehn.org/resolutions.shareholder.php (accessed July 28, 2008).

49. Spivak, "Investors Take Aim at Plastic Products."

50. Janice Barlow, in discussion with the author, November 12, 2007.

51. Geri Barish, in discussion with the author, April 21, 2008. See also "Gene Elevating Breast Cancer Risk Also Causes Prostate Cancer," *Science Daily*, February 9, 2007, http://www.sciencedaily.com/releases/2007/02/070208131722.htm (accessed December 14, 2008).

52. Center for Environmental Oncology, "Devra L. Davis, PhD, MPH," http://www.environmentaloncology.org/staff_davis.htm (accessed July 26, 2008); ibid., "Helping to Make Prevention the Cure for Cancer," http://www.environmentaloncology.org/node/1 (accessed July 26, 2008).

53. Karen Joy Miller, in discussion with the author, November 13 and 14, 2007.

54. Collaboration on Health and the Environment, "History," http://www.healthandenvironment.org/about/history (accessed April 10, 2008).

55. Ibid., "Mission," http://www.healthandenvironment.org/about/mission (accessed April 10, 2008).

56. Ibid., "What Is a Working Group?" http://www.healthandenvironment.org/working_groups/what_is (accessed April 10, 2008).

Index

About the Author

Barbara L. Ley is an assistant professor in the Department of Journalism and Mass Communication at the University of Wisconsin–Milwaukee. She teaches and conducts research on science and culture, the social dimensions of digital technology, and health and the media.

Available titles in the Critical Issues in Health and Medicine series:

Emily K. Abel, *Suffering in the Land of Sunshine: A Los Angeles Illness Narrative*

Emily K. Abel, *Tuberculosis and the Politics of Exclusion: A History of Public Health and Migration to Los Angeles*

Susan M. Chambré, *Fighting for Our Lives: New York's AIDS Community and the Politics of Disease*

James Colgrove, Gerald Markowitz, and David Rosner, eds., *The Contested Boundaries of American Public Health*

Cynthia A. Connolly, *Saving Sickly Children: The Tuberculosis Preventorium in American Life, 1909–1970*

Edward J. Eckenfels, *Doctors Serving People: Restoring Humanism to Medicine through Student Community Service*

Julie Fairman, *Making Room in the Clinic: Nurse Practitioners and the Evolution of Modern Health Care*

Jill A. Fisher, *Medical Research for Hire: The Political Economy of Pharmaceutical Clinical Trials*

Gerald N. Grob and Howard H. Goldman, *The Dilemma of Federal Mental Health Policy: Radical Reform or Incremental Change?*

Rebecca M. Kluchin, *Fit to Be Tied: Sterilization and Reproductive Rights in America, 1950–1980*

Jennifer Lisa Koslow, *Cultivating Health: Los Angeles Women and Public Health Reform*

Bonnie Lefkowitz, *Community Health Centers: A Movement and the People Who Made It Happen*

Ellen Leopold, *Under the Radar: Cancer and the Cold War*

Barbara L. Ley, *From Pink to Green: Disease Prevention and the Environmental Breast Cancer Movement*

David Mechanic, *The Truth about Health Care: Why Reform Is Not Working in America*

Alyssa Picard, *Making the American Mouth: Dentists and Public Health in the Twentieth Century*

Karen Seccombe and Kim A. Hoffman, *Just Don't Get Sick: Access to Health Care in the Aftermath of Welfare Reform*

Leo B. Slater, *War and Disease: Biomedical Research on Malaria in the Twentieth Century*

Rosemary A. Stevens, Charles E. Rosenberg, and Lawton R. Burns, eds., *History and Health Policy in the United States: Putting the Past Back In*

Printed in the United States
218987BV00002B/1/P